'Admission to a psychiatric unit is a terrifying and demoralizing experience for people who feel that they are already standing on a precipice from which there is no return. That is why this is such an important book. The kind of facility being described here holds the possibility of helping people whose lives have been desperately hurt not to jump off that precipice but instead to make life-affirming decisions focused on healing and recovery. For me, this book is about passing the baton to a new generation of people who care about some of the most vulnerable in our culture.'

Sandra L. Bloom, M.D., *author, Creating Sanctuary:*
Toward the Evolution of Sane Societies,
www.creatingpresence.net

'What an important and timely book this is – the first to describe a comprehensive attempt to institute a trauma-informed approach to psychosis on an inpatient unit. It is fascinating to read about the multi-year journey of dedicated clinicians and researchers – and their patients – confronting and overcoming obstacles and learning much personally and professionally in the process – including the crucial importance of the creative art therapies to healing from trauma and psychosis. This pioneering book will provide a blueprint worth its weight in gold for anyone hoping to develop a trauma-informed psychosis unit. May this success story encourage many to try!'

Andrew Moskowitz, Ph.D., *lead editor of Psychosis,*
Trauma and Dissociation (Wiley, 2008, 2019) and
Associate Professor of Psychology at the George
Washington University in Washington, DC

'Workers in public psychiatric settings can find it hard to keep their eyes on the prize of humane, healing treatment, plowed under as they are by funding concerns and ever-increasing regulations and documentation. In this inspiring book, a multi-disciplinary team documents their efforts over the years to transform psychiatric care through a deep understanding of the effects of trauma in the lives of people with serious mental illness. Chapters detail from multiple perspectives how this attention to trauma results in a safer, healthier environment for staff, who can in turn provide compassion and healing for the people in their care. Interestingly, creative arts therapies are a crucial part of the solution, and all staff are considered. The psychiatric system is much in need of this hopeful message, and detailed map of the way forward.'

Julie Kipp, PhD., LCSW, *President of the Executive*
Committee of the International Society for Psychological
and Social Approaches to Psychosis (ISPS)

DEVELOPING TRAUMA INFORMED SERVICES FOR PSYCHOSIS

A multidisciplinary group of clinicians explore the connections between traumatic experiences and psychosis, charting the development of a series of interventions designed for both inpatients and outpatients over the course of two decades.

Developing Trauma Informed Services for Psychosis details how clinicians developed a trauma committee in a public mental health facility and implemented trauma informed policies and practices, including assessments and multimodal treatment options. Chapters outline trauma informed approaches that include individual, group, and family modalities. Emphasis is on core aspects of programming such as building safety, establishing trusting relationships, and empowerment. One survivor's descriptive account as well as service users' and therapists' experiences are brought to life through personal narratives and fictionalised vignettes. This volume advocates for a multidisciplinary approach that fosters the development of unique treatment paradigms and leads to a dynamic interplay between verbal and creative arts therapies.

This book will be of interest to clinicians, administrators, students, caregivers, and anyone interested in the intersection between therapy and the arts.

Kristina Muenzenmaier is associate clinical professor of psychiatry and behavioural sciences at the Albert Einstein College of Medicine, USA. Her clinical and research interests focus on public psychiatry and childhood trauma in people with serious mental illness and psychosis.

Mara Conan was assistant professor of psychiatry and behavioural sciences at the Albert Einstein College of Medicine, USA (2003–2014). She has worked for over 30 years as a psychologist in public psychiatry with individuals who were diagnosed with psychotic disorders.

Gillian Stephens Langdon is an adjunct professor and internship supervisor in the Music Therapy Department at New York University, USA. A pioneer of music therapy, she has worked for over 40 years with people experiencing psychosis and trauma.

Toshiko Kobayashi is an onsite supervisor and guest speaker at New York University. She worked for many years as an art therapist both in the United States and internationally. She developed Expressive Origami Therapy and is president of the Origami Therapy Association. Currently, her focuses are intergenerational trauma and self-care.

Andres R. Schneeberger is an associate clinical professor at the University of California San Diego, Department of Psychiatry, USA. His main clinical and research interest focus is on mental health care delivery, measurement-based care, aggression, coercion and complex traumatisation in minority populations and people with serious mental illness.

THE INTERNATIONAL SOCIETY FOR PSYCHOLOGICAL AND SOCIAL APPROACHES TO PSYCHOSIS BOOK SERIES

Series editor: Anna Lavis

Established over 50 years ago, the International Society for Psychological and Social Approaches to Psychosis (ISPS) has members in more than 20 countries. Central to its ethos is that the perspectives of people with lived experience of psychosis, their families and friends, are key to forging more inclusive understandings of, and therapeutic approaches to, psychosis.

Over its history ISPS has pioneered a growing global recognition of the emotional, socio-cultural, environmental, and structural contexts that underpin the development of psychosis. It has recognised this as an embodied psycho-social experience that must be understood in relation to a person's life history and circumstances. Evidencing a need for interventions in which listening and talking are key ingredients, this understanding has distinct therapeutic possibilities. To this end, ISPS embraces a wide spectrum of approaches, from psychodynamic, systemic, cognitive, and arts therapies, to need-adapted and dialogical approaches, family and group therapies and residential therapeutic communities.

A further ambition of ISPS is to draw together diverse viewpoints on psychosis, fostering discussion and debate across the biomedical and social sciences, as well as humanities. This goal underpins international and national conferences and the journal *Psychosis*, as well as being key to this book series.

The ISPS book series seeks to capture cutting edge developments in scholarship on psychosis, providing a forum in which authors with different lived and professional experiences can share their work. It showcases a variety of empirical focuses as well as experiential and disciplinary perspectives. The books thereby combine intellectual rigour with accessibility for readers across the ISPS community. We aim for the series to be a resource for mental health professionals, academics, policy makers, and for people whose interest in psychosis stems from personal or family experience.

To support its aim of advancing scholarship in an inclusive and interdisciplinary way, the series benefits from the advice of an editorial board:

Katherine Berry; Sandra Bucci; Marc Calmeyn; Caroline Cupitt; Pamela Fuller; Jim Geekie; Olympia Gianfrancesco; Lee Gunn; Kelley Irmen; Sumeet Jain; Nev Jones; David Kennard; Eleanor Longden; Tanya Luhrmann; Brian Martindale; Andrew Moskowitz; Michael O'Loughlin; Jim van Os; David Shiers.

For more information about this book series visit www.routledge.com/The-International-Society-for-Psychological-and-Social-Approaches-to-Psychosis/book-series/SE0734

For more information about ISPS, email isps@isps.org or visit our website, www.isps.org.

For more information about the journal *Psychosis* visit www.isps.org/index.php/publications/journal

DEVELOPING TRAUMA INFORMED SERVICES FOR PSYCHOSIS

A Multidisciplinary Journey Towards Healing

Edited by
Kristina Muenzenmaier, Mara Conan,
Gillian Stephens Langdon,
Toshiko Kobayashi,
and Andres Ricardo Schneeberger

Routledge
Taylor & Francis Group
LONDON AND NEW YORK

Designed cover image: 'Path We Share' © Noriko Yasuda Ito

First published 2023
by Routledge
4 Park Square, Milton Park, Abingdon, Oxon OX14 4RN

and by Routledge
605 Third Avenue, New York, NY 10158

Routledge is an imprint of the Taylor & Francis Group, an informa business

British Library Cataloguing-in-Publication Data
A catalogue record for this book is available from the British Library

ISBN: 978-0-367-51967-4 (hbk)
ISBN: 978-0-367-51971-1 (pbk)
ISBN: 978-1-003-05591-4 (ebk)

DOI: 10.4324/9781003055914

Typeset in Times New Roman
by codeMantra

TO FAYE MARGOLIS

CONTENTS

Acknowledgments   xvii
In Memoriam   xxi
About the Authors   xxiii
Introduction   xxvii
KRISTINA MUENZENMAIER, MARA CONAN, GILLIAN STEPHENS
LANGDON, TOSHIKO KOBAYASHI, AND ANDRES R. SCHNEEBERGER

PART I
Foundations of a Trauma Focused Approach in a
Psychiatric Facility   1

1 **The Relation between Trauma and Psychosis: Historical**
   Background and Theoretical Issues   3
   KRISTINA MUENZENMAIER AND ANDRES R. SCHNEEBERGER

2 **Life Experience Behind and Beside Symptoms**   20
   MARY AUSLANDER

3 **Discovering Trauma Histories in Women with Psychosis**
   Leads to Political Action   31
   KRISTINA MUENZENMAIER, ANDRES R. SCHNEEBERGER, AND
   MARY AUSLANDER

4 **Implementing Hospital-Wide Trauma Assessments** 47
   KRISTINA MUENZENMAIER, MARA CONAN, GILLIAN STEPHENS
   LANGDON, TOSHIKO KOBAYASHI, AND JOSEPH BATTAGLIA

CONTENTS

5 Development of a Trauma Committee: Forming Connections   64
   KRISTINA MUENZENMAIER, GILLIAN STEPHENS LANGDON,
   MARA CONAN, TOSHIKO KOBAYASHI, AND JOSEPH BATTAGLIA

6 Widening the Circle of Care: Trauma Programme for Staff   76
   KRISTINA MUENZENMAIER, TOSHIKO KOBAYASHI,
   AND JOSEPH BATTAGLIA

PART II
Trauma Focused Interventions: From Fragmentation to Integration 95

7 Exploring a Group Therapy Approach for Healing from
   Complex Trauma   97
   MARA CONAN, KRISTINA MUENZENMAIER, GILLIAN STEPHENS
   LANGDON, AND TOSHIKO KOBAYASHI

8 Implementing a Trauma Informed Approach on an Inpatient Unit 116
   KRISTINA MUENZENMAIER, GILLIAN STEPHENS LANGDON,
   TOSHIKO KOBAYASHI, MARA CONAN, AND JOSEPH BATTAGLIA

9 Trauma Informed Care in Outpatient Clinics   136
   MARA CONAN, GILLIAN STEPHENS LANGDON, TOSHIKO
   KOBAYASHI, AND KRISTINA MUENZENMAIER

10 Family Therapy Model for Treating Trauma in
   Serious Mental Illness   155
   MADELEINE SEIFTER ABRAMS AND KRISTINA MUENZENMAIER

11 Towards an LGBTQI+ Affirmative and Trauma Informed
   Approach in People with Psychosis   168
   ANDRES R. SCHNEEBERGER

PART III
Collaboration with Creative Arts Therapies Opens up New
Doors in Trauma Treatment   181

12 Music Therapy: Exploring a Structured Trauma Informed
   Group Therapy Model   183
   GILLIAN STEPHENS LANGDON, GINA KIJEK, AND
   STACIE AAMON YELDELL

CONTENTS

13 **Interweaving Words and Music in a Music-Verbal Therapy Trauma Group** 203
GILLIAN STEPHENS LANGDON

14 **Developing Structured Art Therapy Groups to Treat Complex Trauma** 215
TOSHIKO KOBAYASHI AND KIMBERLY MICHAUD

15 **Folding and Unfolding: Expanding Trauma-Focused Art Therapy** 232
TOSHIKO KOBAYASHI, AMARA CLARK, EUNHONG PARK,
PING-RONG CHEN, AND KAMILA AGI-MEJIAS

16 **Trauma Informed Dance/Movement Therapy: Embodied Moving and Dancing** 251
KELLY LONG

Conclusion 265
KRISTINA MUENZENMAIER, MARA CONAN, GILLIAN STEPHENS
LANGDON, TOSHIKO KOBAYASHI, AND ANDRES RICARDO
SCHNEEBERGER

Index 267

ACKNOWLEDGMENTS

First and foremost, we would like to acknowledge Faye Margolis who has been an integral part of our work throughout the years. She joined the trauma committee early on and has been one of its most ardent supporters. She was eager to start this book project and share her experiences. Not long after, she was diagnosed with a serious illness. She fought long and hard. For decades a dear friend and colleague, she collaborated and conceptualised together with us much of what is written in the book. Her courage and spirit have sustained us throughout this process. By creating community, she inspired us to work together to develop a well-thought-out programme. Her background as an artist and a psychologist encouraged multidisciplinary collaborations. Throughout she weathered the hurdles and enjoyed the gains as our programme evolved. As a therapist, Faye listened carefully and her calming presence and keen attentiveness to emotional states fostered survivors' trust. Her broad understanding of theoretical concepts and her ability to integrate different modes of therapeutic interventions made a nuanced approach possible when working with survivors. She loved sharing her knowledge and providing support and she worked tirelessly teaching trainees and staff across disciplines. As colleagues who worked with her closely, we remember her empathy and her nurturing way of being. She was able to hold us and guide us even in the most challenging situations. The connectedness among members of the trauma committee would not have had the same depth without her. We treasured her as a loving friend.

We are grateful to Andrew Moskowitz, who early on suggested describing our journey throughout the many years we worked with individuals who experienced both trauma and psychosis.

Alison Summers and Andrew Shepherd, who were the editors for the book series of ISPS (International Society for Psychological and Social Approaches to Psychosis) were helpful in the initial conceptualisation of the book and reading the early chapters. Anna Lavis bore with us throughout the lengthy and arduous process of writing by tirelessly reviewing and suggesting improvements.

ACKNOWLEDGMENTS

In the early stages of the programme development, which was in fact part of a much larger movement, Mary Jane Alexander and Janet Chassman were instrumental in their support and their commitment to inclusiveness and fostering collaboration between clinicians, administrators, researchers, and peer networks. We also want to acknowledge colleagues and survivors from the early years of the New York State trauma task force. We learned from each and every one.

Much appreciation goes to our family members especially Jeff, Marv, and Tom while we were engaged in this project.

We thank our mentors, supervisors and colleagues who guided us in working with people who have experienced psychosis. We also thank Dorothy Castille and Bruce Link for their guidance in the research. We are indebted to Joseph Battaglia who navigated administrative channels and was always there to provide input in the development of trauma informed clinical assessments and therapeutic interventions. The contribution of Maia Mammamtavrishvilli, Ekaterini Spei, Madeleine Seifter Abrams, and Patricia Gross who participated in trauma programmes for many years in both a clinical and supervisory capacity were invaluable. They were always available as a source of support.

We also want to acknowledge all the people who participated in the trauma committee throughout the years. Without their help we would not have been able to develop the program. We will not be able to mention each and everybody by name. Many staff from different disciplines and settings joined training sessions and participated in trauma sensitive programming. They contributed with their time, knowledge and commitment. Among this group were individuals whose therapeutic work, ideas and engagement contributed directly to the writing of the book: Ofra Bloch, Rebecca Fleetwood, Lisa Oliveri, Richards Perry, Dorothy Rhodes, and Kenji Takeda.

Much thanks go to the many trainees/residents from psychiatry, psychology, social work, creative arts therapies and interns/externs who led and co-led trauma groups and worked individually with survivors, their families and support networks. Their eagerness, fresh outlook and creativity were an energising force.

An important part of our work was organising and presenting at conferences. We would like to acknowledge Stefan Larkin who facilitated trainings and presentations and countless staff who collaborated in organisational tasks as well as in the presentations.

The book cover was designed by Noriko Yasuda Ito. Thomas Langdon did proofreading. Brian Ferrel helped with the music tracks. Kathy McNulty was an important source of support.

We also wish to acknowledge the important role of peer specialists. Celia Brown was a pioneer in the peer movement whose leadership led to the national and international expansion of peer services. Her caring and passionate voice empowered so many individuals with disabilities to focus on resiliency and recovery. Celia's thoughtfulness, compassion and engagement played an instrumental role in fostering a more insightful and humane mental health practice.

Most importantly, we want to thank the survivors who worked with us and taught us by sharing their joys and sorrows. They entrusted us to walk together through challenges and accomplishments and showed us how to be resilient – and, as one of the survivors in this book demonstrated, to be inspired to ask, "What's next?"

IN MEMORIAM

Just as we were finalizing changes in our manuscript our co-author and dear friend Gillian Stephens Langdon passed away.

Gillian was very dedicated to the writing of this book. Though she was feeling quite ill she was able to review her proofs and make last minute changes to her chapters. Two days later she was admitted to the hospital with a devastating diagnosis. One of the last texts she sent was on 3/15/23, "So glad we got it done." Five days later she died peacefully.

The writing of this book has indeed been a multidisciplinary collaborative effort and Gillian played a major role in this process. Creating connections was extremely important to Gillian. We think about her sensitivity in listening to others, her attunement to emotional expressions, and her ability to compassionately reach out and engage. She brought consistent balance and focus to our meetings.

Gillian demonstrated the many ways in which she could use music and words to establish contact when words alone failed. This initiated the process of incorporating creative arts therapies in trauma informed programming as Gillian encouraged involvement of music, art and dance therapists.

Gillian's dedication to creative arts therapies was reflected in her clinical and administrative work as well as when she taught. In working with service users, she always had an eye towards acknowledging and building on an individual's resources and creating hope in the process. In the music groups she led (which included a service user's band) value was placed on each person's contribution.

She was there not only for service users, but also for colleagues and students. Gillian was a gifted teacher. For many years she was involved in recruiting interns and mentoring students. In this way she left an important imprint for emerging professionals. She was a leader among the creative arts therapists. Her incredible organizational skills, as well as her striving for inclusiveness made her indispensable in creating community.

Gillian cherished her close relationship with family and friends. She followed local community issues as well as more global events. She was an inspiring activist and worked towards creating a healthier environment for people and for the earth. We will always treasure Gillian's spiritual and lyrical quality of being. This, along with her strong belief in standing up for what she believed, was instrumental in helping us to carry on when we were faced with difficult challenges.

We can't put into words how much we miss her. She was an inspiration to all of us. The only way we can celebrate the publication of this book is by remembering her and what a beautiful person she was.

ABOUT THE AUTHORS

Stacie Aamon Yeldell is an award-winning vocalist, speaker, and music psychotherapist with over 15 years of experience in mental health treatment. She holds a Master's degree in music therapy (New York University) and certifications in sound and music healing (Open Center) and vocal psychotherapy (Vancouver Vocal Psychotherapy Institute).

Madeleine Seifter Abrams is the director of family studies for the Department of Psychiatry of Albert Einstein College of Medicine (AECOM) in the Bronx, New York. Her academic interests include serious mental illness, trauma, systems, emerging adults, and underserved populations.

Kamila Agi-Mejias received her Master's degree in art therapy/counselling at the College of New Rochelle, New York. Her internship was work with adult psychiatric inpatient units in New York City. She has worked with many diverse groups including paediatric populations at the Stead Family Children's Hospital in Iowa City.

Mary Auslander is a Trauma Therapist in private practice, ex-psychiatric inpatient, and advocate. She is committed to conceptualisation of symptoms through the lens of unresolved trauma and the connections between PTSD and diagnoses of mental illness. She is a graduate of Columbia University and Smith College School for Social Work, and has a private practice in Damariscotta, Maine.

Joseph Battaglia, psychiatrist, assistant professor of psychiatry and behavioral sciences and director of the Einstein Student Mental Health Center, Albert Einstein College of Medicine, Bronx, New York.

Ping-Rong Chen received her Master's degree from New York University art therapy programme. She is a registered art therapist in United States and Taiwan. She currently works as a counselling supervisor in Taiwan. Her main interests are adapting digital media or non-traditional art mediums and trauma theory in art therapy practices.

Amara Clark is a visual artist and art therapist currently in private practice in Brooklyn, New York. Amara received a Master's degree in art therapy from New York University and is a candidate in psychoanalytic training at the William Alanson White Institute, in NYC.

Mara Conan is a psychologist who worked for over 30 years in a psychiatric centre with individuals who were diagnosed with psychotic disorders. She was an assistant professor of psychiatry and behavioral sciences at the Albert Einstein College of Medicine, USA (2003–2014).

Gina Kijek is a music therapist and a sound therapy practitioner. She received her Master's degree from New York University and has been working with adults in an acute inpatient psychiatric setting for 16 years in New York City.

Toshiko Kobayashi received her Master's degree in art therapy from New York University. She has worked for many years as an art therapist both in the United States and internationally. Her major focus is on intergenerational trauma and self-care. She developed Expressive Origami Therapy and is a president of the Origami Therapy Association.

Gillian Stephens Langdon received her Master's degree in music therapy from New York University where she is currently an adjunct professor and supervisor. She practised for over 40 years as a music therapist pioneering music therapy work with people experiencing psychosis and trauma. She served as director of creative arts therapies and supervisor of music therapy interns and creative arts therapists in New York City.

Kelly Long Kelly Long earned a Master's of Science in dance/movement therapy from the Pratt Institute in Brooklyn, NY. She has been working in inpatient psychiatric centers for more than 10 years and currently serves in an administrative position. She supervises creative arts therapists and teaches graduate students at Sarah Lawrence College.

Kimberly Michaud graduated from New York University with a Master's degree in art therapy, and is currently working at a community-based health care agency for adults in New York City. She is a licensed creative arts therapist and lives and practices in New York City.

Kristina Muenzenmaier studied medicine in Munich, Germany and medical anthropology at the New School for Social Research New York. She completed residency training and served as associate clinical professor of psychiatry at AECOM. She has been working in public psychiatry for many years. Her clinical and research interests focus on childhood trauma in people with serious mental illness and psychosis.

Eunhong Park originally from South Korea, graduated with a Master of Science in art therapy/counselling at College of New Rochelle. She is a project manager at the Origami Therapy Association and provides origami therapy for immigrants and their families and homeless residents in a transitional facility in New York City.

Andres R. Schneeberger received his medical degree from the University of Basel, Switzerland. He did his psychiatry residency training in Switzerland and at Albert Einstein School of Medicine, New York. Currently he is working at the University of California San Diego and holds a faculty position as clinical health science associate professor.

INTRODUCTION

Kristina Muenzenmaier, Mara Conan,
Gillian Stephens Langdon, Toshiko Kobayashi,
and Andres R. Schneeberger

The question that faces us today, perhaps the most pressing question of human evolution, is how do we create and maintain environments now that are truly supportive of life? In awkward words, with
slow and laborious efforts, fitful starts, and many stumbles there
are people out there in every discipline who are struggling to find
and define a new way of being, of learning, of acting, of working,
of playing, of healing the world. Now we need to reach out and find
each other in order to create a community of care, of concern, of
commitment-- in order to create sanctuary.

(Bloom, 1997, p. 257)

Twenty-five years have passed since Sandra Bloom stressed the importance
of creating sanctuary. Given current global circumstances which include
strains on families and communities all over the world, the need to support
victims of trauma remains strikingly apparent today. This book was written to describe a trauma programme that grew out of multicultural and
multidisciplinary collaborations within the context of a trauma committee
in an urban mental health setting in the US. We will provide the reader with
a detailed description of the development of the programme designed for
trauma survivors who also experienced psychosis. By chronicling our journey over a period of two decades beginning in the 1990s, our aim is to focus
on what we considered to be key factors when developing such a trauma
programme. Trauma assessments and treatment paradigms, education and
support programmes for staff as well as implementation of trauma sensitive
policies are several of the topics highlighted. Throughout the book we strive
to address the concerns of service users, involved families and advocates,
clinicians, and administrators. We believe that the book also provides guidance when working with trainees from various professional disciplines.

As we began to assess service users for a trauma history in the early 1990s,
it became very clear that the majority of the individuals we worked with,
both in inpatient and outpatient services, reported severe traumatic experiences. Research findings also began to support our clinical observations

that people who were diagnosed with schizophrenia and schizoaffective disorder (or severe mental illness) have often experienced a multitude of traumatic events, including various and often co-occurring forms of stressful childhood experiences (Muenzenmaier et al., 1993; Mueser et al., 1998; Read, Goodman, Morrison, Ross, & Aderhold, 2004; Muenzenmaier et al., 2014; Chapter 3). It also became clear that symptoms of post-traumatic stress disorder (PTSD) were rarely assessed in persons who exhibited psychosis (Mueser et al., 1998; Muenzenmaier et al., 1993, 2014). In addition, when we started to develop our trauma programme in the late 1990s treatment models were limited particularly in regard to interventions for people who had experienced both trauma and psychosis. With these realisations we were highly motivated to develop trauma assessments and interventions that would address the needs of the people we were working with.

An important focus in the book is the exploration of the connection between trauma and psychosis (Chapter 1). In discussing this relationship, we look beyond traditional diagnoses such as schizophrenia and schizoaffective disorder (Muenzenmaier, Spei, & Gross, 2010; Reiff, Castille, Muenzenmaier, & Link, 2012). A strong motivation for this change is that psychiatric diagnosis seemed to have limited value for understanding and responding therapeutically to the needs of the survivors with whom we worked. In addition to psychosis, a complex array of difficulties and symptoms (such as flashbacks, dissociation, affect dysregulation, numbing, feelings of isolation and self-injurious behaviours) could not be explained by a diagnosis of schizophrenia nor were they taken into consideration in treatment approaches.

The development of trauma informed interventions was central to our psychiatric programme. Throughout the book, we emphasise the relational aspects of our therapeutic interactions and a multidisciplinary team approach. As trauma committee members worked together, we were able to integrate several therapeutic modalities into the trauma informed interventions we developed, including individual, group, milieu, and family therapy approaches. The addition of creative arts therapies provided the unique perspective of combining verbal and nonverbal approaches. With our growing awareness of the psychological needs of traumatised individuals who experience psychosis and the use of a variety of trauma sensitive therapeutic approaches came the flexibility to adjust to the individual needs of the people we were working with.

During the development of our programme we realised that, especially when working from different perspectives and in different settings, we had difficulties seeing the traumatised person as a whole. We often found ourselves discussing concepts of fragmentation and integration. In a sense this was the background theme to our work. As we worked, it became apparent that the fragmentation of an individual's thoughts and feelings is reflected in their life and often re-enacted in treatment, the mental health system, and the community. Therefore, we felt it was essential to be able to integrate the different perspectives, in collaboration with the survivor, in order to begin a process of healing and recovery. Since the trauma committee was both multi-disciplinary and multi-cultural, we hoped to design a programme that would reflect a variety of viewpoints and result in a more integrated and complex understanding of the survivors we worked with. The evolution of specific aspects of our programme is described in detail.

The issues of systemic racism and power differentials are vital to consider in trauma informed therapeutic practices: "It is critical to include the interplay of gender, race, culture, minority status, low socioeconomic status, disability, recent migration history, poverty, violence, and oppression within the therapeutic relationship" (Muenzenmaier et al., 2015, p. 143). This is particularly relevant when working with individuals and groups who have experienced trauma, social and economic stressors and marginalisation. In both the second and third parts of the book where we discuss therapeutic interventions, we make clear that for a therapist, basic to heightened awareness and facilitating a healing process, is humility and ability to attentively listen as survivors tell their stories verbally, physically or through their artistic expression. It is essential that the therapist strives for an empowering relationship in which survivors' concerns are heard, understood and acknowledged. The fostering of community has been of utmost importance in our work and is highlighted in discussions of safe therapeutic environments.

In writing this book, in addition to focus on therapeutic practices, we also consider policy issues within the facility (Chapter 8). Many theorists have noted that the experience of psychiatric hospitalisation as well as psychotic symptoms can both be overwhelming and often compound prior trauma (Mueser, Lu, Rosenberg, & Wolfe, 2010; Jennings, 1994; Chapter 2). We discuss the way in which we responded to this challenge by promoting a trauma sensitive approach within the facility. We believe that in collaboration with survivors, hospital staff (including clinicians, non-clinicians and administrators) need to work together to review policies and practices to become trauma informed and minimise coercion (e.g. seclusion and restraints; Chapter 3). We were intent on promoting an environment in which safe relationships and empowering communication could replace an atmosphere of fear and blame. There was recognition of the importance of staff support (Chapter 6) as well as education (Chapters 8 and 9). The joint efforts of many staff members made it possible to work towards an empowering and less traumatising environment.

It is important to note that our programme was developed in a public institution. Michael Garrett (2019) in *Psychotherapy for Psychosis* indicates that "in great measure, public psychiatry attends to people who have been deeply damaged by their lives, whose emotional scars assume the shape of mental illness" (p. 289). He explains that, in addition to financial reasons, treatment of acute and chronic psychosis requires the integration of many levels of multidisciplinary care, ranging from inpatient to step down programs to outpatient clinics, including an array of agencies, professional disciplines, and support services not easily accessed from or billed for by a private practitioner.

(Garrett, 2019, p. 287)

At the same time, he discusses difficulties encountered in public institutions. In our book we focus on the way we dealt with the challenges that can arise within facilities that are publicly funded (e.g. periods of limited financial and staff resources).

In order to illustrate our work, we include fictionalised vignettes. None of the vignettes describe one specific person, but they are based on common traumatic and psychotic symptoms and life experiences. In addition, to illustrate our journey throughout these years, we provide descriptions of our personal reactions and discoveries. In doing so we hope we can bring to life the practical aspects and dilemmas we faced and the hurdles we were able to overcome. Writing this book allows us to share our experiences and what we have learned from working with people who have experienced trauma and psychosis. Although our work was in a public mental health setting, we believe it is applicable as well to other settings. While we were not always able to achieve our goals, we believe we had an impact in implementing trauma sensitive principles and practices for people with psychosis.

Overview

The book is divided into three main parts:

1. Part I Foundations of a Trauma Focused Approach in a Psychiatric Facility
2. Part II Trauma Focused Interventions: From Fragmentation to Integration
3. Part III Collaboration with Creative Arts Therapies Opens up New Doors in Trauma Treatment.

Part I outlines the beginnings of our awareness of the relation between trauma and psychosis, and the development of the trauma committee and trauma informed interventions. Chapter 1 provides historical background and addresses the theoretical issues that we struggled with when the high prevalence of trauma histories in people with psychosis became apparent. Chapter 2 underlines the importance of including survivors' perspectives. It is an account of a trauma survivor's reflections on her traumatic life experiences, including her navigation of circumstances within the mental health system. Chapter 3 describes some of the early studies regarding prevalence of trauma histories in people with severe mental illness (SMI). The way in which the collaboration between survivors and professionals led to changes in hospital policies and practices is also discussed. In Chapter 4 we describe our interviewing method for assessment of past and current trauma in which special consideration is given to avoiding re-traumatisation. Chapter 5 outlines the formation of a multidisciplinary trauma committee that met weekly and made possible the development and implementation of trauma informed interventions. Chapter 6 focuses on the multiple traumatic experiences and challenges when working in a public mental health facility and highlights the need to provide support services to staff. It specifies hurdles to be overcome and describes the development of a trauma programme for staff.

In Part II we focus on exploration and integration of trauma focused interventions and the trials and errors we experienced in their development. Chapter 7 outlines the development of group therapy approaches for complex trauma for people who experience psychosis. It emphasises the way in which 'multidisciplinary' group therapies, including creative arts therapy modalities, facilitate group cohesion making discussion about the impact of trauma and adoption of new strategies for coping easier. Chapter 8 describes the development of an inpatient unit for traumatised women and the challenges that arise out of this work. Implementation of a comprehensive trauma informed approach in an outpatient setting is described in Chapter 9. Chapter 10 outlines a four-phase family model for working with traumatised families and individuals dealing with SMI. Chapter 11 describes specific hurdles encountered by trauma survivors in the LGBTQI+ affirmative community. The chapter examines the effects of prejudice and discrimination and delineates ways to build safety and trust.

Part III presents unique creative arts therapy approaches to trauma informed treatment illustrated with fictionalised vignettes. Throughout this part the way in which these programmes build relationships and community is explored. The use of specific modules from the educational and cognitive behavioural approaches described in Chapter 7 to focus on symptoms of complex trauma are described for music therapy (Chapter 12) and art therapy (Chapter 14). Examples in each of these chapters illustrate how music, art and origami therapy can provide unique modalities in assisting each trauma survivor according to their specific needs. Chapter 13 presents a music-verbal therapy model interweaving music and verbal elements in healing from trauma. In Chapter 15 a vision of art therapy for trauma treatment is presented that broadens the view of traditional art therapy and includes origami therapy as well as a unique approach of gardening groups. Chapter 16 describes a three-step trauma informed dance/movement therapy process that highlights the important role of body-oriented approaches in healing from trauma.

Background

From the earliest involvement of psychiatry with traumatized patients, there have been vehement arguments about trauma's aetiology. Is it organic or psychological? Is trauma the event itself or its subjective interpretation? Does the trauma itself cause the disorder, or do preexisting vulnerabilities cause it?

(van der Kolk, Weisaeth, & van der Hart, 1996, p. 47)

In the years that we have adopted a trauma informed perspective in working with women and men experiencing psychosis, our ideas have been shaped by a variety of approaches. We have been influenced by psychodynamic/psychoanalytic perspectives of theorists working with individuals who experienced psychosis (e.g. Sullivan, 1953; Fromm-Reichman, 1950; Searles, 1965; Ferenczi, 1980). Attachment research and theory have also been a rich source of understanding how relationship styles (secure, anxious, avoidant, disorganised) are established in childhood and manifested later in life (Bowlby, 1982; Ainsworth, Blehar, Waters, & Wall, 2015). In recent years a possible relationship between disorganised attachment and psychotic processes has been suggested (Berry, Danquah, & Bucci, 2020).

Another major influence has been the growing awareness of clinicians during the 1970s and 1980s of the effects of trauma on mental health both in the context of war trauma (Figley, 1978; van der Kolk, 1984), and sexual assault (influenced by the women's consciousness raising movement) (Courtois, 1988; Herman, 1981). The introduction of the diagnosis of PTSD in the third edition of the *Diagnostic and Statistical Manual of Mental Disorders* (DSM-III; APA, 1980) and the description of the syndrome of complex PTSD (Herman, 1992) have been essential to our understanding of and work with individuals who experience psychotic symptoms.

One of the challenges when working with people who are experiencing psychosis is that it is often difficult to understand the messages that are conveyed in the midst of psychotic expression. Karon and Van den Bos (1981) suggest that it is important to accept that deciphering a person's statement and arriving at a meaningful understanding can be a slow and challenging process.

The most important thing for a therapist to remember is that every one of the symptoms of schizophrenia is meaningful and is embedded in the life history of the patient. There is a difference between something being meaningless and its meaning being obscure.

(Karon & Van den Bos, 1981, p. 63)

Exemplifying a psychodynamic/psychoanalytic approach, Fromm-Reichman (1950) emphasised the importance of life history, including traumatic experiences, and understood hallucinations to be "the unrecognised expression of repressed or dissociated material" (p. 174). Her treatment approach advocates for a 'collaborative model'. She cautions that authoritarian behaviours can re-enact the traumatic experiences in a person's life and asks therapists to become aware of the potential of their own authoritarian tendencies, however these may have become rooted in their own lives.

During the last quarter of the twentieth century and first decades of the twenty-first century the recognition of the effects of trauma upon the body and the mind has led to extensive and rapidly expanding research in neuroscience and deepened our understanding of its complexity. In the 1980's clinicians became interested in determining what impact stressful life circumstances had on body physiology as well as brain chemistry (neuroendocrinology). In subsequent years research started to emerge involving brain scans showing the extent to which traumatic experiences can affect different parts of the brain including changes in the anatomical structure of the hippocampus (van der Kolk, 1996; Bremner et al., 1999; Lanius et al., 2005; Schore, 2005). This was followed by the exploration of brain plasticity and epigenetics (i.e. the way in which lived experience can influence a specific expressions of genes) (Yehuda & Bierer, 2009; Yehuda et al., 2014; Malaspina et al., 2008). Studies examining the relationship between stress and psychotic disorders have implicated the effects of the hypothalamic–pituitary–adrenal (HPA) axis on the hippocampus (Corcoran et al., 2003; Phillips et al., 2006). More recently Malaspina (2022) suggested a relationship between social determinants, stress, and the emergence of psychotic symptoms via the microbiome and immune system dysfunction that could result in hippocampal inflammation.

While the prevailing view in psychiatry during the 1970s was that the underlying cause of mental illness is mostly determined by biological and/or genetic factors these new scientific discoveries, namely that traumatic life circumstances influence body physiology and genetic expressions (including changes on an intergenerational level) led to a major paradigm shift. A dialogue emerged that was dialectic in nature and involved the bidirectional relationship between biological and environmental factors. *The Traumagenic Neurodevelopmental Model Of Psychosis Revisited* (Read, Fosse, Moskowitz, & Perry, 2014) reviews 125 studies supporting direct and indirect connections between early adversities, various biological stress responses and psychotic symptoms and provides helpful suggestions regarding future directions for research and interventions.

During the last three decades many clinicians have stressed the importance of maintaining a neurobiologically based perspective in helping survivors to recover from trauma (Levine, 1997; Siegel, 2007; Ogden, Pain, & Fisher, 2006; van der Kolk, 2006; Frewen & Lanius, 2015; Fisher, 2017). For example, Ogden et al. (2006) describes a sensorimotor approach in which the early emphasis in treatment is on trauma related bodily reactions. They indicate that in this way "it becomes possible to address the more primitive automatic and involuntary functions of the brain that underlie traumatic and post-traumatic responses" (p. 265). The emergence of neurobiological research and related treatment approaches has had a major influence in our understanding of the impact of trauma on the body and important factors to consider in therapeutic interventions.

Throughout the years we attempted to develop a programme to meet this need. Below we briefly discuss the scope of our work and highlight the major focus within each part. In addition, we mention important influences in the development of our therapeutic approach.

Part I: Foundations of a Trauma Focused Approach in a Psychiatric Facility

Beginnings

The early beginnings of trauma informed care in the US were characterised by advocacy work and collaborations between survivors, clinicians, policy makers and researchers. A focus on women's mental health care pointed toward high rates of victimisation experiences and prevalence studies conducted supported those high rates also in women with SMI and psychosis (Muenzenmaier, Meyer, Struening, & Ferber, 1993; Mueser et al., 1998; Read et al., 2004). During a national conference in 1994 'Dare to Vision: Shaping the National Agenda for Women, Abuse and Mental Health Services' survivors voiced concerns about the kind of mental health services provided to women with victimisation histories. A growing feminist movement as well as a psychiatric survivor movement demanded greater attention to be paid to the traumatic experiences of women in the delivery of mental health care in substance abuse as well as psychiatric treatment settings (Center for Mental Health Services, 1995). Questions raised included: What are the particular needs of women in the mental health care system? How can they be best served? Are trauma histories being assessed and taken into consideration in the treatment process? Are reports of trauma being taken seriously and in what way do psychotic symptoms affect the assessment? How do coercive treatment practices affect survivors? What are the clinical guidelines and recommendations for women receiving care in public mental health settings? (Carmen & Rieker, 1998; Levin, Blanch, & Jennings, 1998). The conference marked the beginning of changes in the delivery of mental health care services resulting in implementation of trauma informed policies and programme development in various health care systems within the US (Jennings, 2004).

The first stage at the facility in which we worked to develop a trauma programme started in the late 1990s with assembling a team of clinicians who were interested in addressing the above questions and in participating in a trauma committee. Although the leaders of the trauma committee had expertise in trauma informed care, many of the members did not. Becoming familiar with trauma theories and practices and exploring important steps in assessment of trauma in service users at our facility were the first tasks of the committee.

In the first part of the book we describe our consideration of the connection between childhood trauma and psychosis (Chapters 1–3). The realisation of the extent of traumatic circumstances in the lives of people who experience psychosis led to our quest to understand the impact of trauma in the expression of psychotic symptoms and behaviours (Reiff, Castille, Muenzenmaier, & Link, 2012). In developing our programme an important focus was on dissociative processes (Kluft, 1985; Putnam, 1989). Several clinicians and researchers propose that in the presence of a trauma history certain psychotic symptoms such as auditory hallucinations should be understood as dissociative processes rather than being categorised as positive symptoms of schizophrenia (Kluft, 1987; Ross, Anderson, & Clark, 1994; Read & Argyle, 1999; Moskowitz & Corstens, 2008; Ross, 2008; Moskowitz, Read, Farrelly, Rudegeair, & Williams, 2009). We suggest conceptualising the complex overlap of symptoms in the context of a trauma model in which psychosis, dissociation and PTSD are intertwined and can include re-experiencing, hyperarousal, numbing and avoidance symptoms. Chapter 1 outlines the development of our thinking and includes fictionalised vignettes demonstrating the complexities of symptomatology and our therapeutic approach.

Chapter 2 is a woman's reflections on her traumatic life experiences including her navigation of circumstances within the mental health system. The viewpoint of survivors has been paramount in helping us understand the difficulties and challenges faced by survivors of trauma in a psychiatric service system. The importance of working with survivors in developing programmes based on trauma informed principles is illustrated in Chapter 3. Here we discuss the beginnings of a movement that started to explore the impact of trauma on individuals with psychosis. Local and national collaborations between survivors, advocates and clinicians in the context of larger advocacy movements led to changes in organisational policies and practices in mental health care moving the discussions to a focus on trauma informed care, recovery and peer support.

As we began to develop a trauma programme at our facility in the 1990s several comprehensive models influenced our approach. Among clinicians whose work served as resources for us were Maxine Harris (1998) and her colleagues who stressed the importance of empowerment in working with women with serious mental illness and co-occurring disorders. Staff participating in 'Community Connections' developed groups for traumatised women with histories of mental illness and homelessness as well as didactic videos for staff education. Members of another programme, 'Risking Connection' (Saakvitne, Gamble, Pearlman, & Tabor, 2000) provided a training manual for clinicians working with survivors. It included detailed information and clinical examples that heightened our awareness of important aspects of trauma informed treatment. In addition, Harris and Fallot (2001) edited a book that outlined ways to implement a trauma informed care system in a variety of organisations.

During the early period of our work, the trauma committee came together as a group focused on developing a comprehensive assessment of trauma history and symptoms associated with experiences of trauma (Chapters 4 and 5). One of the resulting policy changes at our facility was not only assessing trauma in the lives of people with psychosis but also how to conduct an interview in a trauma sensitive and empowering manner. This is described in Chapter 4. Training staff was extremely important in the initial stages of developing a trauma sensitive programme at the facility. The formation of the trauma committee that met regularly to discuss assessment and treatment needs is described in Chapter 5. As the assessment process began, the prevalence of trauma history among service users became quite apparent and members of the committee identified important aspects of the assessment process. This included gathering information from the medical record, conducting a trauma assessment interview, and implementing a comprehensive written trauma evaluation including treatment plan recommendations. Chapter 4 focuses on the details of the assessment process while Chapter 5 describes the way in which members of the trauma committee worked together and were committed to supporting one another in a rewarding but often challenging process. We discuss concerns expressed by many of the committee members about triggering strong emotional reactions while conducting trauma focused interviews and how to prevent retraumatisation.

The development of a trauma programme for staff (TPS) was seen as essential in this process. In the course of listening to staff we became aware that there were situations that were overwhelming and traumatising. We also realised the long-term impact of working with trauma survivors. Pearlman & Saakvitne (1995) emphasised the importance of 'vicarious traumatisation' which served as an important guide in the development of our support programme for staff discussed in Chapter 6.

Before we go on to discuss Part II and Part III of the book, in the next section we review the important factors we considered in designing interventions for individuals who have experienced both trauma and psychosis.

Core Aspects of Trauma Treatment Programme

The concept of complex posttraumatic stress disorder (cPTSD)[1] (Herman, 1992; Courtois, Ford & Cloitre, 2009; Courtois & Ford, 2016) has been par-

---

1   In a guideline written by the International Society for Traumatic Stress Studies, it is explained that "Complex PTSD is typically the result of exposure to repeated or prolonged instances of multiple forms of interpersonal trauma, often occurring under

ticularly important in the development of our treatment programme (and this applies to both the predominantly verbal psychotherapies described in Part II as well as the creative arts therapies described in Part III). Herman (1992) describes the complex spectrum of trauma reactions resulting from the devastating effects of childhood trauma. She lists the following categories in her description of cPTSD: alterations in 'affect regulation', 'consciousness', 'self-perception', 'perception of perpetrator', 'relations with others', 'systems of meaning' and 'somatisation'. These processes are discussed throughout the book.

When working with people who have been diagnosed with a psychotic disorder, we believe it is essential, in addition to PTSD, to also assess cPTSD. The finding that the majority of service users at our facility had histories of serious ongoing trauma often beginning in childhood, suggests that these circumstances contributed to a complex array of difficulties including affective, behavioural and bodily disturbances, in addition to psychotic processes. Judith Herman's (1992) groundbreaking work of a three-stage model in the recovery from trauma formed the basis of much of our thinking. Her stages include establishment of 'safety' followed by 'remembrance and mourning' and 'reconnection'. The focus of much of our work centred on the first stage of establishing safety which is also emphasised in the recent publication *Group Trauma Treatment in Early Recovery* (Herman & Kallivayalil, 2019). Our programme includes education about cPTSD and related feelings, cognitions and behaviours and is followed by teaching skill management (tools) to identify and deal with triggers, arousal states, dissociation, numbing, and re-enactment of trauma.

In both the second and third parts of the book we focus on key features of our therapeutic interventions. This includes our attempts to: foster a psychologically and physically safe environment; develop trusting relationships as well as establishing a sense of community; enhance the ability to modulate emotional reactions; provide opportunities that are empowering and result in positive changes in self-perception and self-efficacy; and foster experiences that help instil the belief that recovery is possible. As Koehler and Silver (2009) indicate in discussing psychodynamic treatment of psychosis, "We and the sufferers of psychosis all need time together, regular dependable time, to build our relationships and our bridges back to manageable emotions and everyday living" (p. 218). In the course of our discussion, we provide details about different treatment modalities and different psychiatric settings. We begin this discussion summarising four key factors that are the foundations of our therapeutic approach.

---

circumstances where escape is not possible due to physical, psychological, maturational, family/environmental, or social constraints" (Cloitre et al., 2012).

Educational Components

In our beginning discussions of how to develop interventions for people with trauma and psychosis we started out with an educational model, *Understanding and Dealing with Sexual Abuse* (Muenzenmaier et al., 1998), which we thought would be useful for both trauma survivors and clinicians. The term 'traumatic' has been used to describe a variety of circumstances and in working with survivors an important starting point was discussing the concept of trauma and how we would be approaching the topic. We talked about the kinds of stressful events that we would be focusing on and the possibility that overwhelming childhood experiences can cause long lasting reactions that influence functioning in adulthood. We also explained that not all individuals have similar reactions to a specific overwhelming event.

It was important to convey that the way in which survivors experience their world (e.g. sensations, thoughts, behaviour, belief systems, and emotional responses) can at times be related to their traumatic experiences. It is helpful to know that while the connections are not always obvious there is a growing recognition that psychotic symptoms can also be related to traumatic experiences. When appropriate we encouraged the exploration of the details of auditory hallucination, paranoid delusions or other psychotic symptoms which can provide a window into such a connection (Chapter 1). This realisation can be normalising and another step in the healing process.

Familiarising survivors with a variety of concepts related to trauma was also important. For example, we introduced the topic of 'coping strategies' and talked about the way in which individuals develop skills for negotiating situations that they encounter and that sometimes those strategies developed early in life might not always be effective skills in adulthood. We discussed situations in which a child may have experienced a physically abusive relationship with an adult and learned that the best way to cope was to not fight back and to try to shut out the ongoing experience. To help in understanding this, the ability to 'tune out' and the process of dissociation needed to be explained.

We focused on the concept of complex PTSD and elaborated on psychological and behavioural symptoms that are common when exposed to trauma (e.g. intense emotional reactions and/or numbing of emotions, actively avoiding situations that served as reminder of trauma, self-injury, substance abuse, somatic reactions, impulsivity, having difficulty judging when a situation is unsafe, and difficulties in establishing trusting relationships). In Chapter 7 there is a detailed description of the development of symptom specific group therapy (Shelley, 2006) in which these symptoms are addressed. Because re-experiencing aspects of traumatic circumstances is a common reaction to trauma (e.g. flashbacks, nightmares, hearing voices), we discussed 'triggering' of emotional responses. We explained that following traumatisation a variety of circumstances can set off emotional reactions, but that it is often not clear to the survivor or a therapist what the precipitating factors are. It is noted that a joint process of assessment can help in identifying triggers and developing new coping strategies (Chapter 4).

There also was an emphasis on specific emotional reactions and cognitive distortions related to traumatic experience. Many survivors were able to talk about feelings of guilt, shame, hopelessness, sadness, and isolation (Chapter 7). At the same time, we introduced topics designed to heighten awareness of abilities and resources and encourage acquisition of new skills. Because service users were at different stages in the recovery process, we worked in different ways to introduce concepts and engage survivors. Issues specific to each modality were discussed. With groups it was important to decide which service users would benefit from a specific kind of group (e.g. creative arts therapies and verbal therapies). If, how, and when to reach out to family members to discuss issues related to traumatic experiences was an initial question faced in considering family interventions.

Safety and Establishment of Relationship

The need to establish personal safety and safe relationships as a foundation in the healing process is essential. This also includes establishing a therapeutic relationship (Fromm-Reichman, 1950; Sullivan, 1953; Searles, 1965; Schore, 1997) which is often a difficult and a slow process for individuals who experience psychosis (Karon & Van den Bos, 1981). While establishing a safe alliance with people who experience trauma symptoms is difficult, additional psychotic processes such as delusions and paranoid ideation can make this process even more challenging. In our work in different settings, we emphasised the fostering of a safe community environment which is based on developing trusting relationships as well as the provision of a safe psychological and physical space. Winnicott's (1965) stress on the importance of a therapeutic 'holding environment' in which individuals feel safe is a valuable underpinning to our work, as is Bloom's (1997) emphasis on a safe and empowering therapeutic milieu.

Development of a Positive Sense of Self

In describing the aftermath of cPTSD Herman (1992) suggests that the survivor is left with feelings of 'disconnection' and 'dis-empowerment'. Recovery involves reconnection with others and the possibility of re-establishment of "the psychological faculties that were damaged or deformed by the traumatic experiences" (ibid., p. 133). Feelings of helplessness, shame, guilt, isolation, as well as fragility of a sense of self have often left survivors without a sense of agency and a coherent voice to express themselves. This is compounded when survivors experience periods of psychotic processes, psychiatric hospitalisation and the stigma of being labelled 'crazy'.

An important goal in the second part of the book is to describe the way in which psychological interventions can be transformative (van der Kolk, McFarlane, & van der Hart, 1996) and empowering (Harris, 1998) in terms of helping to work through the difficult feelings survivors are struggling with as well as hesitancy in negotiating challenging life circumstances. We discuss the way in which group experiences allow for the possibility of identifying commonality of experience (Yalom & Leszcz, 2005; González de Chávez, 2009) and instilling awareness that in cases of victimisation the survivor is not responsible for the abuse that was inflicted (Courtois, 1988; Herman, 1992; Herman & Kallivayalil, 2019).

Hearing other survivors describe feelings of guilt, shame, and lack of self-worth as well as obstacles they were able to overcome can lead to a stronger sense of empowerment as well as a belief that recovery is possible. Moreover, by discussing trauma related symptoms a survivor can begin to understand the way in which these symptoms developed. Our focus centres around strategies that are effective in managing symptoms as well as skills in negotiating both practical and interpersonal experiences. The heightening of awareness of accomplishments and resources helps to provide a sense of mastery, agency, and self-worth.

Working with Emotions

Herman (1992) has noted that when working with individuals with symptoms of complex PTSD it is important to help develop strategies for managing periods of hyperarousal and/or hypoarousal. Among the survivors we worked with were many who showed extreme variation in affective states – at times an individual could be extremely agitated and then have periods in which emotions were continuously dampened. Saakvitnes et al. (2000) have made it clear that an important aspect of working with a trauma survivor is to concentrate on skills that involve managing emotions, namely learning how to "recognize, tolerate, modulate, and integrate his/her own feelings" (p. 60). This can be challenging especially when a survivor also experiences psychotic symptoms (e.g. paranoid delusions, hallucinations and disorganised thought). Cloitre, Koenen, Cohen, and Han (2002) developed a two-phase cognitive behavioural model where they outline the importance of building affect regulation skills during the first eight weeks prior to modified exposure work.

The importance of early attachment relationships in affect modulation and brain development was extensively researched by Schore (2005). He studied the effects of trauma and disrupted attachment on the endocrine and autonomic nervous system suggesting that individuals with insecure attachment may have more difficulties managing stressful emotions. Many theorists/clinicians (Schore, 1997; Saakvitnes et al., 2000; Ogden, Pain, & Fisher, 2006; Fisher, 2017) have emphasised that within therapy sessions

survivors and clinicians can work together in a way that heightens awareness of increased emotional intensity and fosters the ability to modulate
these reactions. This in turn makes it possible to talk about and come to
a greater understanding of emotional reactions. Fisher (2017) describes a
variety of techniques when working with dysregulation: "my tone of voice,
pacing of speech, smiling and laughing versus a serious facial expression,
choice of focus (beliefs, affect, body, vulnerability, strength, parts), pro-
jecting a confident energy versus a questioning, more tentative energy"
(p. 57). We also stress that as important as the development of strategies
for managing emotions is a therapist's awareness of what can trigger strong
reactions during therapy sessions (such as discussions related to trauma
and/or family relationships). The ability of the trauma survivor to take in
information can be disabled when in a state of hyper or hypo-arousal (van
der Kolk, McFarlane & van der Hart, 1996). Many theorists (Siegel, 2007;
Ogden, Pain, & Fisher, 2006; Fisher, 2017) have emphasised the importance
of therapists' ongoing assessment of what might cause emotional dysregulation. When working with psychiatric service users it is especially important to consider specific system practices which can trigger traumatic
re-enactments including physical and dental exams, restraints/seclusion,
and nightly checks (Jennings, 1994).

Part II: Trauma Focused Interventions: From Fragmentation to Integration

Below we outline the material covered in each chapter of Part II. In the
course of doing this we summarise the way in which several comprehensive models influenced the way in which our programme developed. In these
chapters we discuss different treatment modalities and include fictionalised
vignettes drawn from individual psychotherapy (Chapters 9 and 11), group
therapy (Chapters 7 and 9) and family therapy (Chapter 10). We also describe the programme in both inpatient and outpatient settings and devote
one chapter (Chapter 11) to discussion about special issues involving a minority population.

The first chapter in this part (Chapter 7) outlines the evolution of the
trauma group programme and the process in which trauma committee
members worked closely in developing different kinds of trauma informed
therapy groups. We describe our journey from an educational to a cognitive
behavioural approach. Cognitive behavioural therapies (CBT) for people
who had a history of psychosis and trauma started to emerge (Mueser, et al.,
2004; Morrison, 2004). In collaboration with the trauma committee a CBT
trained therapist developed a model that focused on symptoms of cPTSD
which we refer to as a Symptom Specific Group Treatment (SSGT) for complex PTSD (Shelley, 2006). We then used elements of the CBT paradigm
with a more process-oriented approach. In addition, we introduced groups

that included both creative arts therapies and verbal components. Using these multimodality and multidisciplinary approaches we were able to be flexible and adjust the groups to the needs of the participants. We felt that a combination of verbal and creative arts therapies provided useful and flexible interventions regarding level of functioning and interests of participants. We also discuss the reasons why group therapy became such an important modality and was adopted in different settings.

Chapter 8 provides a description of an inpatient service designated as a unit for women who have experienced trauma. We were inspired by Sandra Bloom's work on a psychiatric unit in a general hospital setting. *Creating Sanctuary* (Bloom, 1997) outlines an approach to working with trauma survivors by focusing on safety and the development of community in an empowering therapeutic milieu. The description of her model included a combination of treatments such as individual, group, family, creative arts therapies, psychopharmacology as well as supports for staff and systems modifications. In Chapter 8 we discuss our attempts to create a safe unit environment for both service users and staff in a public service system. A fictionalised vignette illustrates the interdisciplinary collaborations on the unit and the integration of the various aspects of treatment.

Chapter 9 discusses the implementation of a trauma informed approach in an outpatient clinic. Both the inpatient and outpatient chapters emphasise the importance of a multidisciplinary-collaborative approach within units as well as networking between units and community agencies. Since in- and outpatient clinicians met on a regular basis during the trauma committee it was easier to share trauma assessments and trauma informed interventions for particular service users with each other and collaborate on treatment plans. Chapters 8 and 9 also describe the development of staff education. In addition, contrasting fictionalised vignettes in the two chapters highlight different therapeutic practices based on the needs of the survivor.

Despite the fact that engaging family members in treatment has been complex, especially when the trauma occurred within the family system, we have found that inclusion of the family in the treatment process has often facilitated recovery in trauma survivors. In Chapter 10 we present a model for working with traumatised individuals and families in which the effects of childhood trauma and serious mental illness both compound the difficulties experienced by the service user and the family. The model was developed through collaborative efforts between two supervisors (one family therapist and one individual therapist) and integrates both modalities.

As our work with survivors of trauma evolved it became obvious that, in addition to people with psychosis, different minority groups were particularly vulnerable to being victims of stressful childhood experiences (Schneeberger et al., 2014). Moreover, many struggled with experiences of discrimination from within their own families and in public. Chapter 11 outlines specific considerations when working with lesbian, gay, bisexual, transgender, queer, and intersex life (LGBTQI) populations. In this chapter there is focus on the complexities in developing a trusting relationship between therapist and service user when working with traumatised LGBTQI survivors suffering from severe mental illness. In addition to extensive self-examination, it was necessary to develop outreach efforts in educating staff as well as service users about human sexuality, sexual orientation, and gender variance.

Part III: Collaboration with Creative Arts Therapies Opens up New Doors in Trauma Treatment

There is a long history of creative arts therapists working with people with psychosis (Harris & Joseph, 1973; Priestley, 1975; Sandel, Chaiklin, & Lohn, 1993). However, interventions that took into account both trauma and psychosis were more infrequent during the last four decades. As we continued to learn more about the impact of trauma on the body (Ogden, Minton, & Pain, 2006; van der Kolk, 2006; Porges, 2010), we began to have a deeper understanding of the contribution creative arts therapies were making in non-verbal and somatic approaches to trauma treatment. As van der Kolk (2006) indicates "For therapy to be effective it might be useful to focus on the patient's physical self-experience and increase their self-awareness, rather than focusing exclusively on the *meaning* that people make of their experience – their narrative of the past" (p. 289). In Porges's description of the 'social engagement system' (in which he identified the neurological process that signals environmental safety as opposed to threat) there is an emphasis on the way in which sound and facial expressions play an instrumental role in assessment of a safe interactive space (Porges, 2010).

Creative arts therapies have an inherent capacity to work with non-linear and complex threads of communication making them an effective tool for treating psychosis and severe trauma (Sutton & De Backer, 2009; Borczon, Jampel, & Langdon, 2010; Killick & Schaverien, 2013; King, 2016; Payne, Koch, & Tantia, 2019; Dieterich-Hartwell & Melsom, 2022). Moreover, they have the potential to foster connection, creativity, and a positive sense of self in both individual and group settings. Music therapy connects in a unique way through sound (e.g. music improvisation and song writing). Group members can experience themselves "in relationship to others on two levels, the *actual*, the very real interaction of his or her sounds with those of others; the *symbolic*, in that the music contains expressions of emotions, thoughts, and memories" (Stephens, 1983, p. 29). Similarly, the two levels of *actual* and *symbolic* efficacies can be experienced by other creative arts therapies interventions. Art therapy creates connections through tangible creative expressions (e.g. drawing, clay modelling, collage, and origami). Dance/movement therapy supports healing by using the body and its resources.

In trauma committee meetings creative arts therapists were supported in their endeavour to incorporate their skills into a more conscious focus on the needs of trauma survivors. In treating trauma survivors' complex manifestations of their traumatic experiences we sought new ways to create safety and interpersonal connection using the unique characteristics of each modality. For example, in music therapy a steady rhythm can create a foundation of predictability for a melodic improvisation or a song that expresses difficult emotions without the survivor feeling overwhelmed (Chapters 12 and 13). Art therapy uses tactile and visual expression to create a predictable and safe environment such as the step-by-step approach in origami or adding a frame drawn around an artwork as well as the careful choice of art media (Chapters 14 and 15). Dance/movement therapy has its own unique way to keep service users physically and emotionally safe through kinaesthetic expression (Chapter 16).

As we began to develop trauma focused groups, we found the structure of the educational and the SSGT models (Chapter 7) concrete places to begin. With the symptoms of trauma as a fundamental basis, creative arts therapists could explore both verbal and non-verbal techniques to promote healing. Music therapists and art therapists began to develop techniques for 12-week modules that were based on complex PTSD symptoms (Chapters 12 and 14). As we became more familiar with the symptoms of trauma and coping strategies we started to explore a more flexible approach. This progression is described for music therapy (Chapter 13) and for art therapy (Chapter 15). In music therapy we began to experiment with a more flexible approach combining words and music in the music-verbal therapy trauma groups. Art therapists began to explore a wide variety of art experiences including the adaptation of origami (Kobayashi, 2004) and gardening in order to meet the individual needs for recovery.

In Chapter 16 the dance/movement therapist presents her 3-step approach to group trauma treatment with each step working towards heightening awareness of one's own body, helping to integrate the fragmented elements of a survivor's experience and strengthening connections within the group.

Being able to offer a variety of multi-modal approaches provides flexibility to adapt to the unique needs and levels of recovery of trauma survivors. Choices of modalities also empowers each person to choose a way of working towards their own recovery. Throughout Part III theoretical backgrounds, approaches, and practices of music, art, and dance/movement therapies are introduced. Fictionalised vignettes illustrate this clinical work combined with several personal experiences written by individual therapists.

Summary

Throughout the book we delve into specific topics: prevalence of trauma in people who also experience psychosis; implementation of assessment and treatment approaches; staff education and support; and implementation of facility wide policies that are sensitive to the needs of trauma survivors. We focus on both inpatient and outpatient settings and emphasise the importance of a multidisciplinary and multicultural collaborative approach.

Fictionalised vignettes are included which provide examples of different treatment modalities (individual, group, and family). Core aspects of our programme include providing information about specific issues related to trauma as well as the development of a safe environment, establishing trusting relationships and a sense of community, emotional regulation and provision of therapeutic opportunities to enhance a positive sense of self. With the inclusion of descriptions of art, origami, music, and dance/movement therapies we introduce the unique contribution of psychotherapeutic approaches that necessitate less verbal interaction and/or allow for the blending of both verbal and nonverbal techniques.

The spirit of our collaborative and multidisciplinary work is illustrated in Chapter 8 where we describe the development of a trauma informed unit and include a fictionalised vignette demonstrating the transformation in a specific service user, Antonia. Antonia's responsiveness to overtures to enter the art therapy room and to gradually more actively engage in verbal interactions with her individual therapist begins to facilitate interactions with peers. Also important is her ability to identify nursing staff on each shift to walk with when she feels unsafe. Antonia is now able to recognise when interactions with others can help her to feel calmer and is able to initiate actions to help in this soothing process. For Antonia her journey toward healing includes individual sessions with a psychologist and with a music therapist, participating in art activities in the art therapy room, attending a music-verbal therapy trauma group, and family sessions. This complex programming allows the disparate pieces of the puzzle of who she is coalesce into a comprehensive picture of the way in which Antonia experiences the world. As staff becomes more aware of her resources as well as limitations, we see a gradual change in her ability to relate to others and the development of skills that enable her to return to the community.

References

Ainsworth, M. D. S., Blehar, M. C., Waters, E., & Wall, S. N. (2015). *Patterns of attachment: A psychological study of the strange situation*, classic edition. New York: Psychology Press.

APA. (1980). *Diagnostic and statistical manual*, 3rd edition (DSM-III). Washington, DC: American Psychiatric Association.

Berry, K. C., Danquah, A. N., & Bucci, S. (2020). Cross-cutting themes and future directions. In K. C. Berry, S. Bucci, & A. N. Danquah (eds), *Attachment theory and psychosis: Current perspectives and future directions*. (pp.270–274). New York: Routledge.

Bloom, S. L. (1997). *Creating sanctuary: Toward the evolution of sane communities*. New York: Routledge.

Borczon, R., Jampel, P., & Langdon, G. S. (2010) Music therapy with adult survivors of trauma. In K. Stewart (ed.), *Music therapy and trauma: Bridging theory and clinical practice* (pp. 39–57). New York: Satchnote Press.

Bowlby, J. (1982). *Attachment*, 2nd edition. New York: Basic Books.
Bremner, J. D., Staib, L., Kaloupek, D., Southwick, S.M., Soufer, R., & Charney, D.S. (1999). Neural correlates of exposure to traumatic pictures and sound in Vietnam combat veterans with and without posttraumatic stress disorder: A positron emission tomography study. *Biology Psychiatry, 45,* 806–816.
Carmen, E. & Rieker, P. P. (1998). Foreword. In B. Levin, A. Blanch, & A. Jennings (eds), *Women's mental health services: A public health perspective.* (pp. xi–xiv). Thousand Oaks, CA: Sage Publications.
Center for Mental Health Services. (1995). *Dare to vision: Shaping the national agenda for abuse and mental health services.* Proceedings of a conference in Arlington, VA, July. Rockville, MD: Center for Mental Health Services.
Cloitre, M., Koenen, K. C., Cohen, L. R., & Han, H. (2002). Skills training in affective and interpersonal regulation followed by exposure: A phase-based treatment for PTSD related to childhood abuse. *Journal of Consulting and Clinical Psychology, 70(5),* 1067–1074. https://doi.org/10.1037/0022-006X.70.5.1067.
Cloitre, M., Courtois, C. A., Ford, J. D., Green, B. L., Alexander, P., Briere, J., Herman, J. L., Lanius, R., Stolbach, B. C., Spinazzola, J., van der Kolk, B. A., van der Hart, O. (2012). The ISTSS expert consensus treatment guidelines for complex PTSD in adults. Retrieved from www.istss.org.
Corcoran, C., Walker, E., Huot, R., Mittal, V., Tessner, K., Kestler, L., & Malaspina, D. (2003). The stress cascade and schizophrenia: etiology and onset. *Schizophrenia bulletin, 29(4),* 671–692.
Courtois, C. A, & Ford, J. D. (2016) *Treatment of complex trauma: A sequenced, relationship-based approach.* New York: Guilford Press.
Courtois, C. A., Ford, J. D., & Cloitre, M. L. (2009). Best practices in psychotherapy for adults. In C. A. Courtois & J. D. Ford (eds), *Treating complex traumatic stress disorders: An evidence-based guide* (pp. 82–103). New York: Guilford Press.
Courtois C. (1988). *Healing the incest wound: Adult survivors in therapy.* New York: Norton.
Dieterich-Hartwell, R., & Melsom, A. M. (eds). (2022). *Dance/movement therapy for trauma survivors: Theoretical, clinical, and cultural perspectives.* New York: Routledge.
Ferenczi, S. (1980). *Final contributions to the problems and methods of psychoanalysis,* 2nd edition. New York: Brunner/Mazel.
Figley, C. R. (1978). *Stress disorders among Vietnam Veterans.* New York: Brunner/Mazel.
Fisher, J. (2017). *Healing the fragmented selves of trauma survivors: Overcoming internal self-alienation.* New York: Routledge.
Frewen, P. A., & Lanius, R. A. (2015). *Healing the traumatized self: Consciousness, neuroscience, and treatment.* New York: W. W. Norton.
Fromm-Reichmann, R. (1950). *Principles of intensive psychotherapy.* Chicago, IL: University of Chicago Press.
Garrett, M. (2019) *Psychotherapy for psychosis: Integrating cognitive-behavioral and psychodynamic treatment.* New York: Guilford Press.
González de Chávez, M. (2009): Group psychotherapy and schizophrenia. In Y. O. Alanen, M. González de Chávez, A. S. Silver, & B. Martindale (eds), *Psychotherapeutic approaches to schizophrenic psychoses: Past, present and future* (pp. 251–266). New York: Routledge.

Harris, M. (1998). *Trauma recovery and empowerment: A clinician's guide for working with women in groups.* New York: Free Press.

Harris, M., & Fallot, R. D. (eds) (2001). *Using trauma theory to design service systems.* San Francisco, CA: Jossey-Bass.

Harris, J., & Joseph, C. (1973). *Murals of the mind.* New York: International Universities Press.

Herman, J. L. (1981). *Father–daughter incest.* Cambridge, MA: Harvard University Press.

Herman, J. L. (1992). *Trauma and recovery.* New York: Basic Books.

Herman, J., & Kallivayalil, D. (2019). *Group treatment in early recovery: Promoting safety and self-care.* New York: Guilford Press.

Jennings, A. (1994). On being invisible in the mental health system. *Journal of Mental Health Administration, 21,* 374–387.

Jennings, A. (2004). *Models for developing trauma-informed behavioral health systems and trauma specific services.* Alexandria, VA: National Association of State Mental Health Program Directors, National Technical Assistance Center for State Mental Health Planning.

Karon, B. P., & Van den Bos, G. R. (1981). *Psychotherapy of schizophrenia: The treatment of choice.* New York: Jason Aronson.

Killick, K., & Schaverien, J. (eds). (2013). *Art, psychotherapy and psychosis.* London, UK: Routledge.

King, J. L. (ed.) (2016). *Art therapy, trauma, and neuroscience: theoretical and practical perspectives.* London: Routledge.

Kluft, R. P. (1987). First-rank symptoms as a diagnostic clue to multiple personality disorder. *The American Journal of Psychiatry, 144,* 293–298.

Kluft, R. P. (1985). *Childhood antecedents of multiple personality.* Washington, DC: American Psychiatric Press.

Kobayashi, T. (2004). *Enrichment origami art therapy with the people at Lower Eastside.* Care Study no. 4. Tokyo, Japan: Index Press.

Koehler, B. & Silver, A. L. (2009). Psychodynamic treatment of psychosis in the USA: Promoting development beyond biological reductionism. In Y. O. Alanen, M. Gonzalez de Chavez, A.L. Silver, & B. Martindale (eds.), *Psychotherapeutic approaches to schizophrenic psychoses: Past, present and future* (pp. 217–232). New York: Routledge.

Lanius, R. A., Williamson, P. C., Bluhm, R. L., Densmore, M., Boksman, K., Neufeld, R. W., et al. (2005). Functional connectivity of dissociative responses in posttraumatic stress disorder: A functional magnetic resonance imaging investigation. *Biological Psychiatry, 57(8),* 873–884.

Levin, B. L., Blanch, A. K., & Jennings, A. (1998). *Women's mental health services: A public health perspective.* Thousand Oaks, CA: Sage Publications.

Levine, P. A. (1997). *Waking the tiger: Healing trauma: The innate capacity to transform overwhelming experiences.* Berkeley, CA: North Atlantic Books.

Malaspina, D., Corcoran, C., Kleinhaus, K. R., Perrin, M. C., Fennig, S., Nahon, D.,... & Harlap, S. (2008). Acute maternal stress in pregnancy and schizophrenia in offspring: a cohort prospective study. *BMC Psychiatry, 8(1),* 1–9.

Malaspina D. (2022). *Trauma and psychosis: Where are we now?* Psychiatry Grand Rounds, Montefiore Medical Center, Albert Einstein College of Medicine, 2 March.

Morrison, A. P. (2004). Cognitive therapy for people with psychosis. In J. Read, L. R. Mosher, & R. P. Bentall (eds), *Models of madness: Psychological, social and biological approaches to schizophrenia* (pp. 291–306). New York: Brunner/Routledge.

Moskowitz, A., & Corstens, D. (2008). Auditory hallucinations: Psychotic symptom or dissociative experience? *Journal of Psychological Trauma, 6(2–3)*, 35–63.

Moskowitz, A., Read, J., Farrelly, S., Rudegeair, T., & Williams, O. (2009). Are psychotic symptoms traumatic in origin and dissociative in kind? In P. F. Dell & J. O'Neil (eds), *Dissociation and the dissociative disorders: DSM-V and beyond* (pp. 521–533). London: Routledge.

Muenzenmaier, K., Sampson, D., Norelli, L., Alexander, K., Stephens, B. & Huckeba, H. (1998). *Understanding and dealing with sexual abuse trauma: An educational group for women.* Albany, NY: New York State Office of Mental Health Trauma Initiative Publication.

Muenzenmaier, K., Spei, K., & Gross, D. R. (2010). Complex posttraumatic stress disorder in men with serious mental illness: A reconceptualization. *American Journal of Psychotherapy 64*, 257–268.

Muenzenmaier, K., Margolis, F., Langdon, G. S., Rhodes, D., Kobayashi, T., & Rifkin, L. (2015). Transcending bias in diagnosis and treatment for women with serious mental illness. *Women & Therapy, 38(1–2)*, 141–155.

Muenzenmaier, K., Meyer, I., Struening, E., & Ferber, J. (1993). Histories of childhood abuse among mentally ill outpatient women. *Hospital and Community Psychiatry, 44*, 666–670.

Muenzenmaier, K., Schneeberger, A., Castille, D., Battaglia, J., Seixas, A., & Link, B. (2014). Stressful childhood experiences and clinical outcomes in people with serious mental illness: a gender comparison in a clinical psychiatric sample. *Journal of Family Violence, 29(4)*, 419–429.

Mueser, K. T., Lu, W., Rosenberg, S. D., & Wolfe, R. (2010). The trauma of psychosis: posttraumatic stress disorder and recent onset psychosis. *Schizophrenia Research, 116(2–3)*, 217–227.

Mueser K. T., Goodman L. B., Trumbetta S. L., Rosenberg S. D., Osher C., Vidaver R, Ausiello, P., & Foy, D. W. (1998). Trauma and posttraumatic stress disorder in severe mental illness. *Journal of Consulting Clinical Psychology, 66*, 493–500.

Mueser, K. T., Rosenberg, S. D., Jankowski, M. K., Hamblen, J. L., & Monica, D. (2004). A cognitive-behavioral treatment program for posttraumatic stress disorder in persons with severe mental illness. *American Journal of Psychiatric Rehabilitation, 7(2)*, 107–146.

Ogden, P., Pain, D., & Fisher, J. (2006). A sensorimotor approach to the treatment of trauma and dissociation. *Psychiatric Clinics of North America, 29*, 263–279.

Ogden, P., Minton, K., & Pain, C (2006). *Trauma and the body.* New York: W. W. Norton & Co.

Payne, H., Koch, S., & Tantia, J. (eds). (2019). *The Routledge international handbook of embodied perspectives in psychotherapy: Approaches from dance movement and body psychotherapies.* New York: Routledge.

Pearlman, L.A.& Saakvitne, K. W. (1995). *Trauma and the therapist: Countertransference and vicarious traumatization in psychotherapy with incest survivors.* New York: Norton.

Phillips, L. J., McGorry, P. D., Garner, B., Thompson, K. N., Pantelis, C., Wood, S. J., & Berger, G. (2006). Stress, the hippocampus and the hypothalamic-pituitary-adrenal axis: implications for the development of psychotic disorders. *Australian & New Zealand Journal of Psychiatry, 40(9)*, 725–741.

Porges, S. W. (2010). Music therapy and trauma: Insights from the Polyvagal Theory. In K. Stewart (ed.), *Music therapy and trauma: Bridging theory and clinical practice* (pp. 3–15). New York: Satchnote Press.

Priestley, M. (1975). *Music therapy in action.* London: Constable & Co.

Putnam, F. W. (1989). *Diagnosis and treatment of multiple personality disorder.* New York: Guilford Press.

Read, J., Fosse, R., Moskowitz, A., & Perry, B. (2014). The traumagenic neurodevelopmental model of psychosis revisited. *Neuropsychiatry, 4(1)*, 65–79.

Read, J., Goodman, L., Morrison, A. P., Ross, C., & Aderhold, V. (2004). Childhood trauma, loss and stress. In J. Read, L. R. Mosher, & R. P. Bentall (eds). *Models of Madness: Psychological, social and biological approaches to schizophrenia* (pp. 223–252). New York: Brunner-Routledge.

Read, J., & Argyle, N. (1999). Hallucinations, delusions, and thought disorder among adult psychiatric inpatients with a history of child abuse. *Psychiatric Services, 50(11)*, 1467–1472.

Reiff, M., Castille, D. M., Muenzenmaier, K., & Link, B. (2012). Childhood abuse and the content of adult psychotic symptoms. *Psychological Trauma: Theory, Research, Practice, Policy, 4(4)*, 356.

Ross, C. A., Anderson, G., & Clark, P. (1994). Childhood abuse and the positive symptoms of schizophrenia. *J Psychiatric Services, 45(5)*, 489–491.

Ross, C. A. (2008). Dissociative schizophrenia. In A. Moskowitz, I. Schaefer & M. Dorahy (eds), *Psychosis, trauma and dissociation: Emerging perspectives on severe psychopathology* (pp. 281–294). Chichester: John Wiley & Sons.

Saakvitne, K. W, Gamble, S. J., Pearlman, L. A. & Tabor, B. T. (2000). *Risking connection: A training curriculum for working with survivors of childhood abuse.* Lutherville, MD: The Sidran Press.

Sandel, S., Chaiklin, S., & Lohn, A. (eds) (1993). *Foundations of dance/movement therapy: the life and work of Marian Chace.* Columbia, MD: Marian Chace Memorial Fund of the American Dance Therapy Association.

Schneeberger, A. R., Dietl, M. F., Muenzenmaier, K. H., Huber, C. G., Lang, U. E. (2014). Stressful childhood experiences and health outcomes in sexual minority populations: a systematic review. *Social Psychiatry and Psychiatric Epidemiology, 49(9)*, 1427–1445.

Schore, A. N. (1997). Interdisciplinary developmental research as a source of clinical models. In M. Moskowitz, C. Monk, C. Kaye, & S. Ellman (eds), *The neurological and developmental basis for psychotherapeutic Intervention* (pp. 1–71). Northvale, NJ: Jason Aronson.

Schore, A. N. (2005). Attachment, affect regulation, and the developing right brain: Linking developmental neuroscience to pediatrics. *Pediatrics in review, 26(6)*, 204–217.

Searles, H. F. (1965). *Collected papers on schizophrenia and other related subjects.* New York: International Universities Press.

Shelley, A.-M. (2006). *Men's trauma manual.* n.l.: Anne-Marie Shelley. Retrieved from www.lulu.com/en/en/shop/dr-anne-marie-shelley/mens-trauma-manual/paperback/product-1yvmnwe.html?page=1&pageSize=4.

Siegel, D.J. (2007). *The mindful brain: Reflection and attunement in the cultivation of well-being.* New York: W. W. Norton and Company.

Stephens, G. (1983). The use of improvisation for developing relatedness in the adult client. *Music Therapy, 3(1)*, 29–42.

Sullivan, H. S. (1953). *The interpersonal theory of psychiatry.* New York: W. W. Norton and Company.

Sutton, J. & De Backer, J. (2009). Music, trauma and silence: The state of the art. *Arts in Psychotherapy, 36(2)*, 75–83.

van der Kolk, B. A. (ed.) (1984). *Post-traumatic stress disorder: Psychological and biological sequelae.* Washington, DC: American Psychiatric Press.

van der Kolk, B. A. (1996). The body keeps the score. Approaches to the psychobiology of posttraumatic stress disorder. In B. A. van der Kolk, A. C. McFarlane, & L. Weisaeth (eds), *Traumatic stress: The effects of overwhelming experience on mind, body, and society* (pp. 214–241). New York: Guilford Press.

van der Kolk, B. A. (2006). Clinical implications of neuroscience research in PTSD. *Annals of the New York Academy of Sciences, 1071(1)*, 277–293.

van der Kolk, B. A., McFarlane, A. C. & van der Hart, O. (1996). A general approach to treatment of posttraumatic stress disorder. In B. A. van der Kolk, A. C. McFarlane, & L. Weisaeth (eds), *Traumatic stress: The effects of overwhelming experience on mind, body, and society* (pp. 417–440). New York: Guilford Press.

van der Kolk, B. A., Weisaeth, L., & van der Hart, O. (1996). History of trauma in psychiatry. In B. A. van der Kolk, A. C. McFarlane, & L. Weisaeth (eds), *Traumatic stress: The effects of overwhelming experience on mind, body, and society* (pp. 47–74). New York: Guilford Press.

Winnicott, D. W. (1965). *The maturational processes and the facilitating environment: Studies in the theory of emotional development.* New York: International Universities Press.

Yalom, I. D. & Leszcz, M. (2005). *The theory and practice of group psychotherapy,* 5th edition. New York: Basic Books.

Yehuda, R. & Bierer, L. M. (2009). The relevance of epigenetics to PTSD: implications for the DSM-V. *Journal of traumatic stress, 22(5)*, 427–434. https://doi.org/10.1002/jts.20448.

Yehuda, R., Daskalakis, N. P., Lehrner, A., Desarnaud, F., Bader, H. N., Makotkine, I., Flory, J. D., Bierer, L. M., & Meaney, M. J. (2014). Influences of maternal and paternal PTSD on epigenetic regulation of the glucocorticoid receptor gene in Holocaust survivor offspring. *American Journal of Psychiatry, 171(8)*, 872–880.

Part I

FOUNDATIONS OF A TRAUMA FOCUSED APPROACH IN A PSYCHIATRIC FACILITY

1

THE RELATION BETWEEN TRAUMA AND PSYCHOSIS

Historical Background and Theoretical Issues

Kristina Muenzenmaier and Andres R. Schneeberger

> I have always viewed symptoms as **communication tools** because in the land of trauma, words which we use in the prevailing spoken language, can't begin to explain the depth and complexity of Pain (and I use capital letter P intentionally). The sufferer must move to another realm of existence, another zone, where communication is expressed in different ways – be it hallucinations or delusions ...
>
> I knew that I must be a witness and find some way to acknowledge, recognize and validate her experience. I wasn't 'entering' her delusions or hallucinations as much as understanding that they simply provided the music to the unspeakable ...
>
> (Ofra Bloch, personal communication, 23 April 2022)

Introduction

This chapter outlines the evolution of our thinking, questioning the utility of traditional diagnoses such as schizophrenia and schizoaffective disorder without taking into consideration trauma related symptomatology and its impact on treatment resistant forms of psychotic disorders. We elaborate on the connections between stressful childhood experiences and psychotic symptomatology (e.g. hallucinations and delusion). In addition, we will consider symptom specific criteria for the dissociative disorders as well as post-traumatic stress disorder (PTSD). While PTSD and dissociative disorders are clearly related to trauma the connection between psychosis and trauma is less obvious. Fictionalised vignettes are presented that suggest an interplay of symptoms associated with all three diagnostic categories. Failing to address the relationship between trauma and psychosis, by not taking into account the complex array of trauma related symptomatology, makes it impossible to understand the specific treatment needs of this population. This prevents people diagnosed with psychotic disorders from receiving trauma informed interventions.

DOI: 10.4324/9781003055914-2

Several decades ago when I started working on a psychiatric inpatient unit as a young clinician in training one major issue stayed in my mind which I will elaborate on with a fictionalised vignette of Brenda.

Brenda exhibited psychotic symptoms that included multi-sensory hallucinations and several different categories of delusions. Her thought process often was disorganized and presented with tangentiality and a loosening of associations. Brenda reported having experienced severe childhood abuse including violent physical and sexual abuse, and neglect (a more detailed description of Brenda is presented later in the chapter). With a re-examination and after knowing her trauma history some of her psychotic symptoms could also be classified as dissociative in nature – such as depersonalization and identity confusion. Therefore, Brenda was presented to a consultant specialising in dissociative disorders. The consultant stated that Brenda's symptoms clearly included delusions. The hallucinations as well were seen to be of a psychotic nature. Therefore, a diagnosis of a dissociative disorder was not warranted. So here I was! While the discussant seemed to be able to clearly differentiate, I was confused. and questioned my clinical judgment. Why would I not be able to accept and confirm to existing clinical categories? In another instance, prior to a conference presentation, when I voiced my uneasiness about this same question, my co-presenter stated that it is not at all difficult to differentiate between psychotic and dissociative symptoms and that when delusions are present it clearly indicates psychosis.

Shortly thereafter, I signed up for a conference on dissociative disorders. The seminar was conducted by a psychiatrist who was treating people with dissociative disorders. I remember how after one of his talks I approached him and described Brenda, her history, and her symptoms. He did not seem to be surprised and explained that psychotic symptoms such as delusions can co-exist with dissociative symptoms. Here was my answer! The acknowledgment of the co-occurrence of psychotic and dissociative symptoms finally validated and contextualized my observations. In the 1980s, the notion that dissociative disorders, in particular Multiple Personality Disorder, are 'iatrogenic' (meaning to be created by the treating psychiatrist/psychotherapist) was widespread in the field of psychiatry (Dell, 1988). The question of what is psychosis, what is dissociation, and whether they can be clearly differentiated puzzled me then and has preoccupied me since that time. This is an important question because in biological psychiatry the treatment for psychosis differs from that of dissociation.

Discussion of the Existing Literature

The relationship between psychosis and trauma has been gaining more attention in recent decades. Studies document the high prevalence of childhood trauma in people with psychosis (Bonoldi et al., 2013; Mauritz, Goossens, Draijer, & Van Achterberg, 2013; Muenzenmaier et al., 2014; Read, van Os, Morrison, & Ross, 2005).

- If prevalence rates of childhood trauma are so high in people exhibiting psychosis should we assume that there might be an association between the two and if so, what kind?

Historically, there have been many attempts to understand and classify psychotic symptoms. Auditory hallucinations, delusions, external influences, thought withdrawal, and thought broadcasting have been seen as a hallmark syndrome of schizophrenia (Andreasen, Arndt, Alliger, Miller, & Flaum, 1995). The *DSM-IV* (APA, 1994) required either two of the criteria to be present, or if two or more voices were conversing with each other, one criterion was sufficient to make the diagnosis of schizophrenia. The latter criterion was dropped in *DSM-5* (APA, 2013). Service users still need to meet a minimum of two criteria (either delusions, hallucinations, disorganized speech, grossly disorganized or catatonic behaviour or negative symptoms) and at least one of the specific positive symptoms (delusions, hallucinations, or disorganized speech) in order to receive the diagnosis of schizophrenia (Mattila et al., 2015).

However, some clinicians have argued that hallucinations present in people with childhood sexual abuse are 'pseudo-hallucinations' and should not be confused with 'true' hallucinations, so as not to wrongly diagnose schizophrenia. (Heins, Gray, & Tennant, 1990). Ellenson (1986) distinguishes hallucinations based on their sensory modalities (visual, tactile, auditory, kinaesthetic, somatic, olfactory) and on their biopsychosocial source (e.g. organic hallucinations resulting from neurological disturbances, functional hallucinations serving a defensive function, etc.). He describes incest related hallucinations to be memory hallucinations which are sensory, can be fleeting or elementary, and represent intrusive recollections of parts of the traumatic event/s and/or related affects.

Read and Argyle (1999) emphasize that by re-categorizing some hallucinations in trauma survivors as pseudo-hallucinations we miss the fact that some psychotic symptoms can be the result of childhood trauma. Since traumatic childhood histories are highly prevalent in people with psychosis as well as dissociative disorders the question arises:

- Do psychotic symptoms co-occur with dissociative symptoms? Or are hallucinations in fact misclassified and should they be seen as dissociative in nature?

An extensive historical review contrasts the development of the concept of hysteria by Charcot and Janet (and others who studied dissociation at the end of the nineteenth century) with the development of Kraepelin's view of psychosis and dementia precox as a biologically based disease (Middleton, Dorahy, & Moskowitz, 2008). Moreover, the authors delineate the influence the concept of dissociation had on Bleuler's classification system of schizophrenia in an attempt to integrate both (ibid.).

While biological psychiatry was dominant for many decades, a renewed interest in dissociation developed in the 1980s when mental health professionals realized the importance of trauma in the development of mental illness. Included among the psychiatrists working with severely traumatized individuals with dissociative disorders in those years[1] were Kluft (1985) and Putnam and Carlson (1998). Kluft (1987) and Ross, Anderson, and Clark (1994) point out that auditory hallucinations and other Schneiderian symptoms (e.g. delusional perception, delusions of control and thought interference) can be due to dissociative processes (e.g. intrusions of alter personalities) and are often observed in people with dissociative disorders. Ross (2004) extends the argument and argues for the inclusion of a dissociative sub-type of schizophrenia in the psychiatric classification system.

In an overview of the theoretical approaches to 'voice hearing', Moskowitz and Corstens (2007) discuss past attempts to differentiate between 'true' and 'pseudo' hallucinations and between 'outside' and 'inside location' of voices. They conclude that no consistent differences could be found between non-patient populations and persons diagnosed with either schizophrenia or dissociative disorders and propose that "hearing voices should be considered a dissociative experience, which under some conditions may have pathological consequences". (ibid., p. 36). They further elaborate that dissociative processes may even underlie delusions (Moskowitz, Read, Farrelly, Rudegeair, & Williams, 2009). Here they propose that so-called bizarre delusions (e.g. delusions of control, thought insertion etc.) frequently found in persons with dissociative identity disorder may be due to the intrusion of alter personalities while so-called non-bizarre delusions (e.g. paranoia) may be the result of 'dissociative flashbacks' expressing the implicit or emotional memory without recall of the actual traumatic event (explicit memory) (ibid.).

Our Longitudinal Research and Qualitative Research

Having been preoccupied with the question of the relationship between trauma and psychosis since the 1980s we thought of ways that we could

---

1   In 1984 Kluft (1985) and Putnam and Carlson (1998) were among the early founding members of the International Society for the Study of Multiple Personality and Dissociation. The Society had a small membership and was seen as marginal by the psychiatric establishment. The society has gone through several name changes and is now the International Society for the Study of Trauma and Dissociation (ISSTD).

try to study and better understand the association between stressful childhood experiences (SCE) and hallucinations and delusions. In a year-long longitudinal study, [2] we interviewed 183 public service users between the ages of 18–65 years who were enrolled in one of seven inner city psychiatric outpatient clinics after their discharge from a psychiatric inpatient facility. Their diagnoses included schizophrenia, schizoaffective disorder, mood disorders, and other mental health problems that significantly impaired socioemotional functioning (Muenzenmaier et al., 2014; Muenzenmaier et al., 2015). We assessed childhood trauma with History of Physical and Sexual Abuse Questionnaire (HPSAQ) (Meyer, Muenzenmaier, Cancienne, & Struening, 1996) at the initial interview. Symptomatology was assessed at the initial interview and at follow-up periods using the following scales: PTSD symptoms with the Posttraumatic Stress Disorder Checklist (PCL) (Blanchard, Jones-Alexander, Buckley, & Forneris, 1996); dissociation with the Dissociative Experiences Scale-Taxon (DES-T) (Bernstein & Putnam, 1986); and hallucinations and delusions both open ended and with the Structured Clinical Interview for the Diagnostic and Statistical Manual of Mental Disorders (SCID) (First & Gibbon, 2004). To measure symptom severity we used the SCID (ibid.) and created a delusion scale (Cronbach's alpha = 0.67) and a hallucination scale (Cronbach's alpha = 0.59). Then we assessed lifetime experience at baseline and occurrence during the last three months at each follow-up point (Muenzenmaier et al., 2015). Moreover, we created a composite stressful childhood experiences (SCE) score with seven categories including childhood abuse and stressful familial environment (see table below) which was modelled after Felitti et al. (1998). The participants showed a high prevalence of stressful childhood experiences, often reporting more than one category of trauma (Table 1.1).

- The questions to answer were – is there a relation between stressful childhood experiences (SCE) and hallucinations and delusions? Is there a dose response? In other words, do the symptoms increase with increased categories of stressful childhood experiences?

The results of an assessment at baseline and follow-up periods (Muenzenmaier et al. 2015) supported our hypothesis that both hallucinations and delusions were related to severity of SCE (dose-response relationship). As the number of co-occurring SCE categories (Figure 1.1) increased so did delusions and hallucinations. The higher the traumatization categories, the

---

2   The longitudinal study conducted between 2003–2006 and commissioned by the New York State Office of Mental Health (NYS OMH) was approved by the institutional review boards of NYS OMH and New York State Psychiatric Institute. The results reported here are a secondary analysis of a pre-existing data set on Assisted Outpatient Treatment (Muenzenmaier et al, 2015).

Table 1.1. Gender differences in types of stressful childhood experiences.
Total *n* = 183 (males, *n* =111, females, *n* =72).

Type of stressful childhood experience	Males (%)	Females (%)	Total (%)	p-value
Emotional abuse/rejection *n* = 177	49.5	56.9	51.4	0.178
Physical abuse *n* = 181	82.7	65.3	75.4	0.013
Sexual abuse *n* = 179	17.6	40.3	26.2	0.001
Witnessing of sexual or physical abuse *n* = 177	38.3	36.1	36.6	0.501
Mental illness in primary caretaker *n* = 181	34.9	20.8	29.3	0.036
Substance abuse in primary caretaker *n* = 183	52.3	38.9	47.0	0.053
Arrest history in immediate family *n* = 176	39.8	30.9	36.4	0.149

Source: Muenzenmaier et al. (2014)

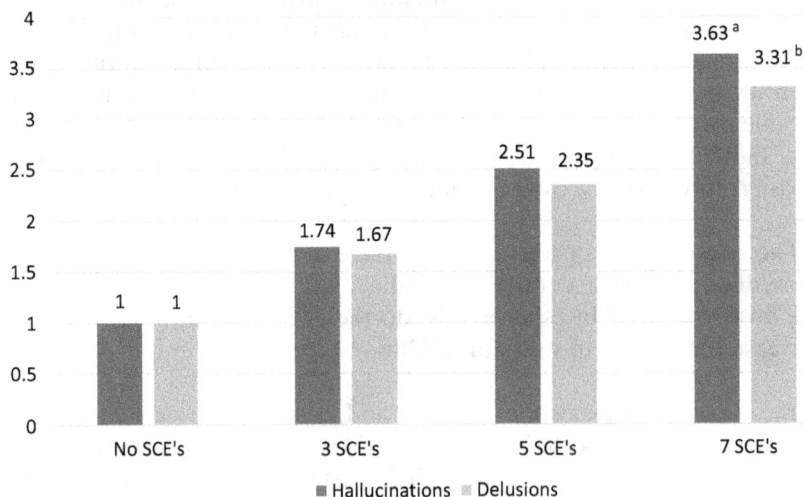

Figure 1.1. Predicted incidence rate ratios showing a dose–response relationship between stressful childhood experiences (SCE) and reports of life-time experience of delusions and hallucinations. Negative binomial regression (via generalized estimating equations) adjusting for sex, education, age, marital status, race/ethnicity, psychiatric diagnosis (Axis I), and assisted outpatient treatment status. [a]Dose–response association significant at *p* < 0.001. [b]Dose–response association significant at p < 0.001.

higher was the symptom severity as measured by hallucination and delusion scales.

Now that we could show a 'dose-response', the next question was whether dissociation mediates that relation? In other words, could the increase in hallucinations be due to the fact that more categories of stressful childhood experiences (SCE) lead to more hallucinations via dissociative symptoms? And what about the delusions? Was this also the case for delusions? Felitti and colleagues found in their groundbreaking work that adverse childhood experiences were related to many deleterious health outcomes in adulthood including delusions and hallucinations (Felitti et al., 1998; Whitfield, Dube, Felitti, & Anda, 2005). Moreover, they postulated that traumatic experiences in childhood could lead to different types of impairments enabling health-risk behaviours (Figure 1.2).

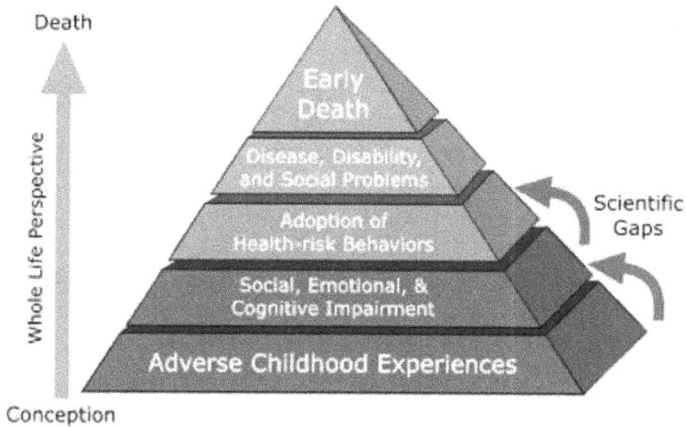

Figure 1.2. Potential influences throughout the lifespan of adverse childhood experiences.
Source: Felitti et al. (1998)

We found that after we controlled for dissociation, delusions continued to be independently associated with SCE but not hallucinations. While dissociation seemed to mediate the perceptual disturbances, this was not the case for delusions.

These results supported our clinical impressions. After clinically working with trauma survivors for many years we understood that hallucinations as well as delusions were often related to childhood trauma. But how could we understand the connection between delusions and SCE if it was not through the pathway of dissociation. Are there different ways of thinking that can explain why delusions are increased in people who have experienced childhood trauma?

Prior studies had already indicated that the content of hallucinations and delusions might be of relevance and related to the traumatic experiences (Read et al., 2005). In an attempt to validate our clinical impressions, we decided to conduct a qualitative study with a sub sample of 30 participants (Reiff, Castille, Muenzenmaier, & Link, 2012). We were interested in finding out whether in fact experiences of childhood sexual or physical abuse as measured by the HPSAQ (Meyer et al., 1996) affected the content of hallucinations and delusions. We conducted two different analyses. A 'trauma relevant symptom score' was created by coding and comparing trauma related characteristics in the content of both hallucinations and delusions in participants who reported childhood trauma. The nine items included in the measure were: threat, somatic/ tactile, olfactory, or kinetic sensations, real person involved, fear, malevolence, sexuality, and memories. The results showed that participants who had experienced childhood sexual or physical abuse had a higher score of trauma relevant symptom characteristics than those who had not.

The second analysis (Reiff et al., 2012) was based on narratives about interpersonal interactions in a multiple case study using a modified approach of the Core Conflictual Relationship Theme (CCRT). We tried to identify common relationship themes occurring in both traumatic experiences and psychotic symptoms and were able to show a high congruence. For example, one of the themes was reluctance to disclose the abuse for fear of not being believed either by the caretaking adults regarding the abuse or later by the health care providers regarding the psychotic symptoms. We concluded that in order to provide trauma informed treatment for people with psychosis the content of psychotic symptoms was paramount to both diagnosis and treatment.

Clinical Description

The fictionalized vignette of Brenda described at the beginning of this chapter will clarify the importance of considering both delusions and hallucinations in a trauma context. In fact, the description of Brenda appears to indicate the overlap between PTSD, dissociation, and psychosis rather than viewing each category as a separate entity. Moreover, we begin to see that the hallmark symptoms of PTSD such as reexperiencing, hyperarousal, numbing and avoidance can be expressed in both psychotic as well as dissociative thought processes, including hallucinations and delusions.

Vignette 1

An African American woman in her mid-50s, Brenda had been repeatedly hospitalized in various psychiatric hospitals during the previous 20 years with only short stays in the community in between. Over the years she had received a variety of different diagnoses starting with bipolar disorder, then schizophrenia, chronic, paranoid, and schizoaffective disorder. She also had a history of substance abuse including alcohol, crack, marijuana, and heroin.

Her childhood history included extensive and long lasting sexual and physical abuse and neglect. She was raised by her father and his girlfriend and felt unwanted and uncared for. When she was returned to her birth mother she was exposed to the chaotic life style of substance abuse behaviours including her mother's substance abusing/ drug dealing boyfriends. Brenda reported that over the years she was sexually abused repeatedly, resulting in her first pregnancy as a teen with a subsequent abortion. Brenda reported to also have been physically abused by her birthmother.

Brenda exhibits positive and negative symptoms of schizophrenia that do not respond to psychotropic medications and are seen as 'treatment resistant'. She presents with a whole array of hallucinations and delusions some of them fixed, others fluctuating according to states of anxiety and terror. In addition to these delusions and hallucinations, she also exhibits negative symptoms as well as a formal thought disorder, justifying a diagnosis of schizophrenia.

On the unit generally she is isolative, shows little affect and is observed to be talking to herself. Several times a week she comes running back to the unit in terror reporting that she just has been stabbed. At other times she reports that she is being poisoned and that she has been raped. During those times she is extremely frightened. She describes that her body is being operated on and that parts of her brain have been removed and that her blood was exchanged from white to black, hence her true skin colour is white, not black. At times, she reports seeing snakes crawling out of her vagina.

During interviews she mentions that she was born in Portugal and that she is waiting for papers that can prove her identity; at other times she states that she was President Kennedy's mistress; she considers herself to be a famous writer and to be independently wealthy.

Description of Delusions[3] and Hallucinations[4]

In her mental status exam Brenda clearly exhibited **paranoid and grandiose** delusions. The **paranoid delusions** and feelings of being attacked both physically and sexually are extremely frightening and put her in a state of terror.

---

3 False beliefs, based on incorrect inference about external reality.
4 False sensory perceptions not associated with real external stimuli, it is a psychotic disturbance only when associated with impairment of reality testing.

Her **grandiose delusions** make her feel important and powerful. They are related to finding her papers in order to prove her identity and high social status.

In her **somatic delusions** both paranoid and grandiose ideations are present. She feels that her body has been violated and that an exchange of her body fluids from white to black resulted in a change of her racial identity. With regard to her gender identity, she describes it to be neutral, but fluid, with an ability to change from a man to a woman and from a woman to a man.

Moreover, she exhibits another delusional belief in which she considers her birth mother not to be her real mother but an imposter (Capgras syndrome).[5] She also has the delusional conviction that other people in her environment are not their real selves but are imposters who assume the role of the person they impersonate. Her false beliefs include her ability to read people's minds and the belief that she has machines in her brain.

Brenda also reported several different kinds of **hallucinations.** The nature of her hallucinations are less fixed than her delusions and encompass numerous sensory modalities including visual/olfactory and somatic/kinaesthetic. Here too we can see the alternation between paranoid/frightening voices and voices with grandiose content trying to make her feel important. While the frightening voices torment and threaten to perform science on her, other voices soothe her and tell her how to regain her wealth. Still others run commentaries on her behaviours, or are nagging and judgmental, or tell her to hurt herself.

The visual/olfactory and somatic/kinaesthetic hallucinations include: Seeing people performing various sexual activities; seeing snakes coming out of her vagina; feelings of people violating her body including taking her guts out.

Discussion

It is clear that Brenda has an extensive trauma history that began in childhood. Our fundamental question is therefore, how do we understand her symptoms? Is it helpful to categorize and differentiate her symptoms as dissociative or psychotic? Or is it more meaningful to understand all of the above symptoms in the context of a complex trauma disorder that includes overlapping symptoms of PTSD, psychosis, and dissociation?

Brenda's delusions and hallucinations and her perceptions about her body seem to be related to her traumatic experiences. The content of her delusions is painful and retraumatizing. Somatic and intrusive re-experiencing alternates with dissociative detachment where she sees herself as an automaton without

---

5   A psychiatric syndrome in which a person believes that a friend, spouse, parent, or other close family member has been replaced by an impostor, it is often associated with impairment in reality testing and seen as occurring with schizophrenia.

feelings. Her flashbacks are triggered by sensory perceptions such as smelling drugs or observing sexual acts. She is terrified that her body once again will be violated, a feeling triggered by thoughts and observations of sexual stimulation and by medical interventions. The flashbacks happen in the present and bring her back to past traumatic experiences. Along with the flashbacks there is a loss of reality and a significant distortion of her present environment. Paranoid delusions are triggered and distort the present by continuing the cycle of fear and terror leading themselves to the re-experiencing and perpetuation of her past traumas. Brenda's flashbacks are at once dissociative and psychotic. The content of her delusions, hallucinations and flashbacks express her pain, fear, and helplessness. But she also has grandiose delusions that soothe her and make her feel powerful, rich and famous.

Brenda also exhibits Capgras syndrome, claiming that her birth mother is not her real mother and that she was born in Portugal as a white child; that she is honourable, powerful, and wealthy, with plenty of money and property; that she is married to Kennedy. Instead of seeing herself as a battered and frightened child she expresses grandiose beliefs by defending herself against the neglect and trauma that led to feelings of worthlessness and the fragmentation of her identity, likely to be both of a psychotic and dissociative nature. While dissociation distances her from her painful and neglectful childhood experiences, grandiose delusions make her feel special and fill in the gap in self-worth. In her narrative she is a wealthy and famous white woman who has never lost her identity and self-worth. Thus, psychosis and dissociation can be seen as intertwined and connected to her traumatic past and fragmented sense of self.

Focus groups (Alexander, Muenzenmaier, Battaglia, Conan, & Spei, 2001) that we designed to understand the interaction between PTSD and hallucinations and delusions strongly suggest that there are two pathways, an *intrusive* and an *avoidant* pathway that can lead to psychosis.

The *intrusive* pathway in PTSD consists of the re-experiencing of traumatic memories or flashbacks. Those flashbacks can also be expressed in delusions and hallucinations. Memories, fragments of memories or feelings associated with the trauma are perceptually distorted and may include tactile, auditory, visual, olfactory or kinaesthetic sensory modalities. The content is often of a paranoid nature and accompanied by fear and anxiety (fear can trigger paranoid ideation and/or paranoid ideation can trigger fear). Those perceptual disturbances can be associated with or without loss of the current reality. While in a dissociative flashback the person returns to the current reality after the flashback, in a psychotic flashback the current reality is transformed into a delusional world and remains distorted even after the flashback subsides.

The *avoidant* pathway consists of avoidance of internal and external reminders of trauma-negative dissociative symptoms. While some of the voices can be interpreted as representing memories or memory fragments of past traumatic experiences (i.e. hearing the voice of the abuser), in the *avoidant* pathway voices are designed to avoid the re-experiencing by creating another reality. These perceptual distortions often have a soothing function and are filling in the gaps created by the avoidance of feeling the pain. They are often more complex and can be seen as an elaboration and re-interpretation of painful realities (e.g. soothing voices who advise her to get her wealth back).

Vignette 2

The following fictionalized vignette demonstrates a more dissociative pattern of functioning. Monica's beliefs alternate between being fixed and appearing psychotic in nature to being mere soothing fantasies. Her voices and beliefs fluctuate depending on the level of anxiety. At times Monica expresses some understanding of her traumatic experiences. She is able to acknowledge that her voices give her what is missing in her real life. She observes that listening to these voices takes a lot of time and that afterwards she feels even worse when she realizes that her reality has not changed.

> *she remembers how she and her mother were evicted from their apartment when she was young and how the voices she was hearing reassured her then that they would be getting another apartment.*
>
> *... at other times or during her hospital stays the voices would give her specific telephone numbers and when she would call those numbers her children would not answer her.*
>
> *... often at night she would be visited by her 'good parents' in heaven who love and respect her and they would ask her to come and join them.*

In all of the above statements Monica's voices are an attempt to transform her painful reality (i.e. getting an apartment, speaking to her children, having caring parents). Monica feels her imaginary parents hugging and soothing her and wants to join them in heaven where she will be happy and safe. She has this fantasy usually at night. She hears their warm and caring voices talking to her. At times of increased anxiety and tension those imaginary parents become a fixed and delusional entity and she strongly holds on to the belief that her biological parents are not her real parents, but those in heaven are. This belief then cannot be challenged; it is fixed and accompanied with suicidal ideation that has led to several serious suicide attempts.

Numbing and avoidance of intrusive thoughts and pain can lead to the creation and rebuilding of a world which is no longer painful but makes a person feel better about themselves. Those dissociative states can fluctuate and shift between periods when people do not experience them at all or regard them as fantasy or they can become a fixed delusional belief system. Monica's dissociative symptoms fluctuate according to her mood states and crystallize into a fixed belief system when her anxiety level increases. These beliefs then function as a rigid shield (delusions) in a desperate attempt to avoid painful reality by soothing her and making her feel that she is loved and an important person (grandiosity).

The example of Monica illustrates the transition from dissociative experiences designed to soothe to a fixed delusional belief system that includes Capgras syndrome.

At one time Monica reported that a few days after she was taken off medication she experienced the return of her delusions and paranoid ideation. Inside herself she had a 'terrible fear'. She felt that she had to suppress and conceal her feelings. She did not believe that what was happening to her was real. She attributes this denial of her reality as leading to the appearance of her 'symptoms'. She states that what we define as 'symptoms' for her are 'feelings'. She thinks that at times of stress some people retreat into delusions because they could not deal with their reality. They were pushed over the edge and stayed there unable to return. She emphasizes that her delusions of 'feeling special' appear during stressful times when she has difficulties coping with her current reality.

In one meeting she expressed that the medication helps her get relief from the threatening voices but not from the flashbacks that overwhelm her and cannot be controlled.

We propose that it is essential to understand a person's complex array of psychotic symptoms and behaviours in the context of a trauma model where PTSD, dissociation, and psychosis overlap. The confusing interplay of re-experiencing, hyperarousal, numbing and avoidance can be expressed in all of the different categories and includes hallucinations and delusional thought processes. While we are not always able to distinguish and differentiate between the different existing diagnostic categories, we can attempt to identify elements of each and describe how they are intertwined with each other. They can be part of a confusing cycle of re-experiencing; or be avoidance of painful re-experiencing by numbing and dissociation; or filling in and trying to make sense of the existing gaps in memory and reality by constructing an imaginary delusional belief systems that can soothe but also trigger and re-traumatize. Psychotic experiences can be triggered by sensory experiences, feelings, thoughts and can represent flashbacks, memories or memory fragments of past traumatic experiences (e.g. hallucinations, paranoid and somatic delusions) or be a delusional elaboration of a person's current or past reality; they can be seen as coping mechanisms such as attempts to soothe and avoid painful realities (e.g. Capgras syndrome and grandiose delusions); and the delusions themselves can also trigger flashbacks (e.g. paranoid and somatic). Depending on the intensity and content of the experience the goal is to avoid pain and suffering by constructing and reconstructing imaginary worlds that take over the emptiness and/or pain by numbing or soothing and recreating a delusional world whereby reality is avoided at all cost.

The fluidity of transitions from delusions to dissociative symptoms and back to delusions (depending on states of distress) can be observed in severely traumatized persons. The categorical nature of the psychiatric diagnostic classification system of the DSM has severely limited our understanding. It is important to see the connections between different states resulting from deep and underlying pain, in order to understand the defensive and creative nature of thoughts, feelings and behaviours and how they serve to undo and lessen suffering and create meaning. The broad range of intertwining symptoms of PTSD, dissociation and psychosis can make treatment challenging. In particular, the fixed delusional states are less translucent and more resistant to interventions.

Therapeutic Implications

For Brenda, the goal for treatment is first and foremost to restore safety and calm. During the times of her flashbacks and paranoid ideations, her delusional beliefs are fixed and immutable. But when she feels safe, sometimes she is able to connect her past experiences with the current reality and differentiate between flashbacks and voice hearing. In one meeting she expresses that the medication helps her get relief from the threatening voices but not from the flashbacks that overwhelm her and cannot be controlled.

Establishing safety cannot be achieved without the development of a trusting relationship with a therapist. This is a long and arduous process. While Brenda is mostly isolative and withdrawn, sometimes she comes running back to the unit in an agitated state of terror screaming that she is being stabbed and that they are trying to kill her. One time her therapist happens to be there. She responds to Brenda in a calm way and reassures her that she is safe. By validating Brenda's fears (independent of whether it originated from a delusional belief or not) the therapist is able to quiet the threatening voices, the agitation and the hyperarousal.

Brenda feels understood and trusts her therapist to keep her safe. During the times when she feels overwhelmed she has no insight and seems to be protected by a rigid delusional armour. At other times she is able to explore the triggers and connections to her past traumata. However, the delusions surrounding her identity and grandiosity are not amenable to interpretation. We propose that rather than giving Brenda a diagnosis of schizophrenia and treating the symptoms with medications alone, it is possible to examine the connections between her trauma history and her behaviours, her hallucinations and her delusions in the context of a healing therapeutic relationship. There are periods in which the therapeutic relationship helps her dispense with both her psychotic and dissociative defences. At such times she is able to connect with her therapist and other survivors in contexts where she feels safe. It is then that we are able to explore the relationship between trauma, dissociation and psychosis.

Conclusion

The problem is not only whether dissociative processes underlie psychosis but that trauma is rarely addressed when psychosis is present, thus preventing people diagnosed with psychotic disorders from receiving trauma informed interventions (Read, Hammersley, & Rudegeair, 2007; Read, Harper, Tucker, & Kennedy, 2018; Tucker, 2002). In fact, the diagnostic system of the *DSM-5* (APA, 2013) tends to parcel out the different aspects of a person and unlike *ICD 11* (World Health Organization, 2021) does not include complex PTSD as an independent diagnosis (Cloitre et al., 2018). As a result, the survivor ends up being related to as if they are a fragmented entity. This perpetuates the fragmentation resulting from severe traumatization. The hope is that we can improve our understanding of complex trauma related symptoms in the context of each particular survivor's experience and that we are able to empathically connect. Recognizing trauma related characteristics in the content of symptoms is often a beginning step for clinicians in being able to recognize trauma-related illness. And it is by understanding the connection between trauma, the symptom expression, and the symbolic representation that both the survivor and the clinician will be able to create a new narrative that can lead to healing.

Rather than seeing symptoms as something to simply medicate away we advocate for a deeper understanding of the protective defences and the creation of new reality as meaningful communications in the context of a safe and healing therapeutic relationship. These newly found perspectives serve to enrich our work with mental health treatment teams and reduce bias, stigma, and limitations associated with psychiatric diagnoses.

References

Alexander, M. J., Muenzenmaier, K., Battaglia, J., Conan, M., & Spei, E. (2001). *Trauma, psychosis and PTSD*. Workshop presented at the 6th Annual Mastering the Key Connection: Clinical Training Conference on Trauma Services in the Public Mental Health System, Albany, NY.

Andreasen, N. C., Arndt, S., Alliger, R., Miller, D., & Flaum, M. (1995). Symptoms of schizophrenia: Methods, meanings, and mechanisms. *Archives of General Psychiatry*, *52*(5), 341–351.

APA. (1994). *Diagnostic and Statistical Manual of Mental Disorders: DSM-IV.* Washington, DC: American Psychiatric Association.

APA. (2013). American Psychiatric Association: Diagnostic and Statistical Manual of Mental Disorders, Fifth Edition. Arlington, VA: American Psychiatric Association.

Bernstein, E. M., & Putnam, F. W. (1986). Development, reliability, and validity of a dissociation scale. *Journal of Nervous and Mental Disease, 174(12)*, 727–735.

Blanchard, E. B., Jones-Alexander, J., Buckley, T. C., & Forneris, C. A. (1996). Psychometric properties of the PTSD Checklist (PCL). *Behaviour Research and Therapy, 34(8)*, 669–673.

Bonoldi, I., Simeone, E., Rocchetti, M., Codjoe, L., Rossi, G., Gambi, F., ... Fusar-Poli, P. (2013). Prevalence of self-reported childhood abuse in psychosis: A meta-analysis of retrospective studies. *Psychiatry Research, 210(1)*, 8–15.

Cloitre, M., Shevlin, M., Brewin, C. R., Bisson, J. I., Roberts, N. P., Maercker, A., ... Hyland, P. (2018). The International Trauma Questionnaire: Development of a self-report measure of ICD-11 PTSD and complex PTSD. *Acta Psychiatrica Scandinavica, 138(6)*, 536–546.

Dell, P. F. (1988). Professional skepticism about multiple personality. *Journal of Nervous and Mental Disease, 176(9)*, 528–531.

Ellenson, G. S. (1986). Disturbances of perception in adult female incest survivors. *Social Casework, 67(3)*, 149–159.

Felitti, V. J., Anda, R. F., Nordenberg, D., Williamson, D. F., Spitz, A. M., Edwards, V., ... Marks, J. P. (1998). Relationship of childhood abuse and household dysfunction to many of the leading causes of death in adults: The Adverse Childhood Experiences (ACE) study. *American Journal of Preventive Medicine, 14(4)*, 245–258.

First, M. B., & Gibbon, M. (2004). The structured clinical interview for DSM-IV axis I disorders (SCID-I) and the structured clinical interview for DSM-IV axis II disorders (SCID-II). *Comprehensive Handbook of Psychological Assessment, 2*, 134–143.

Heins, T., Gray, A., & Tennant, M. J. A. (1990). Persisting hallucinations following childhood sexual abuse. *Australian and New Zealand Journal of Psychiatry, 24(4)*, 561–565.

Kluft, R. P. (1985). *Childhood antecedents of multiple personality.* Philadelphia, PA: American Psychiatric Publisher.

Kluft, R. P. (1987). First-rank symptoms as a diagnostic clue to multiple personality disorder. *The American Journal of Psychiatry, 144*, 293–298.

Mattila, T., Koeter, M., Wohlfarth, T., Storosum, J., van den Brink, W., de Haan, L., ... Denys, D. (2015). Impact of DSM-5 changes on the diagnosis and acute treatment of schizophrenia. *Schizophrenia Bulletin, 41(3)*, 637–643.

Mauritz, M. W., Goossens, P. J., Draijer, N., & Van Achterberg, T. (2013). Prevalence of interpersonal trauma exposure and trauma-related disorders in severe mental illness. *European Journal of Psychotraumatology, 4(1)*, 19985.

Meyer, I. H., Muenzenmaier, K., Cancienne, J., & Struening, E. (1996). Reliability and validity of a measure of sexual and physical abuse histories among women with serious mental illness. *Child Abuse & Neglect, 20(3)*, 213–219.

Middleton, W., Dorahy, M. J., & Moskowitz, A. (2008). Historical conceptions of dissociation and psychosis: Nineteenth and early twentieth century perspectives on severe psychopathology. In A. Moskowitz, I. Schäfer, & M. J. Dorahy (eds), *Psychosis, trauma and dissociation: Emerging perspectives on severe psychopathology* (pp. 9–20). Hoboken, NJ: Wiley-Blackwell.

Moskowitz, A., & Corstens, D. (2007). Auditory hallucinations: Psychotic symptom or dissociative experience? In S. N. Gold & J. D. Elhai, (eds.), *Trauma and serious mental illness* (pp. 35–63). Binghamton, NY: Haworth Press.

Moskowitz, A., Read, J., Farrelly, S., Rudegeair, T., & Williams, O. (2009). Are psychotic symptoms traumatic in origin and dissociative in kind? In P. Dell & J. O'Neill (eds), *Dissociation and the dissociative disorders: DSM-V and beyond* (pp. 521–533). New York, NY: Routledge.

Muenzenmaier, K., Schneeberger, A. R., Castille, D. M., Battaglia, J., Seixas, A. A., & Link, B. (2014). Stressful childhood experiences and clinical outcomes in people with serious mental illness: a gender comparison in a clinical psychiatric sample. *Journal of Family Violence, 29(4)*, 419 429.

Muenzenmaier, K., Seixas, A. A., Schneeberger, A. R., Castille, D. M., Battaglia, J., & Link, B. G. (2015). Cumulative effects of stressful childhood experiences on delusions and hallucinations. *Journal of Trauma Dissociation & Dissociation, 16(4)*, 442–462.

Putnam, F. W., & Carlson, E. B. (1998). Hypnosis, dissociation, and trauma: Myths, metaphors, and mechanisms. In B. J. D & M. C. R (eds), *Progress in psychiatry, No. 54. Trauma, memory, and dissociation*. Philadelphia, PA: American Psychiatric Association.

Read, J., & Argyle, N. (1999). Hallucinations, delusions, and thought disorder among adult psychiatric inpatients with a history of child abuse. *Psychiatric Services, 50(11)*, 1467–1472.

Read, J., Hammersley, P., & Rudegeair, T. (2007). Why, when and how to ask about childhood abuse. *Advances in Psychiatric Treatment, 13(2)*, 101–110.

Read, J., Harper, D., Tucker, I., & Kennedy, A. (2018). Do adult mental health services identify child abuse and neglect? A systematic review. *International Journal of Mental Health Nursing, 27(1)*, 7–19.

Read, J., van Os, J., Morrison, A. P., & Ross, C. A. (2005). Childhood trauma, psychosis and schizophrenia: a literature review with theoretical and clinical implications. *Acta Psychiatrica Scandinavica, 112(5)*, 330–350.

Reiff, M., Castille, D. M., Muenzenmaier, K., & Link, B. (2012). Childhood abuse and the content of adult psychotic symptoms. *Psychological Trauma: Theory, Research, Practice, Policy, 4(4)*, 356.

Ross, C. A. (2004). *Schizophrenia: Innovations in diagnosis and treatment*. Binghamton, NY: Haworth Maltreatment and Trauma Press.

Ross, C. A., Anderson, G., & Clark, P. (1994). Childhood Abuse and the Positive Symptoms of Schizophrenia. *J Psychiatric Services, 45(5)*, 489–491.

Tucker, W. M. (2002). How to include the trauma history in the diagnosis and treatment of psychiatric inpatients. *Psychiatric Quarterly, 73(2)*, 135–144.

Whitfield, C. L., Dube, S. R., Felitti, V. J., & Anda, R. F. (2005). Adverse childhood experiences and hallucinations. *Child Abuse & Neglect, 29(7)*, 797–810.

World Health Organization. (2021). *International statistical classification of diseases and related health problems*, 11th edition. Washington, DC: World Health Organization. Retrieved from https://icd.who.int/.

2

LIFE EXPERIENCE BEHIND AND BESIDE SYMPTOMS

Mary Auslander

Prologue

Every time I've been asked to tell the story of how I first came to be psychiatrically hospitalised and diagnosed with mental illness, I find it difficult to get much beyond the first day and the nine more of my first admission. Not only are the details of that momentous occasion vivid to me, but they determined so much of how and where I spent the next decade of my then young life, my twenties, and much of the next decade as well. There is something about the 'age of onset' theory (Kessler et al., 2005) that was once, and often still is, disturbing in its focus on biology out of the context of developmental tasks one faces, especially in one's late teens and early twenties in our society.

Trauma disrupts development in myriad ways and so does treatment that does not consider the whole of a person – the who, what, where, and why of them rather than the visible behaviour alone. If one is being viewed through the medical model psychiatric lens, this is defined as symptoms (Read, Bentall, & Fosse, 2009). The bio-psycho-social model (Borrell-Carrió, Suchman, & Epstein, 2004) does more and is yet incomplete. The trauma lens includes all of these and whether one suffered 'small-t or big-T trauma' (i.e. minor car accident to regular beatings as a child), what happened to us needs to be the foundation of our exploration. "What's wrong with you?" is best replaced with "What happened to you?" (Jennings, 1994) and then, combined with our bio-psycho-social development, primarily relational, our environmental influences, cultural contexts (colour, class, gender, etc.), and yes, our genetic endowment, we can be seen as whole and only then begin to organise our priorities for healing the pain we present with over time.

The first 72 hours of my first admission to a psychiatric unit are significant because they held the last clear view of a whole, albeit fragmented, self before the shroud of medications wrapped my body, feelings, and thoughts in a thick container in which I essentially completed the process of dissociation that I had begun in order to survive my life experiences thus far. This unconscious strategy was necessary to survive the priorities of the psychiatric

   DOI: 10.4324/9781003055914-3

system with its extra-legal power and mandate to keep society safe from those labelled with mental illness. It was necessary to survive my new invisibility as a person who knew she needed help and was then convinced she knew nothing about what she needed, and certainly had no expertise, even or perhaps especially, about herself.

Once I get through the telling of the first admission, including the much longer, coerced-voluntary admission within two months of the first discharge, and how my career as a mental patient was launched (Goffman, 1959; Goffman, 1968), I then rush through the next nine years to get to the part where I said, "No more". I said this then without realising I was now *invisibly* stigmatised from without and within (Goffman, 1986) and still laden with all my original unprocessed trauma and shame. Now I would have another layer to add to what I often called my "stigma collection" – a decade of psychiatric trauma to process. I used to say it took another decade to "undo" what that layer created, but like childhood trauma, especially interpersonal abuse and/or neglect, there is no undoing. There is simply the long work of healing, a life's worth. In fact, I often say to clients that, in addition to being a rehearsal for the "next life", healing is what our lives are for.

My Story

The first time I wandered out of my class in the old three-year diploma programme in nursing I was enrolled in, I was already well-rehearsed in dissociation. That word was not in my vocabulary at the time, nor did it seem known to my out-patient psychotherapist. When I called for a between sessions visit, I couldn't find words to describe what was happening, but I repeated on the phone and later in her office something about feeling paralysed, not being able to return to my dorm room or school, needing to start over, and having no place to go. The bright and clearly caring psychiatric social worker, whom I wanted to become instead of myself, did her best to explore where and with whom I could go for the night, if not longer. I didn't realise she was likely assessing my potential for suicide as my refrain became "I don't know" or "I cannot go back". Our appointment was probably around five or six o'clock. Somewhere between seven and eight, my therapist suggested the only other alternative she knew was the hospital, I was terrified, relieved, and silent. Before nine she was walking me out of the clinic, accompanying me to her car which she then drove around the corner, almost past the nursing school I had left earlier in the day, to just across the street where the mental health centre stood, complete with a short-term in-patient evaluation unit. I had looked out of my dorm window at it since starting nursing school in September 1971, recalling the previous academic year and the sliding scale sessions I had attended as an out-patient, assigned to a psychiatric resident on whom I developed a crush. For the length of his residency, we spent often wordless 50-minute hours, trained as he was, it seemed, to say as little as possible.

When I got to the in-patient evaluation unit, my current therapist spoke quietly with the staff without me. She then wished me well, said goodnight, and left. Soon a nurse in street clothes showed me a room and said she would come back with some medicine to help me sleep. I said that I didn't think I would have trouble sleeping this night, and she replied, "We've heard you have been having trouble sleeping." It was lost on me then how significant this first dismissal of my own words was, but I wanted to assume that they knew best. I had not considered medicine for what was happening to me; I had hoped that being asked questions and talking through as best I could what I thought and felt would be helpful, although I didn't know how. The nurse returned with a pill in a cup and some water. Our eyes met and some-how, I knew right away that I was expected to comply. So, I did.

The next morning, I was awakened by another staff person and could barely open my eyes. My head and mouth felt full of cotton and it took some time to realise where I was. I had a notebook with me and little else. There must have been an offer of breakfast and I was told a group I was expected to attend was happening shortly thereafter. Later I was pressured to contact my parents who had lived right outside of the city until six months before when my dad's job transferred him to another state a couple of hours away. I explained I was on my own, nearly 22 years old, and they needn't be in-volved. This was the second time I was given a "choice" – whether or not to contact them – that evolved into something other than choice, one of the first hints I had that signing into this unit said to those in charge that I didn't know best about myself at all.

My refrain of not knowing what was wrong or what to do was the best I could share in any group that day. That night I did have trouble sleeping and at 2 a.m. I wanted to talk to someone about the thoughts spinning in my mind and the fear filling my body. I was told it wasn't time to talk, that talking occurred during the day in groups with strangers, and that now was the time to sleep. I was offered medicine and this time I was able to refuse. It seemed odd to me that the staff on duty at night were not available to talk, that even though I was there in a crisis, dealing with it had business hours. The next morning, I was called to the nurses' station where a cup with pills awaited me. When I asked what they were for, I was told that they would help with racing thoughts. I wondered aloud whether there was another way to deal with my thoughts and the "explanation" was repeated, as if I were hard of hearing. Within another two days, another pill appeared in the cup and I didn't bother to ask what it was for. The next day the staff said that if I didn't call my parents, they would.

Within another day or two, with four younger children at home, one not even three years old, two states away, my distraught and confused par-ents appeared on the unit for a "four-way meeting". It was made clear that

I needed to be discharged to somewhere and that since I wasn't going to return to nursing school I needed to get a job. Somehow, it was decided that I could stay with my grandmother who was still in the area while I searched for an apartment and a job. By now I was feeling the effects of the medications: dry mouth, slow to form thoughts through a fog that had thickened behind my eyes, and a slight tremor that I was told would likely pass. The meds were increased somewhere in the middle of the 10 days I was on the unit; ten days was the maximum one could be there. On the last day my stunned and generous grandmother took me to her apartment and within a week I had a job working the 3–11 shift at a nursing home, a second-hand Volkswagen Beetle, and a room in a large apartment with three people I didn't know. I had a feeling the medications weren't helping me; I couldn't form sentences easily and I had an anxious edge around my body beyond which was a constant din of ideas and lines of advice I couldn't get to. I thought I had better keep taking those meds, that I must be way sicker than I knew or they wouldn't have been prescribed.

This happened in February 1972. At the end of March, I did turn 22, and in mid-April, I came home one night in that kind of mist early spring often holds as the temperature warms in the midday then drops after dark. The street lamps had auras with prisms around them and the scent of my favourite flowering shrubs was thick in the humidity. I knew it was one of my favourite kind of nights and that I could not feel anything like what I used to when I found something beautiful.

When I got upstairs to the apartment, I created a story on the phone with the ex-boyfriend who helped precipitate my crisis, half wanting to punish him and half wanting to dare myself to do something drastic. After I told him I had taken all my pills, I did take them. He panicked and said he would meet me at the hospital. With one part of me on the ceiling overseeing my every move, and a now familiar voice that told me repeatedly I was crazy and unforgiveable reaching an unprecedented pitch, my body took me to the car which I drove to the emergency room.

In the emergency room I was given something to make me vomit and pressured to give a name of someone who could be contacted. A new friend, who had also left nursing school within months, rallied as if she'd known me for years. She kept the boyfriend from seeing me and held my head while I wretched up the pills. The next day I was back on the evaluation unit I had left not even two full months before. The meds I had taken all of were again dosed out twice a day. When I mentioned I didn't think they were helping me and possibly worsened my condition, I was told that wasn't the issue. The issue was what I had done, it was deemed a suicide attempt, and it was suggested that I go into a longer-term psychiatric unit. I said I would think about it and I did. I had scared myself, yet fully believed that being cut off from life in society and people I knew would be worse. I made a good case for seriously attending out-patient therapy, getting back to work (where they'd held my low-level job), and staying in touch with family. This option, something I thought I had been encouraged to formulate, turned out not to be a real choice. The as it was ultimately made clear, was between voluntarily entering the in-patient psychiatric unit in the big teaching hospital to which this evaluation unit was connected, or be involuntarily committed to the state institution on the basis of having committed the crime of attempting suicide.

So that is how I became a mental patient, as existed in the vernacular then and which we ex-patients retain the right to call ourselves. If any of you have read or seen *Girl Interrupted*, you might be aware of how easy it was to be hospitalised as a white middle-class young woman in 1972 (Kaysen, 1994). Way easier than getting out. Even once discharged, getting "out" was not just a matter of being outside the locked doors. An identity was applied and adopted in such an experience and regardless of doubts about its validity, diagnoses of mental illness by their nature say that one does not have a trustworthy mind. This identity is reinforced by fear of losing one's freedom and of treatments less reversible than medications (like shock treatment or psychosurgery).

I entered into psychiatric care with sincere hope I could work through what ailed me. I was open to understanding how I worked emotionally, relationally, cognitively, and neurologically, but my most critical need was to tell my story of how I got to where I was.

The first two-part hospitalisation was about being labelled and medicated. Those were the offerings of psychiatric care and whether or not they truly applied to my difficulties was not explored. The fact that I was admitted was proof that I was mentally ill. The "treatment" was not about understanding how this had happened or what had hurt me or how limited my coping strategies were. It wasn't about how young and sheltered I'd been or how lost I was out in the adult world where my transition plan of college exploded in a pregnancy and decision not to make one more decision that might hurt, no less create, another human being.

Between these first hospitalisations and the next five years I struggled without being hospitalised. I took the medications for about a year after being discharged, ironically, on Independence Day in 1972. I worked temporary jobs and saw my therapist. I became more and more depressed, almost immobile. My therapist suggested that I had missed my adolescence and needed to retrieve it. Thus, I gave up the minimal life I had working and living on my own and went to live with my parents and sisters in a place I'd never known except to visit after they moved. I sat silent and smoking and attempted to sleep more than was possible. My parents could only finally tell me that I had to work and pay some rent, so I found a certification course and job as a nursing assistant at a nearby hospital. (I had yet to admit nursing was wrong for me or that I never would go back to nursing school.)

I worked evening shifts and signed up for classes at a community college. I finally decided to stop taking medication without guidance and within a month or so afterward my mood began to soar. It wasn't known then that abrupt cessation of a tricyclic antidepressant could trigger mania, including psychosis. My own reasoning said that it was the major tranquiliser, anti-psychotic med since I considered that the suppressing agent.

Being so low for so long and then suddenly soaring actually gave me hope. The first episode lasted a few weeks. I hardly slept, I talked non-stop, my mind burst with ideas, I lost 15 pounds. Then just as suddenly as I soared, I plummeted. It is the rapid cycling that withdrawal of Tofranil causes and can become self-perpetuating. Not one mental health professional I inter-acted with knew that information which was documented approximately a decade later.

My parents were flummoxed, whatever therapist I had was ineffectual, I got married and divorced in one year, and took an overdose in the aftermath. I was found by the police and taken to the local hospital where I had worked.

Pause

I am, nearly 40 years later, amazed at how difficult it is to revisit these times. It is like deliberately inducing flashbacks of how the hospitalisations added layers of trauma to my already traumatised self.

I agreed to enter in-patient psychiatric care believing that I would get help with the psychological pain I was in and guidance about healing the wounds of my adolescence and young adulthood.

I was medicated within two days of becoming an in-patient and was ques-tioned primarily about symptoms and functionality, rather than about the context of my life and what had led me to this point. Neither the side effects of the medications nor the fact that they worsened my confusion, exhaus-tion, and brain fog were considered relevant to discuss.

I had been sexually abused by an older child at the age of six and later exploited through my teens by a friend of my parents for whose children I babysat. I lived a double life with my parents and their friends, their chil-dren, and my younger sisters, with male and female friends, and the nuns in high school. At age 19, while away from home at an all-women's Catholic college, and shortly before my mother gave birth to my youngest sister, I began to grow a baby whom I relinquished for adoption when he was five days old.

Again, in the hospitals, nothing I thought was important about my story was considered relevant (Bloom, 2013). I was urged time and again to accept that I was mentally ill and the probability that I would need medication for the rest of my life and to limit my ambitions.

I managed to stay out of the hospital for five years between the first two-part admission and the second. I had never been manic until ceasing to take

Tofranil so when it happened, I was then labelled with manic depression in addition to borderline personality disorder (Jones, Steinberg, & Chouinard, 1984; Ali & Milev, 2003). The self-perpetuating rapid-cycling episode with manic periods often had "psychosis" mixed in. In retrospect, my delusions were often flashbacks and my "hallucinations" vivid memories that I attempted to relive in order to change their outcome.

Following a disastrous short-lived marriage to a recent widower with three children, I moved back to the city where I was first hospitalised to distance myself from the divorce. I proceeded to be hospitalised four more times within four years. A trial of lithium landed me in an extreme toxic state. Tegretol set off an extreme allergic reaction. Deals about what I would take or be given were broken in scenes of being force-medicated with Haldol in the hall in front of patients and staff. The in-patient stays lasted for the duration of what my insurance would pay for. There was one special hospital where I was transferred against my will where I actually had hope of getting help, but my insurance ran out and I had to leave after thirty days just as I had to from the big teaching hospital where I was hospitalised most often. There would be a rush to give me passes to go outside hospital walls so it could be in the record that I had done so before discharge.

The last hospitalisation began when the police brought me to an emergency room at a small community hospital close to where I had been living with my parents again. I had taken their car after they took the keys to mine. The police found me trespassing where I had been trying to retrace the steps that led to my marriage. Never having been hospitalised from my parents' home before, *I woke up* not only to the aftermath of heavy medication, but to the pattern of each in-patient experience worsening my state of mind and health, destroying any continuity I had in work or living on my own. The small community hospital psych unit worked to my advantage since they had no real security or legal staff. I decided I had to leave before staff would discharge me and had a law degree talk with the nurses while I signed myself out after just six days. This was possible, in part, because I was not medicated beyond the first night on that unit. I had been allowed my right to refuse and I used it.

The colloquial definition of insanity – doing the same thing over and over and expecting a different result – finally became clear to me. Only years later did I learn that repetition and disconnection were at the heart of unresolved trauma.

For the first time after a hospitalisation, I managed to keep my job and determined to put one foot in front of the other to learn how to live an everyday life regardless of mood, memories, or psychiatric opinion.

I emerged from the last hospital in January 1981. It occurred to me in March that I had taken the job I was in because it offered tuition assistance for college. I applied in the nick of time to five universities in New York City and was accepted to all of them. Thus began seven years of what I called my

26

"alternative institutionalisation". I switched jobs to one at the university I attended to take advantage of their tuition benefit and to cut out the commute between work and school. My life consisted of full-time work, coursework, weekends of study, and daily coping with what we would now call symptoms of PTSD, accompanied by severe anxiety, mood fluctuations, flashbacks, near paralytic depressive days, undiagnosed attention deficit and hyperactivity disorder (ADHD), deep bouts of shame, and chronic self-loathing.

I had made a pact to live until a natural death; suicide was no longer an option. The first three friends I met through work and school had all been hospitalised in their young lives. Another had had a baby out of wedlock and relinquished her for adoption. Another was a survivor of a concentration camp, full of post-traumatic stress and determined to get her degree. I swore off intimate relationships, a partially successful campaign, and was drawn to people's stories as if they were instructional scripts about chronically normal people for me to learn from: how to bring one's head up from the pillow and show up for work and school every day without screaming, leaving the classroom, or missing the subway stop for home in a fugue state. Therapeutically, I worked for years with an older interpersonal analyst who, despite a traumatic sexual transgression, refused to treat me as someone mentally ill and normalised almost everything I felt and did. Like quite a number of survivors, relationships with abusers can be complicated at best. He was the first person to suggest that I focus on what was "right" about me vs. what was wrong. Working through his exploitation as another layer of trauma did not erase his faith in my sanity and value.

Synchronicities began to be noticeable not only in those I met, but in the courses and teachers I worked with. I learned to sense a cycle in myself that might lead to hypomania and to temper myself with deliberate shifts in sleep, food patterns, and activities. It was the hardest work of my life and years later, when I realised I could no longer dissociate when I was in pain, I knew I had accomplished true integration.

In my sixth year of working my way through school, I realised I was actually close to finishing a degree. I had been fortunate to study my psychiatric experience from some distance: by taking microsociology courses about the history of mental illness and American medicine. My senior research paper was on the then fledgling National Alliance for the Mentally Ill and my sociology professors were eager for me to explore more closely my own experiences as a psychiatrically labelled person.

To do that, I decided I had to enter the field itself (the belly of the beast) to see what allowed individuals trained as psychiatrists and mental health professionals to blind themselves to the life experiences of someone in pain and instead label the pain "mental illness" in need of medications and/or more drastic treatments. With wanting to do better than what was done to me, I entered a master's programme in clinical social work, offering in my application the lived experience of being on the other side (and later learning that I was the first applicant to have owned that truth before attending the programme).

Never had I felt so exposed in my history of being diagnosed mentally ill as I did on the campus of the finest and most rigorous social work school in the country. Every day there were references made, most often by other students, to the plight of those who needed help, those who required diagnosis, and subsequent guidance of those who knew better. Certain diagnoses sparked particular disdain. Two of them were mine.

While I had been "out" as a former psychiatric patient in my application, no one in my classes knew my history. I confided in a couple of professors that I was sometimes uncomfortable with discussions in class to the point of feeling I had to speak out, which I sometimes did, without self-reference. I counted on compassion and empathy arising once insensitivity or judgmental thinking had been revealed. I was the voice of reminding people that any one of us could be in the position of being diagnosed and even treated against our will.

One evening I was attempting to sort out my reading assignments according to a standard of how likely I was to be upset by reminders of my "patienthood" ("triggered" wasn't yet a word in my vocabulary). I chose to read something I was sure fit the bill of being far from my experience and thus potentially upsetting only on an intellectual level. The article, by Denise Gelinas (1983) was called "The Persisting Negative Effects of Incest", and it contained a definition of incest that included as perpetrators close adults in family-like positions of responsibility for the young person who might be victimised. It also described what the effects of incest perpetrated on a child or teen might look like diagnostically. Many of the symptoms and difficulties uncannily matched my own experience in my late teens and early twenties.

I sat in my room stunned. I had always considered what happened over several years with my parents' closest friend my responsibility and sin. Hadn't I been "in love" with the man whose children I babysat, and hadn't I confided in him my deepest secrets? Wasn't it my decision to allow him to respond to me sexually when I finally professed my love? No matter that I did so fully expecting him to pat me on the head and tell me why it was a flattering fantasy never to be enacted. No matter that I split in two that night and developed the talent of living a double life: one with my parents and siblings (and his wife and children), another with him in the car on elongated rides home from babysitting and sometimes right amid family gatherings.

Suddenly the shame and confusion of those years collided in my mind with the experience of growing a baby I was convinced I could not raise. The second split in my internal existence loomed large in my realisation: that I had fractured to be a "woman of the world" and fractured again to survive being a birth-mother, that ended five days later as I left that baby behind in the hospital.

After relinquishing my infant, I spent a year wandering about in a low-level job and as someone's roommate before deciding that nursing school would solve everything: my parents' dream for me (or so I thought), a lesser financial investment, a job I could do anywhere in the world. No one was going to pay for college or therapy; I could solve it all by entering what was then still a trade school, unattached to college credits and full of practical experience. That's how I ended up in nursing school, having little idea of what nursing entailed, but believing that taking care of others on a physical level would keep me grounded and out of the psychological muck I often found in my own mind.

Two chemistry failures and one affair with a patient later, I started wandering out of my classes. The longing to erase the last decade of my life and to start anew was strong. Part of how I had decided to grow the baby (and let him go) was seeing how poor my decisions had proved to be until then. Now I could only stop dead in my tracks to keep from making a further mess of my life. Knowing I could not stay in nursing school, but believing it was still my only choice, I went to my therapist and sat paralysed in her office until she suggested the almost welcome solution: psychiatric hospitalisation. Wouldn't that just be exactly what I needed to sort out the past and begin again in the present. So, I believed, so fervently I went back a total of seven times. And so, I learned – and grew and backtracked and went in circles and leapt forward.

I went from clinical work with teens and adults in New York City clinics, to being the first NYC Director of Consumer Affairs in the New York State Office of Mental Health, to consulting with the US Center for Mental Health Services, travelling as a speaker and trainer around the country, to settling in Maine, where the first dedicated Office of Trauma Services was created within the state department. It didn't last long – now "everyone knows about trauma". So, I took my ideas about groups for women survivors of childhood sexual abuse to the community and started a private practice with a sliding fee scale. I am called "the trauma lady" and, to some who have seen my practice description or looked me up on the internet, I am "the therapist who has been on the other side".

References

Ali, S., & Milev, R. (2003). Switch to mania upon discontinuation of antidepressants in patients with mood disorders: A review of the literature. *The Canadian Journal of Psychiatry, 48*(4), 258–264.

Bloom, S. L. (2013). *Creating sanctuary: Toward the evolution of sane societies.* New York: Routledge.

Borrell-Carrió, F., Suchman, A. L., & Epstein, R. M. (2004). The biopsychosocial model 25 years later: Principles, practice, and scientific inquiry. *The Annals of Family Medicine, 2*(6), 576–582.

Gelinas, D. J. (1983). The persisting negative effects of incest. *Psychiatry, 46(4)*, 312–332.

Goffman, E. (1959). The moral career of the mental patient. *Psychiatry, 22(2)*, 123–142.

Goffman, E. (1986). *Stigma: Notes on the management of spoiled identity* (1st Touchstone edition). New York: Simon & Schuster.

Goffman, E. (1968). *Asylums: Essays on the social situation of mental patients and other inmates*. Harmondsworth: Penguin.

Jennings, A. (1994). On being invisible in the mental health system. *Journal of Mental Health Administration, 21(4)*, 374–387.

Jones, B. D., Steinberg, S., & Chouinard, G. (1984). Fast-cycling bipolar disorder induced by withdrawal from long-term treatment with a tricyclic antidepressant. *The American Journal of Psychiatry, 141(1)*, 108–109.

Kaysen, S. (1994). *Girl, interrupted*. New York: Vintage Books.

Kessler, R. C., Berglund, P., Demler, O., Jin, R., Merikangas, K. R., & Walters, E. E. (2005). Lifetime prevalence and age-of-onset distributions of DSM-IV disorders in the National Comorbidity Survey Replication. *Archives of General Psychiatry, 62(6)*, 593–602.

Read, J., Bentall, R. P., & Fosse, R. (2009). Time to abandon the bio-bio-bio model of psychosis: Exploring the epigenetic and psychological mechanisms by which adverse life events lead to psychotic symptoms. *Epidemiology and Psychiatric Sciences, 18(4)*, 299–310.

3

DISCOVERING TRAUMA HISTORIES IN WOMEN WITH PSYCHOSIS LEADS TO POLITICAL ACTION

Kristina Muenzenmaier, Andres R. Schneeberger, and Mary Auslander

During the 1970s and 1980s in the US feminist approaches (Webster & Dunn, 2005) brought women's victimisation experiences to the forefront of political and mental health discussions. Clinicians started observing the psychological effects of rape trauma (Burgess & Holmstrom, 1974) and childhood sexual abuse (Burgess, Groth, Holmstrom, & Sgroi, 1978; Herman & Hirschman, 1981) on women's mental health. During the same time period mental health workers realised the emotional impact of war trauma on soldiers returning from the Vietnam War (Haley, 1974). This led to collaborations between clinicians, war veterans, survivors of sexual assault, and journalists joining in social and political activism (Bloom, 2000; Brownmiller, 1994; Herman, 1992; Lifton, 1992). An evolving and shifting awareness of the impact of trauma on mental health led to changes in the psychiatric diagnostic classification system (Shatan, Haley, & Smith, 1977) and post-traumatic stress disorder (PTSD) was added as a newly conceptualised diagnosis in 1980 to the third edition of the *Diagnostic and Statistical Manual of Mental Disorders* (APA, 1980).

There was also a clearer understanding of short-term as well as long-term effects of psychological trauma and a realisation that trauma responses to a single incident differed from those of ongoing and multiple traumas (e.g. childhood sexual assault, combat, torture etc.) (Herman, 1992; Herman, Perry, & Van der Kolk, 1989; Herman, Russell, & Trocki, 1986; Terr, 1991; van der Kolk, McFarlane, & Van der Hart, 1996). Veterans and rape victims started to speak out and the silence surrounding disclosure of stigmatising victimisation experiences was slowly broken (Brownmiller, 1975; Schatzow & Herman, 1989).

In a major victory the Victims of Crime Act was passed in 1984 acknowledging the rights of victims to receive monetary compensation. The Governor of New York State signed an Executive Order in 1989 establishing the

DOI: 10.4324/9781003055914-4

Governor's Task Force on Rape and Sexual Assault (Avner, 1990). In 1993 the Center for Mental Health Services (CMHS) received a congressional mandate to focus on women's mental health issues resulting in examining sexual and physical abuse in women with serious mental illness (SMI).

Nationally and internationally, professional organisations emerged whose main interest was in addressing the psychological effects of trauma. In 1984 the International Society for Trauma and Dissociation (ISSTD)[1] was established followed by the International Society for Traumatic Stress Studies (ISTSS)[2] in 1985. While the diagnosis of PTSD was now validated in many studies (Lyons, Gerardi, Wolfe, & Keane, 1988) clinicians observed that the psychological effects of long-term interpersonal violence extended beyond simple PTSD (Briere, 1988; Herman et al., 1989; Terr, 1991). In *Trauma and Recovery*, Herman (1992) described a complex array of seque-lae she had observed in women survivors of childhood sexual abuse. The syndrome of 'complex PTSD' encompasses somatic, cognitive, affective and behavioural disturbances including relationship difficulties, identity distur-bances and altered belief systems. Despite a field trial showing support for the validity of complex adaptations to long term interpersonal violence (van der Kolk, Roth, Pelcovitz, Sunday, & Spinazzola, 2005) complex PTSD was not adopted in the DSM as an independent diagnosis. Instead, Disorders of Extreme Stress Not Otherwise Specified (DESNOS) was added to the DSM-IV in 1994 and is described solely as an associated descriptive fea-ture of PTSD (APA, 1994). While the children's diagnostic categories in the current DSM-5 (APA, 2013) do include Developmental Trauma Disorder describing the complex adaptation to early trauma, the adult section still does not. In contrast the current World Health Organization (WHO) classi-fication system ICD-11 (WHO, 2018) added the diagnosis of complex PTSD which combines the core symptoms of PTSD and three additional domains of affective dysregulation, negative self-concept and disturbances in rela-tionships (Brewin et al., 2017), thus updating the older classification system (ICD-10) that had included a diagnosis of PTSD as well as a diagnosis of Enduring Personality Change After Catastrophic Events (F62.0) (WHO, 1992) with the latter having been infrequently applied in clinical practice (Maercker, 2021). Numerous studies have supported the validity of both PTSD and cPTSD diagnoses in ICD-11 (Cloitre et al., 2018; Hyland et al., 2017; McElroy et al., 2019). Of particular interest are findings in a recent study showing a co-morbidity between psychotic symptoms and the ICD-11

---

1 The International Society for Trauma and Dissociation (ISSTD) was established in 1984 as the International Society for the Study of Multiple Personality and Dissociation, then in 1994 was named the International Society for the Study of Dissociation until in 2006 it became the International Society for Trauma and Dissociation.

2 The International Society for Traumatic Stress Studies (ISTSS), originally named The Society for Traumatic Stress Studies, was established in 1985 in Washington, DC.

diagnosis of cPTSD in people who were exposed to trauma (Frost, Louison Vang, Karatzias, Hyland, & Shevlin, 2019).

In the early 1980s and after finishing a master's degree in cultural anthropology at the Graduate Faculty of the New School for Social Research in New York City I began residency training in psychiatry. The people I were tasked to work with as a clinician was predominantly an inner-city population. Many belonged to minority groups, some were recent immigrants, and the majority lived in some of the lowest income communities in the city. Many had been confined in long-term psychiatric inpatient settings and were diagnosed either with a psychotic disorder (e.g. schizophrenia) or with an affective disorder (e.g. bipolar disorder or major depression). At times I found it difficult to determine the most appropriate diagnosis and I observed that throughout a person's psychiatric history the chart diagnoses frequently changed and shifted (e.g. schizophrenia, schizoaffective disorder and affective disorders as well as personality disorders such as borderline). The psychiatric terms and the diagnostic puzzles were confusing.

While I wanted to learn the state of the art in psychiatry, I also wanted to understand people's lives and how they come to be confined to a psychiatric inpatient unit. It was these people that I wished to understand fully as human beings not just as patients with a diagnosis and I felt a split that was hard to reconcile. While working with and trying to grasp the various diagnostic categories, the underlying human experiences were in the background and thus were eluding me. I started with some basic anthropological questions: How did immigration, poverty, and trauma affect people's lives? What was it like to grow up in another country and move to New York from the Caribbean, Latin America, Africa, Europe, Asia, or the Middle East? What was it like for a mother to come here and work as a nanny or domestic worker leaving behind her own children? What was it like for a child to grow up in NYC in poverty and have to struggle with economic issues, often with parents spending long hours out of the house working several jobs in order to make ends meet? What was it like to grow up in a household where family members might have had substance abuse problems, or where they may witness domestic violence and/or experience physical and sexual violence? Many reported having grown up with the sound of gun shots at all hours of the night and/or having lost a friend or family member to gun violence. What is the impact or ripple effect of the incarceration of a family member on that family member or the family itself? What impact did this have on the mental health of children and adults? Why did they end up being hospitalised on a psychiatric unit?

The beginning of my understanding of the psychological sequelae of trauma due to child abuse, rape, poverty, immigration/refugee experiences, street violence, and belonging to a minority group (Herman, 1992; Meyer, 1995; Read, 2004) were in sharp contrast to the prevailing bio-genetic model of mental illness such as schizophrenia (Read, Bentall, & Fosse, 2009). In the early 1980s I attended my first American Psychiatric Association (APA) meeting and remember feeling out of place. One of the presentations was on the psychopharmacology of borderline personality disorder. The room was filled with a huge crowd spilling out in the hallway in the hope of learning to prescribe the right medications that would then control and treat 'difficult to manage' clients who presented with affective dysregulations, lack of impulse control and acting out behaviours.

This medical approach stood in sharp contrast to my work in public psychiatry where I was confronted with the realisation that many of the people I treated had experienced or witnessed trauma during their childhood. This could include childhood sexual abuse, rape, physical abuse, neglect, domestic violence, and separation from a parent either due to illness, death, or placement in foster care. However, in my training at the time there was little in the curriculum that would have educated me about the impact of stressful life experiences upon people's mental health, nor did psychiatric assessments routinely inquire about trauma or trauma related symptoms.

Realisation: Extent of the Problem

At the time, existing research on childhood abuse showed mostly two main branches of research: one was about family violence and included physical abuse and domestic violence (Gelles & Straus, 1987); the other developed out of the feminist movement and focused on rape culture and incest (Herman, 1992; Russell, 1986; Wyatt & Powell, 1988). Yet in listening to women's stories it became clear that the various kinds of childhood abuse such as neglect, physical and sexual abuse often overlapped. Moreover, existing studies confirmed that childhood trauma may play a significant role in the clinical presentation of women with psychosis (Beck & Van der Kolk, 1987; Briere & Zaidi, 1989; Bryer, Nelson, Miller, & Krol, 1987; Carmen, Rieker, & Mills, 1984; Craine, Henson, Colliver, & MacLean, 1988; Jacobson, Koehler, & Jones-Brown, 1987).

However, the situation was complicated by the fact that people with psychosis were often disbelieved when they reported childhood trauma. Instead, their reports were seen as unreliable or in this particular population as delusional constructs (Carver, Morley, & Taylor, 2017). If women who had reported rape were often discredited and/or not believed how then could a psychiatric patient labelled with a psychotic disorder be believed and understood to have trauma as a fundamental experience?

This led to the writing of a proposal to study the prevalence of childhood abuse histories and their co-occurrence rates in women with serious mental illness. The goal was to develop a questionnaire in order to evaluate whether reports of trauma and abuse are valid and can be reliably assessed in women with psychosis. The Childhood Trauma Questionnaire (CTQ) was designed specifically for this population. It was carefully structured and started with open-ended questions leading to a funnel design (Meyer, Muenzenmaier, Cancienne, & Struening, 1996; see also Chapter 4 for more information on how to do a trauma assessment). Seventy-eight women who were enrolled in a psychiatric outpatient clinic in New York City and many of whom had a diagnosis of schizophrenia or schizoaffective disorder participated in the research study after giving informed consent (Muenzenmaier, Struening, Ferber, & Meyer, 1993). Some clinicians and researchers expressed their doubt about this proposal. Researchers were concerned about the validity of reports from people with psychosis and clinicians were afraid that the experience of the interview itself would be traumatic and destabilising. We also were concerned and did not want to do harm or trigger suicidal ideations or psychotic decompensations. When we began to assess the trauma history, we were surprised and encouraged how many women disclosed traumatic experiences and often expressed relief at being listened to and heard. This seemed to support the veracity of their disclosures. Some of the women reported to have shared this information for the first time.

The results of the study showed that reports of trauma and abuse can be validly and reliably assessed in women with psychosis. We found a high test-retest reliability for physical abuse and sexual abuse (kappa of 0.63 for PAB and 0.82 for SAB) and a high consistent validity when assessed by an independent clinical interview (agreement of 75% for PAB and 93% for SAB) (Meyer et al., 1996). Moreover, we found that the majority of the women who were enrolled at the clinic reported not just high rates of childhood neglect (22%), physical abuse (51%), and sexual abuse (45%) but also high co-occurrence rates among all of the three categories, with 70–94% of the women reporting at least one additional category of abuse or neglect (Muenzenmaier et al., 1993). Women who disclosed childhood abuse exhibited higher rates of depressive and psychotic symptoms as well as increased rates of sexual victimisation in adulthood when compared to those who did not report abuse. Women with a history of neglect had a threefold increase of adult homelessness. While our earlier prevalence study included only women, later studies documented that men as well had high rates of childhood trauma (Mauritz, Goossens, Draijer, & Van Achterberg, 2013; Muenzenmaier et al., 2014).

Despite the high prevalence, the majority of the abuse histories were not identified (Muenzenmaier et al., 1993). Only 20% of the women who reported CPAB and 32% who reported sexual abuse were identified as such in the chart or by the treating psychiatrist and a mere 10% reported that they had received any counselling or treatment for it. Only one woman was diagnosed with a secondary trauma related diagnosis of PTSD. Craine et al. (1988) found in a similar population that two out of three people he interviewed met criteria for PTSD, but none had received that diagnosis. Other studies documented similar findings (Mueser et al., 1998; Rose, Peabody, & Stratigeas, 1991). We therefore concluded that in this population the long-term outcomes of severe and complex childhood trauma were not being assessed nor interventions offered. Moreover, the complexity of the experiences including the stigma suffered from both serious mental illness and repeated traumatisation was widely neglected by most of the mental health community.

Political Networking: Bottom-up and Top-down

New York State Trauma Initiatives

In the early 1990s we submitted a grant proposal in collaboration with the New York State Office of Mental Health (NYS-OMH) to develop a trauma-based intervention for women with sexual abuse histories who had experienced psychosis. The intervention included educational as well somatic components. Unfortunately, trauma treatment for people with psychosis was not widely established and concerns were raised about the safety of interventions in this population. However, the noted importance of the prevalence studies (above) marked the beginning of a collaboration between NYS-OMH and other public psychiatric service systems on issues regarding childhood sexual abuse in people diagnosed with SMI. This resulted in the creation of a new position of 'Coordinator of the Sexual Abuse Survivors Initiative' within NYS-OMH. The coordinator of the initiative reached out to interested and committed people from the NYS-OMH, the NYS Mental Health Association and various community-based agencies. They organised state-wide meetings and promoted a dialogue between clinicians, consumer/survivor/ex-patient (C/S/X)[3] (Auslander, 1990), administrators, researchers and other interested parties looking for guidance in working with sexual abuse survivors. Over the subsequent years the initiative developed into a state wide trauma task force (NYS Trauma Initiative) that met on a regular basis.

The multidisciplinary committee included an extensive peer network and collaborated in a joint effort to develop guidelines for standards of care for sexual abuse survivors which extended to other C/S/X in the mental health system. Jointly we developed recommendations on: how to do trauma assessments; how to avoid coercive practices in clinical work such as forced medication, restraint and seclusion; how to develop trauma sensitive and trauma informed programmes throughout the state both for in- and

---

3   For in depth discussion of terminology of Consumer/Survivor/Ex-patient (C/S/X) we refer
    to Auslander (1990, p. 31). In other words, in mental health systems consumers are users
    (more in Europe) & consumers (C) in trauma-informed settings. 'Survivor' stood then
    for 'psychiatric survivor', the 'S' is now most often used in reference to trauma survivors;
    and those labelled with mental illness are most frequently both. Many are ex-patients or
    psychiatric survivors as well.

outpatient services; and made recommendations on education and training for all staff. C/S/X shared their experiences and took part in the decision-making process regarding trauma sensitive policies (Chassman, 1995). Feedback on what was helpful and what was re-traumatising was essential in moving forward with the work.

In the mid-nineties the task force was supported by the mental health commissioner of New York State who became aware of the high preva-lence of trauma histories in the lives of C/S/X. The political networking was successful because it included C/S/X and clinicians organising from the bottom up by developing trauma sensitive policies and practices which then were supported and enforced from the top down. Now representa-tives of each facility attended state-wide meetings that outlined and dis-cussed specific topics regarding the impact of childhood abuse on both women as well as men and re-traumatising practices within the mental health care system. Empowerment of survivors, sharing of experiences and ongoing collaborations led to an expansion of trauma committees, trauma training workshops and conferences both in individual facilities and on a state-wide level. The advocacy of the task force and the political activism helped establish a trauma sensitive approach within NYS and included revisions of policies regarding trauma assessments, restraint/ seclusion, retraumatising practices, and trauma-informed interventions. This empowering and collaborative activism led to important changes in the practices of mental health care in NYS.

Local, National, and International Initiatives in Changing the Dialogue on Mental Health Care

Major developments were now taking place on the local level, but also na-tionally and internationally. Discussions initiated by the survivor movement and hearing voices movement brought to the forefront a focus on recovery and peer support (Chamberlin, 1995; Romme & Escher, 1989).

The results of a long-term study in Vermont showed that more than half of the participants diagnosed with schizophrenia either improved or recov-ered, bringing a more positive outlook to mental health (Harding, Brooks, Ashikaga, Strauss, & Breier, 1987). Deegan (1988) wrote about her lived experience of recovery. Recovery was now being redefined and described from a C/S/X perspective (Ralph, 2000; Ralph & Corrigan, 2005). After the first peer-run healing centre had been established in the United States (Chamberlin, 1978), other self-help models emerged and included alternative approaches to psychiatric hospitalisations (Chamberlin, 1995; Dumont & Jones, 2002). Survivor movements started playing important roles in service delivery and organisational policies (Fisher, Penney, & Earle, 1996; Yanos, Primavera, & Knight, 2001).

The first national conference in 1994, 'Dare to Vision: Shaping a National Agenda for Women, Abuse and Mental Health Services',[4] was pivotal in changing the dialogue on women's mental health care. The participants were culturally diverse, came from various backgrounds (e.g. C/S/X, family members, clinicians, administrators, researchers, advocacy groups, etc.) and different service systems (e.g. mental health, homelessness, criminal justice, substance abuse, family services, etc.). The conference centred on issues related to women's mental health care and empowered C/S/X to express their vision on mental health services and recovery-oriented programmes (Levin, Blanch, & Jennings, 1998). Presentations on mental health care delivery included topics such as cultural sensitivity, substance abuse, childhood trauma, re-traumatisation experiences within the mental health system, and limited resources.

The discussions between the various groups coming together under one umbrella were at times heated and difficult. They also were essential in laying the groundwork in recognising the shortcomings and problems within the psychiatric service delivery system. By delegitimising C/S/X's claims of sexual abuse, neglect and physical abuse, the cycle of traumatisation continued. It was far easier to objectify and label a woman as 'borderline' than try to understand and empathise with the pain and cruelty inflicted upon her. Not only was the C/S/X not helped, the hurt was perpetuated.

In a very powerful talk one of the presenters spoke about the violent sexual abuse which her daughter had suffered as a three-year old child. In her paper (Jennings, 1998) she mentions that Anna was seen as a difficult child and started acting out when she was very young. Her first psychiatric hospitalisation occurred at the age of 13. Anna had received numerous diagnoses that included schizophrenia and borderline personality disorder and was seen as being non-responsive to treatment. After many years of repeated psychiatric hospitalisations Jennings learned that her daughter had been violently sexually abused by a babysitter as a child. She spoke of Anna's sexual victimisation and the related symptoms which were not recognised for many years by her or the treating mental health professionals. She spoke of her own despair as a mother and pointed out the many ways the psychiatric service system had failed her daughter by repeating and re-enacting Anna's traumatic experiences. Rather than fostering healing and recovery the early abuse was replicated by institutional re-traumatisation practices such as seclusion and restraint, not being believed, being blamed, shamed, and stigmatised. This also reinforces another dimension of feelings of powerlessness and neglect. At the age of 32 Anna died by suicide in a California State Psychiatric facility.

---

4   The conference was funded by the Center of Mental Health Services and co-sponsored by the Human Resource Association of the Northeast, Arlington, Virginia.

The conference was important in that it marked the beginning of a collaboration of C/S/X, mental health professionals, researchers, administrators, and advocates and was aimed at improving the delivery of mental health care services. Moreover, the shift to a trauma paradigm instilled a new approach to women's mental health practices and led to a growing awareness about victimisation experiences of C/S/X both inside and outside psychiatric institutions.

Local Level

The first NYS Trauma Conference was put forward in 1996 'Mastering the Key Connection: Sexual Abuse Survivors Diagnosed with Serious Mental Illness' bringing attention to the fact of high rates of sexual abuse histories in this population. Follow up conferences were addressing themes such as 'Safety and Recovery', 'Preparing a State Mental Health System to Recognize and Treat Trauma', etc. All conferences continued to be reflective of the Statewide Trauma Initiative and included clinicians, C/S/X, researchers, and policy makers as organisers and presenters. In the mid-1990s there was great excitement when after one of the conferences, the Mental Health Commissioner requested executive and clinical directors of NYS to institute trauma work groups at every psychiatric centre (OMH Quarterly, 1996). This of course validated existing trauma committees and now there was a mandate to develop new ones in every facility. The tasks of the local trauma committees paralleled those of the NYS trauma task force and included trauma assessments and trauma informed policies for each facility. The trauma task force felt inspired and empowered to shape the agenda in the state. There was also active participation and networking going on with dedicated people from other states and the sharing of information and recommendations regarding trauma informed policies and trauma assessments (Carmen et al., 1996; OMH Quarterly, 1996; National Association of State Mental Health Program Directors, 1998; Jennings, 2004).

Training manuals for trauma informed interventions were developed (Miller & Guidry, 2001; Najavits, 2002; Saakvitne, Gamble, Pearlman, & Lev, 2000). C/S/X were instrumental in raising important concerns regarding trauma sensitive practices and policy recommendations. From C/S/X's experiences, such as those described by Mary Auslander (see Chapter 2), we learned how psychiatric hospitals can be re-traumatising when instead they should be promoting healing and recovery in a safe setting. Training manuals for trauma informed interventions addressing the needs of survivors were being developed (Miller & Guidry, 2001; Najavits, 2002; Saakvitne, Gamble, Pearlman, & Lev, 2000).

Advocates, researchers, service users, and service providers participated as active members in committees, conferences, and trainings. Together with C/S/X we developed and piloted an instrument for assessing recovery from

Table 3.1. Recommendations for new trauma policy guidelines.

1. Acknowledgement
   a) that a high number of people with severe mental illness have a trauma history including sexual and physical abuse
   b) that circumstances under which they live (e.g., poverty, homelessness, institutional environments) can put them at continuing risk of violence
   c) that some current therapeutic interventions can be retraumatizing such as seclusion, restraints, involuntary medication.
2. Routine inquiry of trauma history for all service users.
3. Understanding of the impact of sexual and physical abuse trauma so that trauma informed treatment can be implemented.
4. Goal to provide a safe and therapeutic environment.
5. Elimination of four-point restraints in the spread-eagle position if person to be restrained has a history of sexual abuse.
6. Honoring of preferences expressed regarding gender of staff assigned to 'constant observation'.
7. Validation and empowerment by including service users in treatment options.

Source: partially adapted and developed with input of Chassman (1995); Carmen et al. (1996); OMH Quarterly (1996), and the National Association of State Mental Health Program Directors (1998)

sexual abuse (Alexander, Muenzenmaier, Dumont, & Auslander, 2005). Many of the collaborative projects were supported by NYS and included the Center for the Study of Issues in Public Mental Health, Nathan Kline Institute, which was instrumental in funding and moving the work forward.

It was a stimulating and profoundly interesting time to participate in these empowering collaborations that were fundamental in changing the delivery of mental health care services in NYS.

There is one thing that is bugging me – about how after the Dialogues on Recovery, and within the movement seeking compassionate versus coercive treatment, we later realised that we, the ex-patients ourselves, did not discuss our ignored histories of trauma as a critical issue. It was so ignored that we, too, were acculturated to consider it unimportant.

This so struck me that I reconvened several of the original dialogue participants, without the psychiatrists, for a day's discussion that was also recorded & edited for further use.

I do talk, of course, in chapter two about wanting to unravel those events in my life, but it is different from "getting" how integral trauma was and how the psychiatric experience repeated and added to the trauma already borne within.

There were so many aspects of my later experiences, working as an advocate in committees, etc., that I could travel down the path of ...

National Level

On a national level the President's New Freedom Commission on Mental Health (USA, 2003) included childhood trauma in the recommendations for research projects and evidence-based practices, and the National Association of State Mental Health Program Directors discussed the importance of developing trauma informed services in state mental health systems (Blanch, 2003). The creation of the Center on Women, Violence and Trauma was instrumental in the development of trauma informed care systems both on the national and the state level (Jennings, 2004). In 2006, as the National Center for Trauma Informed Care, it became part of the Substance Abuse and Mental Health Services Administration and was pivotal in supporting research and programme developments of trauma informed care on a national level. The Substance Abuse and Mental Health Services Administration (SAMSHA) report wrote extensively on existing trauma informed health care systems and trauma specific services documenting that the number of states developing trauma specific mental health care services more than doubled from 15 to 31 during the period of 2004–2007 (SAMSHA, 2008). Training programmes now incorporated curricula for clinicians in training in assessments and treatment of trauma (Courtois & Gold, 2009; Ferrell, Melton, Banu, Coverdale, & Valdez, 2014; Kosman & Levy-Carrick, 2019; Schneeberger et al., 2012). Our work in the trauma committee attempted to support this work on the local and state level even under difficult circumstances. Despite major gains in implementing trauma informed care in different states and service systems in the US (e.g. schools, residential treatment centres, and the larger health systems) people with psychosis still do not receive the attention they deserve. In a recent review of 13 studies from five different countries Read, Harper, Tucker, and Kennedy (2018) found that people with psychosis are least likely to be assessed for traumatic experiences and referred to trauma treatment. Therefore, we continue to advocate for routine assessments of trauma histories and related symptoms in people with psychosis as well as to develop and implement trauma specific services for this population both nationally and internationally.

Conclusion

The last three decades have brought major changes in mental health care services for trauma survivors in the US. On the national and state level trauma informed care was implemented in many different systems due to the extensive commitment and organising done by C/S/X, mental health care providers, advocates, administrators, politicians, and policy makers. Consumers' voices were heard in individual facilities but also on a national level. This also included guidance on trauma informed peer support (Blanch, Filson, Penney, & Cave, 2012). On an international level a movement of voice hearers ('the Maastricht approach') has developed regional and international networks in order to confront stigma, develop support, focus on recovery as well as guide professionals on how to work with C/S/X and voice hearers (Corstens, Escher, & Romme, 2008; Romme & Escher, 2000).

However, despite a growing general awareness of the impact of trauma and the developments of trauma informed care in many places and settings, there still remains a great need to expand routine trauma assessments and trauma informed interventions in particular for people experiencing psychosis. This must also include an understanding of the connections between trauma, PTSD, complex PTSD, dissociation, and psychosis.

References

Alexander, M. J., Muenzenmaier, K., Dumont, J., & Auslander, M. (2005). Daring to pick up the pieces in the puzzle: A consumer-survivor model of healing from childhood sexual abuse. In R. O. Ralph & P. W. Corrigan (eds), *Recovery in mental illness: Broadening our understanding of wellness* (pp. 207–232). Washington, DC: American Psychiatric Association.

APA. (1980). *Diagnostic and statistical manual of mental disorders: DSM-III.* Washington, DC: American Psychiatric Association.

APA. (1994). *Diagnostic and statistical manual of mental disorders: DSM-IV.* Washington, DC: American Psychiatric Association.

APA. (2013). *Diagnostic and statistical manual of mental disorders: DSM-5*, 5th edition. Arlington, VA. American Psychiatric Association.

Auslander, M. W. (1990). Voices from the ex-patient movement: psychiatric survivors unite and heal: a project based upon an independent investigation. Master's thesis, Smith College School for Social Work, Northampton, MA.

Avner, J. I. (1990). *Rape, sexual assault, and child sexual abuse: Working towards a more responsive society: Final report submitted to Governor Mario M. Cuomo.* New York State Division for Women.

Beck, J. C., & Van der Kolk, B. (1987). Reports of childhood incest and current behavior of chronically hospitalized psychotic women. *The American Journal of Psychiatry, 144(11)*, 1474–1476.

Blanch, A. K. (2003). *Developing trauma-informed behavioral health systems: A report by the National Technical Assistance Center for State Mental Health Planning.* Alexandria, VA: National Association of State Mental Health Program Directors.

Blanch, A., Filson, B., Penney, D., & Cave, C. (2012). *Engaging women in trauma-informed peer support: A guidebook.* Alexandria, VA: National Center for Trauma-Informed Care.

Bloom, S. L. (2000). Our hearts and our hopes are turned to peace. In A. Y. Shalev, R. Yehuda, & A. C. McFarlane (eds), *International handbook of human response to trauma* (pp. 27–50). New York: Kluwer Academic.

Brewin, C. R., Cloitre, M., Hyland, P., Shevlin, M., Maercker, A., Bryant, R. A., ... Rousseau, C. (2017). A review of current evidence regarding the ICD-11 proposals for diagnosing PTSD and complex PTSD. *Clinical Psychology Review, 58*, 1–15.

Briere, J. (1988). The long-term clinical correlates of childhood sexual victimization. *Annals of the New York Academy of Sciences, 528(1)*, 327–334.

Briere, J., & Zaidi, L. Y. (1989). Sexual abuse histories and sequelae in female psychiatric emergency room patients. *The American Journal of Psychiatry. 146(12)*, 1602–1606.

Brownmiller, S. (1975). *Against our will: Men, women and rape.* New York: Simon & Schuster.

Brownmiller, S. (1994). *Seeing Vietnam, encounters of the road and heart.* New York: HarperCollins.

Bryer, J. B., Nelson, B. A., Miller, J. B., & Krol, P. A. (1987). Childhood sexual and physical abuse as factors in adult psychiatric illness. *The American Journal of Psychiatry, 144(11)*, 1426–1430.

Burgess, A. W., Groth, N., Holmstrom, L. L., & Sgroi, S. M. (1978). *Sexual assault of children and adolescents.* New York: Lexington Books.

Burgess, A. W., & Holmstrom, L. L. (1974). Rape trauma syndrome. *American Journal of Psychiatry, 131(9)*, 981–986.

Carmen, E. H., Rieker, P. P., & Mills, T. (1984). Victims of violence and psychiatric illness. In P. P. Rieker, E. H. Carmen, & T. Mills (eds), *The gender gap in psychotherapy* (pp. 199–211). Boston, MA: Springer.

Carmen, E., Crane B., Dunnicliff, M., Holochuck, S., Prescott L., Rieker, P., Stefan, S., & Stromberg, N. (1996). *Massachusetts Department of Mental Health task force on the restraint and seclusion of persons who have been physically or sexually abused: Report and recommendations.* Boston, MA: Massachusetts Department of Mental Health.

Carver, L., Morley, S., & Taylor, P. (2017). Voices of deficit: Mental health, criminal victimization, and epistemic injustice. *Illness, Crisis & Loss, 25(1)*, 43–62.

Chamberlin, J. (1978). *On our own: Patient-controlled alternatives to the mental health system.* New York: McGraw-Hill.

Chamberlin, J. (1995). Rehabilitating ourselves: The psychiatric survivor movement. *International Journal of Mental Health, 24(1)*, 39–46.

Chassman, J. (1995). *Proceedings from a forum on individuals diagnosed with serious mental illness who are sexual abuse survivors.* Albany, NY: New York State Office of Mental Health.

Cloitre, M., Shevlin, M., Brewin, C. R., Bisson, J. I., Roberts, N. P., Maercker, A., ... Hyland, P. (2018). The International Trauma Questionnaire: development of a self-report measure of ICD-11 PTSD and complex PTSD. *Acta Psychiatrica Scandinavica, 138(6)*, 536–546.

Corstens, D., Escher, S., & Romme, M. A. (2008). Accepting and working with voices: The Maastricht approach. In A. Moskowitz, I. Schäfer, & M. J. Dorahy (eds), *Psychosis, trauma and dissociation: Evolving perspectives on severe psychopathology* (pp. 319–331). Oxford: Wiley-Blackwell.

Courtois, C. A., & Gold, S. N. (2009). The need for inclusion of psychological trauma in the professional curriculum: A call to action. *Psychological Trauma: Theory, Research, Practice, and Policy, 1(1)*, 3.

Craine, L. S., Henson, C. E., Colliver, J. A., & MacLean, D. G. (1988). Prevalence of a history of sexual abuse among female psychiatric patients in a state hospital system. *Psychiatric Services, 39(3)*, 300–304.

Deegan, P. E. (1988). Recovery: The lived experience of rehabilitation. *Psychosocial Rehabilitation Journal, 11(4)*, 11–19.

Dumont, J., & Jones, K. (2002). Findings from a consumer/survivor defined alternative to psychiatric hospitalization. *Outlook, 3(Spring)*, 4–6.

Ferrell, N. J., Melton, B., Banu, S., Coverdale, J., & Valdez, M. R. (2014). The development and evaluation of a trauma curriculum for psychiatry residents. *Academic Psychiatry, 38*(5), 611–614.

Fisher, W. A., Penney, D. J., & Earle, K. (1996). Mental health services recipients: Their role in shaping organizational policy. *Administration and Policy in Mental Health and Mental Health Services Research, 23*(6), 547–553.

Frost, R., Louison Vang, M., Karatzias, T., Hyland, P., & Shevlin, M. (2019). The distribution of psychosis, ICD-11 PTSD and complex PTSD symptoms among a trauma-exposed UK general population sample. *Psychosis, 11*(3), 187–198. doi:10.1080/17522439.2019.1626472.

Gelles, R. J., & Straus, M. A. (1987). Is violence toward children increasing? A comparison of 1975 and 1985 national survey rates. *Journal of Interpersonal Violence, 2*(2), 212–222.

Haley, S. A. (1974). When the patient reports atrocities: Specific treatment considerations of the Vietnam veteran. *Archives of General Psychiatry, 30*(2), 191–196.

Harding, C. M., Brooks, G. W., Ashikaga, T., Strauss, J. S., & Breier, A. (1987). The Vermont longitudinal study of persons with severe mental illness, II: Long-term outcome of subjects who retrospectively met DSM-III criteria for schizophrenia. *American Journal of Psychiatry, 144*(6), 727–735.

Herman, J. L. (1992). *Trauma and recovery: the aftermath of violence-from domestic abuse to political terror.* New York: Basic Books.

Herman, J. L., & Hirschman, L. (1981). *Father–daughter incest* (Vol. 12). Cambridge, MA: Harvard University Press.

Herman, J. L., Perry, J. C., & Van der Kolk, B. A. (1989). Childhood trauma in borderline personality disorder. *The American Journal of Psychiatry, 146*(4), 490–495.

Herman, J. L., Russell, D., & Trocki, K. (1986). Long-term effects of incestuous abuse in childhood. *The American Journal of Psychiatry, 143*(10), 1293–1296.

Hyland, P., Shevlin, M., Brewin, C. R., Cloitre, M., Downes, A., Jumbe, S., ... Roberts, N. P. (2017). Validation of post-traumatic stress disorder (PTSD) and complex PTSD using the International Trauma Questionnaire. *Acta Psychiatrica Scandinavica, 136*(3), 313–322.

Jacobson, A., Koehler, J. E., & Jones-Brown, C. (1987). The failure of routine assessment to detect histories of assault experienced by psychiatric patients. *Psychiatric Services, 38*(4), 386–389.

Jennings, A. (1998). On being invisible in the mental health system. In B. L. Levin, A. K. Blanch, & A. Jennings (eds), *Sexual abuse in the lives of women diagnosed with serious mental illness* (pp. 161–180). Thousand Oaks, CA: Sage Publications.

Jennings, A. (2004). *Models for developing trauma-informed behavioral health systems and trauma specific services.* Alexandria, VA: National Association of State Mental Health Program Directors, National Technical Assistance Center for State Mental Health Planning.

Kosman, K. A., & Levy-Carrick, N. C. (2019). Positioning psychiatry as a leader in trauma-informed care (TIC): the need for psychiatry resident education. *Academic Psychiatry, 43*(4), 429–434.

Levin, B. L., Blanch, A. K., & Jennings, A. (1998). *Women's mental health services: A public health perspective.* Thousand Oaks, CA: Sage Publications.

Lifton, R. J. (1992). *Home from the war: Learning from Vietnam veterans.* Boston, MA: Beacon Press.

Lyons, J. A., Gerardi, R. J., Wolfe, J., & Keane, T. M. (1988). Multidimensional assessment of combat-related PTSD: Phenomenological, psychometric, and psychophysiological considerations. *Journal of Traumatic Stress, 1(3)*, 373–394.

Maercker, A. (2021). Development of the new CPTSD diagnosis for ICD-11. *Borderline Personality Disorder and Emotion Dysregulation, 8(1)*, 1–4.

Mauritz, M. W., Goossens, P. J., Draijer, N., & Van Achterberg, T. (2013). Prevalence of interpersonal trauma exposure and trauma-related disorders in severe mental illness. *European Journal of Psychotraumatology, 4(1)*, 19985.

McElroy, E., Shevlin, M., Murphy, S., Roberts, B., Makhashvili, N., Javakhishvili, J., ... Hyland, P. (2019). ICD-11 PTSD and complex PTSD: structural validation using network analysis. *World Psychiatry, 18(2)*, 236.

Meyer, I. H. (1995). Minority stress and mental health in gay men. *Journal of Health and Social Behavior*, 38–56.

Meyer, I. H., Muenzenmaier, K., Cancienne, J., & Struening, E. (1996). Reliability and validity of a measure of sexual and physical abuse histories among women with serious mental illness. *Child Abuse & Neglect, 20(3)*, 213–219.

Miller, D., & Guidry, L. (2001). *Addictions and trauma recovery: Healing the body, mind and spirit*. New York: W. W. Norton & Co.

Muenzenmaier, K., Schneeberger, A. R., Castille, D. M., Battaglia, J., Seixas, A. A., & Link, B. (2014). Stressful childhood experiences and clinical outcomes in people with serious mental illness: a gender comparison in a clinical psychiatric sample. *Journal of Family Violence, 29(4)*, 419–429.

Muenzenmaier, K., Struening, E., Ferber, J., & Meyer, I. (1993). Childhood abuse and neglect among women outpatients with chronic mental illness. *Psychiatric Services, 44(7)*, 666–670.

Mueser, K. T., Goodman, L. B., Trumbetta, S. L., Rosenberg, S. D., Osher, F. C., Vidaver, R., ... Foy, D. W. (1998). Trauma and posttraumatic stress disorder in severe mental illness. *Journal of Consulting Clinical Psychology, 66(3)*, 493–499.

Najavits, L. (2002). *Seeking safety: A treatment manual for PTSD and substance abuse*. New York: Guilford Publications.

National Association of State Mental Health Program Directors. (1998). *Executive summary: Responding to the behavioral healthcare issues of persons with histories of physical and sexual abuse*. Alexandria, VA: National Association of State Mental Health Program Directors.

OMH Quarterly. (1996). Abuse: Connecting the past with present symptoms. *OMH Quarterly, 2*, 13–15.

Ralph, R. O. (2000). Recovery. *Psychiatric Rehabilitation Skills, 4(3)*, 480–517.

Ralph, R. O., & Corrigan, P. W. (2005). *Recovery in mental illness: Broadening our understanding of wellness*. Washington, DC: American Psychological Association.

Read, J. (2004). Poverty, ethnicity and gender. In J. Read, R. Bentall, R. Bentall, & L. Mosher (eds), *Models of madness: Psychological, social and biological approaches to schizophrenia* (pp. 161–194). Abingdon: Routledge.

Read, J., Bentall, R. P., & Fosse, R. (2009). Time to abandon the bio-bio-bio model of psychosis: Exploring the epigenetic and psychological mechanisms by which adverse life events lead to psychotic symptoms. *Epidemiology and Psychiatric Sciences, 18(4)*, 299–310.

Read, J., Harper, D., Tucker, I., & Kennedy, A. (2018). Do adult mental health services identify child abuse and neglect? A systematic review. *International Journal of Mental Health Nursing, 27(1)*, 7–19.

Romme, M. A., & Escher, A. D. (1989). Hearing voices. *Schizophrenia Bulletin, 15(2)*, 209–216.

Romme, M. A., & Escher, S. (2000). *Making sense of voices: A guide for mental health professionals working with voice-hearers (includes interview supplement)*. Mind Publications.

Rose, S. M., Peabody, C. G., & Stratigeas, B. (1991). Undetected abuse among intensive case management clients. *Psychiatric Services, 42(5)*, 499–503.

Russell, D. E. H. (1986). *The secret trauma: Incest in the lives of girls and women*. New York: Basic Books.

Saakvitne, K. W., Gamble, S., Pearlman, L. A., & Lev, B. T. (2000). *Risking connection: A training curriculum for working with survivors of childhood abuse*. Baltimore, MD: Sidran Press.

SAMSHA. (2008). *Models for developing trauma-informed behavioral health systems and trauma-specific services*. Alexandria, VA: National Center for Trauma Informed Care.

Schatzow, E., & Herman, J. L. (1989). Breaking secrecy: Adult survivors disclose to their families. *Psychiatric Clinics of North America, 12(2)*, 337–349.

Schneeberger, A. R., Muenzenmaier, K., Abrams, M., Antar, L., Leon, S. R., Ruberman, L., & Battaglia, J. (2012). Comprehensive trauma training curriculum for psychiatry residents. *Academic Psychiatry, 36(2)*, 136–137.

Shatan, C., Haley, S., & Smith, J. (1977). *Johnny comes marching home: The emotional context of combat stress. Concepts for the new Diagnostic and Statistical Manual (DSM–III) of Mental Disorders*. Paper presented at 'Can time heal all wounds? Diagnosis and Management of post-combat stress', American Psychiatric Association, Toronto.

Terr, L. (1991). Childhood traumas: An outline and overview. *American Journal of Psychiatry, 148*, 16–20.

van der Kolk, B. A., McFarlane, A. C., & Van der Hart, O. (1996). A general approach to treatment of posttraumatic stress disorder. In B. A. van der Kolk, A. C. McFarlane, & L. Weisaeth (eds), *Traumatic stress: The effects of overwhelming experience on mind, body, and society* (pp. 417–440). New York: Guilford Press.

van der Kolk, B. A., Roth, S., Pelcovitz, D., Sunday, S., & Spinazzola, J. (2005). Disorders of extreme stress: The empirical foundation of a complex adaptation to trauma. *Journal of Traumatic Stress: Official Publication of the International Society for Traumatic Stress Studies, 18(5)*, 389–399.

Webster, D. C., & Dunn, E. C. (2005). Feminist perspectives on trauma. *Women & Therapy, 28(3–4)*, 111–142.

WHO. (1992). World Health Organization: The ICD-10 classification of mental and behavioural disorders: clinical descriptions and diagnostic guidelines. *Weekly Epidemiological Record= Relevé épidémiologique hebdomadaire, 67(30)*, 227–227.

WHO. (2018). *The ICD-11 classification of mental and behavioural disorders: clinical descriptions and diagnostic guidelines*. Washington, DC: World Health Organization.

Wyatt, G. E. E., & Powell, G. J. E. (1988). *Lasting effects of child sexual abuse*. Thousand Oaks, CA: Sage Publications.

Yanos, P. T., Primavera, L. H., & Knight, E. L. (2001). Consumer-run service participation, recovery of social functioning, and the mediating role of psychological factors. *Psychiatric Services, 52(4)*, 493–500.

4

IMPLEMENTING HOSPITAL-WIDE TRAUMA ASSESSMENTS

Kristina Muenzenmaier, Mara Conan, Gillian Stephens Langdon, Toshiko Kobayashi, and Joseph Battaglia

During the late 1990s, as we initiated a process of assessing trauma history, we developed an understanding of the way in which asking questions in a measured way, and being attentive to a service user's emotional responses, made it possible to begin discussion about traumatic experiences. We gradually became more confident that many people with psychosis were able to talk about these circumstances without becoming too overwhelmed. Leaders of the trauma committee made it very clear that the way in which difficult topics were approached was extremely important. There was a great deal of thoughtful and sensitive discussions in the development of a trauma assessment form. In addition, we talked about ways to encourage service users to let the interviewer know when they were feeling uncomfortable. During committee meetings, role-playing exercises helped the interviewers to practise how to ask difficult questions and be attuned to the interviewee. I began to assess trauma with service users that I had a therapeutic relationship with in either individual or group therapy. I felt that I would be more aware of nuanced reactions among people who I knew fairly well. All interviews were conducted in individual sessions. There was a great deal of variation in people's reactions. Several made it clear that they were not comfortable with the nature of some or most of the questions. Others indicated that they had not been asked about their traumatic experiences prior to this interview and felt that it was helpful to talk about it. Many were interested in discussing the general topic of trauma and were curious how it could have affected their lives. One individual suggested a growing belief that it was not simply about him 'being crazy', but that what was important to consider was the way in which 'his life was crazy'. Although some appeared quite engaged, there were others who responded to inquiry in a non-emotional way. Several people in

DOI: 10.4324/9781003055914-5

this latter group would repeatedly go back to discussing specifics of a particular experience describing unnerving circumstances with an absence of emotional expression (i.e. a disconnection between thought and emotion). What most impressed me was that, after participating in a trauma interview, many service users became more comfortable talking about trauma in individual psychotherapy sessions. I suppose this was also due to my increased comfort in talking about emotionally charged life experiences.

Later in this chapter two fictionalised vignettes are presented that describe the way in which information gathered during trauma assessment interviews was used in ongoing individual psychotherapy sessions. Assessing readiness for continued exploration of traumatic events was based on the way in which questions were responded to in terms of both content and emotional reactions.

Introduction

As outlined in chapter one high rates of childhood trauma in people with psychosis were not only apparent in our clinical work but were also supported by research that began to be published in the 1980s and 1990s (Goodman, Rosenberg, Mueser, & Drake, 1997; Jacobson & Richardson, 1987; Muenzenmaier, Struening, Ferber, & Meyer, 1993; Mueser et al., 1998; Rose, Peabody, & Stratigeas, 1991). There was, however, at that time very little information about trauma histories in service users' medical records in the psychiatric facilities we worked in. Moreover, trauma was rarely taken into account in treatment planning. We saw an urgent need to develop and implement trauma assessments at our workplace. By the mid-1990s and with the support of the administration we were able to develop training for staff members of various disciplines in the use of the trauma assessment. Important aspects of the interviewing process included respect, understanding, empowerment, and care for the survivors with a special emphasis on avoiding re-traumatisation. It was enlightening and encouraging to see the extent to which survivors were willing to share and disclose their experiences. In order to heighten the awareness of the connection between trauma and survivors' behaviours and symptomatology hospital-wide educational meetings were held. This led to identifying needed changes resulting in a more trauma sensitive environment and the implementation of various trauma informed treatment approaches.

Studies Demonstrating High Rates of Childhood Abuse

In the early 1990s several studies in New York State (NYS) documented high rates of childhood abuse in people with serious mental illness (Rose, Peabody, & Stratigeas, 1991; Muenzenmaier, Struening, Ferber, & Meyer, 1993). A state funded intensive case management programme found high rates of undetected sexual and physical abuse in enrollees (Rose, Peabody, & Stratigeas, 1991). All the participants were chronic users of psychiatric emergency room and acute care services. In another study, 65% of 78 women interviewed in a NYS psychiatric outpatient facility reported childhood abuse with high co-occurrence of neglect, sexual and/or physical abuse (Muenzenmaier, Struening, Ferber, & Meyer, 1993). There was no documentation of abuse reported by the treating clinicians in the first study and only 25–33% in the latter.

Research over the last 40 years has consistently confirmed reports of high rates of childhood abuse and traumatic experiences in people with psychiatric histories (Briere, Woo, McRae, Foltz, & Sitzman, 1997; Carmen, Rieker, & Mills, 1984; Craine, Henson, Colliver, & MacLean, 1988; Goodman, Rosenberg, Mueser, & Drake, 1997; Kendler et al., 2000; Muenzenmaier et al., 2014; Mueser et al., 1998; Scott, Ross, Dorahy, Read, & Schäfer, 2019). However, assessing trauma in people with psychosis has been, and continues to be, frequently overlooked (Moskowitz, Dorahy, & Schäfer, 2019; Read & Fraser, 1998; Read, Hammersley, & Rudegeair, 2007; Read, Harper, Tucker, & Kennedy, 2018; Scott et al., 2019; Tucker, 2002). Moreover, PTSD and dissociative symptoms are neither consistently evaluated nor are treatment resistant symptoms of psychosis and/or depression assessed in the context of a trauma history. This is especially the case in public psychiatry settings (Goodman, Rosenberg, Mueser, & Drake, 1997; Grubaugh, Zinzow, Paul, Egede, & Frueh, 2011; Muenzenmaier et al., 2014; Muenzenmaier, Struening, Ferber, & Meyer, 1993; Mueser et al., 1998; Schneeberger, Dietl, Muenzenmaier, Huber, & Lang, 2014; Tucker, 2002). This is despite the fact that some of the psychotic symptoms seem to be directly connected to a person's traumatic experience (Hammersley, Burston, & Read, 2004; Read & Argyle, 1999; Read, van Os, Morrison, & Ross, 2005; Reiff, Castille, Muenzenmaier, & Link, 2012; Ross, Anderson, & Clark, 1994; see also Chapter 1). Scott et al. (2019) make clear the fundamental importance of trauma assessments in providing treatment to psychiatric service users. They indicate that irrespective of diagnosis individuals should "be routinely asked about childhood adversities, so that meaningful formulations of their difficulties can be made and appropriate treatment plans developed" (p. 149).

It is important to note that in the United States treatment approaches in psychiatry during the last 40 years have been mostly based on a medical model (Deacon, 2013; Jarvis, 2007) which differs from a 'traumagenic neurodevelopmental model' (Read, Perry, Moskowitz, & Connolly, 2001). As a result, routine assessments of trauma histories and trauma informed interventions, in particular in people with psychosis, are very limited (Frueh et al., 2009; Goodman et al., 1997; Lu et al., 2009; Nishith, Mueser, & Morse, 2015; Posner, Eilenberg, Harkavy Friedman, & Fullilove, 2008; Read et al., 2007; Rose et al., 1991; Rosenberg et al., 2001; Tucker, 2002).

Implementing Trauma Assessment

The lack of attention paid to trauma histories in people with psychotic disorders led to the organising of national and state-wide trauma conferences and meetings in the United States starting in the early 1990s (see Chapter 3). Mental health professionals and survivors felt it was imperative to provide trauma informed guidelines for psychiatric practices (Carmen et al., 1996; Jennings, 1994, 2004) since standard psychiatric evaluations did not routinely assess stressful childhood experiences. Through the persistence of organisational efforts in the formation of a New York State (NYS) Trauma Task Force (OMH Quarterly, 1996) and the support of the National Association of State Mental Health Program Directors (Blanch, 2003) (as mentioned in Chapter 3), we developed a collaborative culture among clinicians, trauma survivors and administrators (Jennings, 2004). Thus, trauma sensitive practice began to be instituted in the late 1990s in NYS, including the mandate for trauma assessments and revisions of policies such as restraint and seclusion.

General guidelines on trauma informed care, newly adopted trauma policies and mandatory trauma assessments led to increased awareness about stressful childhood experiences in people with psychosis (Carmen et al., 1996; Jennings, 2004). During the implementation process in the late 1990s we were concerned that the mandatory requirements would cause additional burdens among staff, resulting in either superficial compliance with paperwork and/or feeling emotionally taxed. Clinicians identified several issues and concerns: lack of training; questioning of usefulness since trauma informed treatment approaches did not yet exist; decompensation and destabilisation of vulnerable individuals; re-traumatisation of trauma survivors and time constraints. Thus, we stipulated that intensive training was a prerequisite for anybody conducting trauma assessments since the process can be overwhelming and trigger difficult emotional responses.

Aware that asking questions about trauma and resulting disclosures could be retraumatising to the survivors we recognised that it also could be stressful for the interviewer. Our goals were to be supportive to both. We therefore developed training programmes (Schneeberger et al., 2012) and trauma assessment guidelines to promote a safe environment for both during and after the assessment process (see below summary of guiding principles prepared for this chapter). We taped mock interviews but also developed role plays. During the role plays clinicians could practise as interviewees or as interviewers. This greatly improved the understanding of the intricacies of such a difficult interviewing process and one's own reactions and feelings in both roles. After the role plays, questions for all participants were posed:

- What part of the interview was difficult and why?
- Did the interviewee feel supported? Why and why not?
- Did the interviewee feel empowered to not answer questions when uncomfortable to do so?
- Did the attitude of the interviewee shift? When and why?
- How did the interviewer feel throughout the interviewing process?
- What helped in being able to move through the interview in a safe way?
- What happened during the interview when vulnerabilities and victimisation experiences were disclosed?
- Was there too much detail elicited or not enough?
- Did the interviewee feel safe during the interview?
- What were the observations of the committee members?

Forming Connections

For the training programmes we selected clinicians who were willing to participate regularly in meetings, and were interested in learning how traumatic experiences affected their clients. We invited clinicians from all units (day, evening, and night staff) and disciplines which included people of different genders and ethnic backgrounds. We advised the administration not to make mandatory assignments since clinicians have their own histories and stressors and might not be able to assess details of traumatic experiences given their current circumstances (e.g. dealing with difficult situations at home or in the work place). As we were opposed to clients feeling coerced to answer questions or to participate in a trauma programme, we felt those guidelines should also apply to staff. Because the voluntary aspect was essential, clinicians could participate if they were interested but nobody was forced to join. This is how the trauma committee was formed, resulting in a small group of dedicated people who believed in the importance of this work. We learnt that the involvement of individuals across different disciplines and cultural backgrounds was a major asset of the committee.

It is a challenging task to perform culturally sensitive trauma assessments. What matters is not only the translation of the questions into another language but also the perception and the meaning of the questions in a specific cultural context. The openness of the interviewer and her/his ability to understand and connect with people from different cultural backgrounds form the foundation upon which rests the ability to question and bear witness to difficult and painful traumatic experiences. The fictionalised vignette below describes one such attempt.

Since I belonged to the trauma committee, I was trained in doing trauma assessments on different units. I was often contacted to conduct an assessment for service users. Mr. T. did not speak English well, was easily triggered and showed rageful behaviours. He was very frustrated and felt that nobody believed him. Since Mr. T refused to speak with his therapist, I was called in to do a trauma assessment.

Like Mr. T, I happen to be a non-native English speaker. We sat together and started a conversation about what languages we each spoke and which language he preferred to speak in. He disclosed that he spoke French in addition to English. I tried out French with him and since I also had studied French as a young girl, I asked very simple questions in French. He responded, seemingly surprised that an Asian therapist could speak French. As we continued, he disclosed to me that he had been severely beaten and demeaned as a child. He seemed to feel validated by my listening to his story and as a result he became less confrontational afterward. He continued to connect with me in the following weeks. The encounter made me reflect on how to develop an intervention that could be helpful and also culturally sensitive to trauma survivors. This inspired the development of my first origami trauma group for men (see Chapter 15).

The staff box below illustrates how specific life circumstances can impact and affect one's ability to engage in trauma assessments.

In the late 1980s we had interviewed 78 women with SMI regarding their childhood abuse histories for a prevalence study. The majority of the women responded by expressing surprise and most seemed relieved to be able to talk to somebody about their traumatic childhood experiences. It became obvious that many had experienced childhood abuse often with co-occurring neglect, as well as physical and sexual abuse. A follow up study was planned to assess the past trauma histories of men. Based on my clinical experience, I suspected that sexual abuse was also under-assessed and under-reported in men. We knew that, in a society where men are more likely to be looked at as perpetrators rather than victims, it was important that the questions asked be adapted and reframed. Once, rather than viewing his experience as sexual abuse, a man told me proudly that as an eleven-year-old boy he was sexually 'initiated' by an older woman.

However, we ended up changing our mind about the follow up study. I had a newborn at home and found I could not proceed with the interviewing. Although listening to trauma histories is always difficult and painful, at this point in my life, it was so much more distressing. I felt emotionally closed and realised that I had to protect not only my feelings, but also the image of a safe world for my baby. I had to delay the project for a later time since I was unable at that stage in my life to listen empathically to the traumatic narratives of the people we had planned to interview.

Guidelines for Trauma Assessments

Review of Records

There is a series of steps to doing a trauma assessment. It is important to review the medical record, taking note of information that has been gathered about personal, developmental and social history as well as psychiatric history. Summaries, which provide information about past admissions as well as the current admission, are extremely helpful for gathering details about a service user's history. A major goal of this chart review is to determine if there is information about traumatic experiences including: physical or sexual abuse in childhood and adulthood; neglect; domestic violence; removal from the home; foster care placement; running away from home; homelessness; and substance abuse.

It is also important to review descriptions of behaviours and symptoms mentioned in the chart in order to determine whether some are suggestive of PTSD, dissociation and/or complex PTSD (e.g. self-injurious behaviours, assaultive/violent behaviours towards self or others, impulse control difficulties, dissociative symptoms, substance abuse, and promiscuity). Multiple diagnoses given over a period of time, as well as treatment resistance, could be clues to a trauma history and seen as attempts to explain the syndrome while neglecting the trauma. A thorough trauma assessment could lead to a diagnostic re-conceptualisation. In addition, identification of events that lead to decompensation can provide information about the kinds of circumstances that trigger strong emotional reactions and may be related to past traumatic circumstances (e.g. flashbacks).

Trauma Interview

The most important part of the interview process is to be able to connect with the interviewee in an empathic manner. The interviewer should be able to listen in a non-judgmental way and to be able to hear and process the traumatic materials that might emerge. The interviewer also needs to be understanding and accepting of where the interviewees are in their own healing process. At the start of the interview, it is important to explain the process and be clear that if the discussion is making them uncomfortable, they can stop the interview at any time. It is also important to empower the trauma survivor to be able to decide how much to disclose and when, and that they are aware that questions do not have to be answered. This can help in ensuring that a past experience of coercion is not repeated.

In conducting the interview, it is best to start with general open-ended questions (Alexander & Muenzenmaier, 1998; Read, Hammersley, & Rudegeair, 2007) that can be asked in a social assessment: Where and how did you grow up? Who belonged to your family or lived with you for a period of time? How many rooms were in the apartment/house? Where did you sleep? How were feelings such as love, anger and frustration expressed? It is important to be aware of legal implications and not ask leading questions on whether or not there were incidents of physical or sexual abuse. While the service user may have actually experienced such abuse, they might not categorise it this way. Instead, it is preferable to ask the following types of questions: How were you disciplined when you did something wrong? What happened? How often? Who did it? Have you seen anybody else being disciplined/punished? What would you say was the worst incident? This can be followed up with more specific questions about the actual events, the frequency of particular experiences and people involved.

After inquiry about physical abuse, the next step would be inquiry about sexual abuse as well as other stressful events experienced and/or witnessed. For example, to open discussion about sexual abuse one might inquire "Did anyone from your family ever play with you or touch you in a way that made you feel uncomfortable?" As with questions about physical abuse, this can be followed up with questions about specific incidents. At the end of the interview, the interviewer can assess and make a judgment as to whether the reported events meet the criteria for abuse (for detailed trauma assessment questions see Meyer, Muenzenmaier, Cancienne, & Struening, 1996). If the interview is becoming too stressful, more detailed questions regarding the event (e.g. the relationship to perpetrator and gender of perpetrator) should be avoided and perhaps be addressed at a later time. The interview should not be treated as a legal quest for truth but instead should be conducted in a supportive and therapeutic manner and be seen as a first step in the healing process. Throughout the interview, it is important to check frequently how the person is doing and at the end of the interview, there needs to be a debriefing and assessment as to whether it is safe for them to leave the room (Alexander & Muenzenmaier, 1998). If the person is hospitalised one might want to ask for permission to speak with the treatment team and/or the treating therapist. Any concerns regarding safety need to be reported.

Sometimes service users disclose that this is not the first time that they have talked about their experiences. It is helpful to inquire about what that

Table 4.1. Interviewing guidelines.

1	For each survivor the interview can be the initial step of an ongoing process of dealing with the trauma and/or the resulting symptoms.
2	During the interview, it is extremely important to develop a rapport with the interviewee and establish a safe and comfortable environment. Prior and throughout the interview the survivor needs to feel empowered to let the interviewer know when and if she/he is uncomfortable with the interview process and the questions asked and be offered to terminate the interview at any point.
3	Questions about traumatic experiences can be included into a more general discussion of past history.
4	Whenever possible it is important to try to gather concrete information (for example, kind of event/s, frequency, duration, severity, age, perpetrator, and witnessing).
5	If direct inquiry about traumatic experiences is not possible/advisable, helpful information can be gathered by asking about specific coping strategies and PTSD or complex PTSD symptoms. This can be followed-up with questions about the circumstances that particular feelings, behaviors and thoughts, are associated with. The next step would be identifying ways of dealing with these symptoms (e.g. self-soothing as a way to counteract dysregulated affect).
6	There are different decision points throughout the interview in terms of the kinds of questions asked.
7	It is important to ask open-ended rather than leading questions that then can be followed up with more detailed and structured questions.
8	The pacing of the interview is extremely important. The assessment form has several sections. Interviews can be completed over several sessions. One way of dividing sessions is to do some, but not all sections in one interview (e.g. if a service-user feels reluctant or has difficulty in answering questions).
9	Though it is recommended that the assessment be done on intake, it is important to evaluate readiness. This can include discussions with the service user and the treatment team providers if possible. Sometimes the service user may decide not to be interviewed or she/he may not be stable enough (e.g. in a dissociated or regressed state, actively psychotic or cognitively impaired).
10	At the end of the interview, it is very important to do a debriefing with the interviewee. This includes a check-in asking about emotional reactions to the interview and making sure the interviewee is/feels safe when they leave the interview.

experience was like. Negative consequences including feelings of guilt and shame, or threats and punishments may have shut down any further attempt to talk about the experience. This information can provide the clinician with a better understanding of what issues might come up in early treatment.

In general, while the interview can be stressful, most of our interviewees expressed feelings of relief at being able to talk about their upsetting experience/s, sometimes for the first time in their lives. The importance of disclosure rather than imposed silence is pointed out by Lister (1982) as a secondary and 'neglected dimension of trauma'.

Table 4.1 above is a summary of the interviewing guidelines and was put together for this chapter based on conversations with trauma committee members, the facility's administration as well as members from the NYS trauma task force (see Chapter 3).

Three-Part Trauma Assessment Write-up

Part I: Trauma History

The initial section is designed to summarise information that has been gathered in terms of trauma history. The focus is on childhood trauma such as physical abuse (including domestic violence), sexual abuse and neglect. Information for this section is based on information gathered in a review of medical records as well as the trauma assessment interview. It includes examples of different kinds of physical abuse (e.g. having been beaten with an object, burned, or threatened with a gun), and space to indicate "when" (e.g. childhood or adolescence) and "by whom" (e.g. parents or partner). In the section concerning sexual abuse, the initial question asks about being touched "in a way that made you feel uncomfortable" and an example of a probing questions to a "no" response, "or is there anything that happened that made you feel ashamed or bad about yourself?". In addition, there are questions to differentiate whether the experience was with a family member or non-family member. Moreover, while in the assessment there is an emphasis on childhood trauma, it is essential to also inquire about other traumatic experiences experienced or witnessed that may have happened during the lifespan and can include fire and natural disasters as well as interpersonal violence such as rape, physical assault and stalking.

Part II: Symptomatology

This part of the assessment is divided into three sections. We came to view these sections as a very important part of the interview process. We found it particularly helpful in therapeutic work with survivors.

In the first section there is a list of symptoms (e.g. flashbacks, panic attacks, self-injurious behaviours, difficulties with impulse control, and trust issues), many of which can be associated with a trauma history rather than acute psychotic symptoms. Standardised instruments (e.g. PCL and DES) can be added as needed in order to assess PTSD and/or dissociation in the further evaluation of trauma related symptomatology (Bernstein & Putnam, 1986; Blanchard, Jones-Alexander, Buckley, & Forneris, 1996).

The information is designed to provide information to understand the way in which service users' trauma history has influenced their clinical presentation. It reflects a view that certain symptoms can be conceived of as 'coping strategies' developed to get through very traumatic circumstances (e.g. substance abuse, hypervigilance, dissociation, and numbness). In working with survivors, it is important to explain what coping strategies are, emphasising that while they were helpful at one time in terms of dealing with overwhelming experiences, they may no longer be useful in handling current situations.

The second section focuses on what makes the service user feel better. We have found it to be useful for survivors to identify ways in which they can calm themselves when in a state of tension. The information can be used to develop an action plan in terms of specific self-soothing techniques (e.g. deep breathing exercise, listening to music, exercise, and walking with staff).

In the third section there is a list of factors which may heighten emotional reactivity (e.g. being touched, being isolated, and being yelled at). The concept of 'triggering' is explained to the interviewee. One of the purposes of gathering this information is to help survivors understand that their 'psychiatric symptoms' often are related to their trauma history and that specific stimuli in the environment may cause them to become overwhelmed because of past disturbing experiences.

The following fictionalised vignette describes a survivor's trauma history in which Part II of the assessment form was most important in influencing the ongoing therapeutic work. In this example, the service user and clinician were in agreement that it would be better to not delve into specifics concerning traumatic experience.

Charles was a 70-year-old man who at times experienced intense anxiety. He always came to the clinic well dressed and was very respectful in manner. He attended the clinic once every four weeks and met with me in individual psychotherapy sessions. He had been employed throughout his adult life and often in sessions he would talk about problems with his supervisor and his desire to retire. Based on background information in his case records, it seemed clear that as a child, he had dealt with a series of threatening circumstances, but we rarely talked about this during his session. Charles's mother had suffered from heart problems and was often unable to take care of the family and household responsibilities. During one of these periods Charles was placed in a foster home. Past records indicated that this was a very difficult time for Charles. I had known about this history but had hesitated to focus on this in sessions because I was concerned about how he would react. During the trauma interview, he talked about some of his difficult experiences when I asked about his childhood. He described the violent beatings he had experienced in the foster home, but indicated that he was not angry at his father (who worked full-time

and could not work and manage things at home) or his mother for be-
ing unable to care for him. He also disclosed that at 18 he was raped
by two teenage boys. As he talked about these extremely difficult ex-
periences, he showed no emotional reaction. At one point, he indicated
that it was best for getting along in the world to accept life's circum-
stances and that when dealing with other people he tried not to 'rock
the boat'.

In the next therapy session, I checked in about whether Charles had
any thoughts about the trauma interview and he said he did not. In
therapy sessions that followed we continued to talk about his present
circumstances. My belief was that given his desire to limit his clinic
attendance and his fear of change in his current circumstances, a sup-
portive rather than a psychologically exploratory approach should
continue. He did respond positively during sessions when we focused
on considering different ways he could handle a variety of situations
(e.g. issues at work). He learned to recognise the gradual build-up
of feelings of anxiety, and developed ways to self-soothe and ground
himself. In the course of treatment, a growing sense of agency was an
important achievement.

Part III: Treatment Recommendations

In this part, the clinician provides information on treatment recommendations. It is designed to provide information in a way that can be readily
adapted to the treatment plan. It has sections for statement of problems, the
goal of interventions, and specific methods that can be utilised. This may include: further assessments (e.g. identifying triggers of flashbacks, aggressive
behaviour, or incidents of self-injury); individual therapy in which service
user has the opportunity to develop a trusting relationship; discussion with
the treatment team about ways to provide an environment that feels safe to
the individual; and referral to a trauma group in which a major objective is
to provide a feeling of safety and containment when engaged in interactions
with other people.

The following fictionalised vignette demonstrates the way in which the
information gathered during the trauma assessment interview, including
details of trauma history, influenced the focus during individual therapy
sessions. In this example the survivor, though at times very much affected
by discussion about difficult circumstances, wanted to explore family issues
and the therapist felt that it would be helpful to do so.

Karen had several psychiatric hospitalisations beginning in late ad-
olescence. Her hospitalisations were based on violent behaviour to-
wards both herself and others, as well as delusional thoughts including
paranoid ideation. She participated in a facility programme designed

to provide work experiences based on a service user's skills and as a first step in seeking employment. She believed that other service users in the programme were planning to gang up against her. This was based on the belief that the regular employees in the department favoured her over other programme clients. She heard a voice telling her that she had to fight back. Though Karen had limited education and learning deficits which were likely related to her chaotic childhood background, she was quite verbal and could describe past circumstances in a way that made clear the details of situations as well as her emotional reactions. During the assessment interview she talked about her family and described the behaviour of both of her parents and her older brother. In this segment of the interview, both angry and loving feelings emerged. She initially discussed incidents that she had mentioned to other people. She was terrified of her father who had often been drunk and at such times would 'rage' at her mother, both verbally and physically. She indicated that there were also some situations that she had never told anyone about, but then continued and described a sexual relationship with her older brother. She explained that although she had not wanted to have sex with him and tried to stop him, she did like the money and gifts that he gave her. She blamed herself for the role she had played and tried to block thinking about what happened between them. She never told her parents. Karen had had no recent contact with her family, indicating that she did not even know if they were alive. Because I was seeing Karen weekly in individual therapy, we were able to discuss details of these overwhelming experiences in an ongoing way. We were able to explore her conflicted feelings towards her brother. She developed an understanding of the very disturbing situation she had been put in and gradually was able to voice her anger at him. Gradually her feelings of guilt decreased. She talked about incidents with other people which left her feeling hurt and which often resulted in anger and at times physical aggression. It was helpful for her when a connection was made between feelings of hurt, shame, guilt, and anger. She was able to identify specific kinds of experiences that induced strong emotional reactions and could describe feelings she experienced when she took actions that she later regretted. She could also explore the way in which early life experiences might be influencing her current behaviour. With growing insight, she was able to consider grounding strategies that helped her to modulate her responses to other people.

Conclusion

As clinicians become comfortable conducting a trauma interview designed to identify specific traumatic events as well as related symptoms, the importance of focusing on the specific needs of survivors is more readily recognised. The process of trauma assessment training is essential in increasing clinical awareness of the way that traumatic experiences affect psychological development. It is also a first step in developing competency in working with survivors. It is crucial as well to the goal of establishing a trauma sensitive environment throughout the facility.

Moreover, the assessment often marks the beginning of a process of collaboration between the clinician and the survivor. Together they can identify situations which elicit memories of past traumatic events and emotional responses that are difficult to manage. The appropriate depth of gradual exploration of memories, thoughts and feelings related to traumatic experiences needs to be carefully assessed in treatment. At times rather than focusing on the traumatic experiences themselves it might be more helpful to begin identifying trauma related symptoms and behaviours. Moreover, it is of critical importance to review effective strategies such as grounding techniques and safety plans as part of the assessment.

References

Alexander, M. J., & Muenzenmaier, K. (1998). Trauma, addiction, and recovery: Addressing public health epidemics among women with severe mental illness. In B. Levin, A. Blanch, & A. Jennings (eds), *Women's mental health services: A public health perspective* (pp. 215–239). Thousand Oaks, California: Sage Publications.

Bernstein, E. M., & Putnam, F. W. (1986). Development, reliability, and validity of a dissociation scale. *Journal of Nervous and Mental Disease, 174(12)*, 727–735.

Blanch, A. K. (2003). *Developing trauma-informed behavioral health systems. A report by the National Technical Assistance Center for State Mental Health Planning.* Alexandria, VA: National Association of State Mental Health Program Directors.

Blanchard, E. B., Jones-Alexander, J., Buckley, T. C., & Forneris, C. A. (1996). Psychometric properties of the PTSD Checklist (PCL). *Behaviour Research and Therapy, 34(8)*, 669–673.

Briere, J., Woo, R., McRae, B., Foltz, J., & Sitzman, R. (1997). Lifetime victimization history, demographics, and clinical status in female psychiatric emergency room patients. *The Journal of Nervous Mental Disease, 185(2)*, 95–101.

Carmen, E., Crane, B., Dunnicliff, M., Holochuck, S., Prescott, L., Rieker, P., Stefan, S., & Stromberg, N. (1996). *Massachusetts Department of Mental Health task force on the restraint and seclusion of persons who have been physically or sexually abused: Report and recommendations.* Boston, MA: Massachusetts Department of Mental Health.

Carmen, E., Rieker, P. P., & Mills, T. (1984). Victims of violence and psychiatric illness. In *The gender gap in psychotherapy* (pp. 199–211). Boston, MA: Springer.

Craine, L. S., Henson, C. E., Colliver, J. A., & MacLean, D. G. (1988). Prevalence of a history of sexual abuse among female psychiatric patients in a state hospital system. *Psychiatric Services, 39(3)*, 300–304.

Deacon, B. J. (2013). The biomedical model of mental disorder: A critical analysis of its validity, utility, and effects on psychotherapy research. *Clinical Psychology Review, 33*(7), 846–861.

Frueh, B. C., Grubaugh, A. L., Cusack, K. J., Kimble, M. O., Elhai, J. D., & Knapp, R. G. (2009). Exposure-based cognitive-behavioral treatment of PTSD in adults with schizophrenia or schizoaffective disorder: A pilot study. *Journal of Anxiety Disorders, 23*(5), 665–675.

Goodman, L. A., Rosenberg, S. D., Mueser, K. T., & Drake, R. E. (1997). Physical and sexual assault history in women with serious mental illness: Prevalence, correlates, treatment, and future research directions. *Schizophrenia Bulletin, 23*(4), 685–696.

Grubaugh, A. L., Zinzow, H. M., Paul, L., Egede, L. E., & Frueh, B. C. (2011). Trauma exposure and posttraumatic stress disorder in adults with severe mental illness: A critical review. *Clinical Psychology Review, 31*(6), 883–899.

Hammersley, P., Burston, D., & Read, J. (2004). Learning to listen: Childhood trauma and adult psychosis. *Mental Health Practice, 7*(6), 18–21.

Jacobson, A., & Richardson, B. (1987). Assault experiences of 100 psychiatric inpatients: Evidence of the need for routine inquiry. *The American Journal of Psychiatry, 144*(7), 908–913.

Jarvis, G. E. (2007). The social causes of psychosis in North American psychiatry: A review of a disappearing literature. *The Canadian Journal of Psychiatry, 52*(5), 287–294.

Jennings, A. (1994). On being invisible in the mental health system. *The Journal of Mental Health Administration, 21*(4), 374–387.

Jennings, A. (2004). *Models for developing trauma-informed behavioral health systems and trauma-specific services.* Alexandria, VA: National Association of State Mental Health Program Directors, National Technical Assistance Center for State Mental Health Planning.

Kendler, K. S., Bulik, C. M., Silberg, J., Hettema, J. M., Myers, J., & Prescott, C. A. (2000). Childhood sexual abuse and adult psychiatric and substance use disorders in women: An epidemiological and cotwin control analysis. *Archives of General Psychiatry, 57*(10), 953–959.

Lister, E. D. (1982). Forced silence: A neglected dimension of trauma. *American Journal of Psychiatry, 139*(7), 872–876.

Lu, W., Fite, R., Kim, E., Hyer, L., Yanos, P. T., Mueser, K. T., & Rosenberg, S. D. (2009). Cognitive-behavioral treatment of PTSD in severe mental illness: Pilot study replication in an ethnically diverse population. *American Journal of Psychiatric Rehabilitation, 12*(1), 73–91.

Meyer, I. H., Muenzenmaier, K., Cancienne, J., & Struening, E. (1996). Reliability and validity of a measure of sexual and physical abuse histories among women with serious mental illness. *Child Abuse Neglect, 20*(3), 213–219.

Moskowitz, A., Dorahy, M. J., & Schäfer, I. (2019). *Psychosis, trauma and dissociation: Evolving perspectives on severe psychopathology.* Hoboken, NJ: John Wiley & Sons.

Muenzenmaier, K., Schneeberger, A. R., Castille, D. M., Battaglia, J., Seixas, A. A., & Link, B. (2014). Stressful childhood experiences and clinical outcomes in people with serious mental illness: A gender comparison in a clinical psychiatric sample. *Journal of Family Violence, 29*(4), 419–429.

Muenzenmaier, K., Struening, E., Ferber, J., & Meyer, I. (1993). Childhood abuse and neglect among women outpatients with chronic mental illness. *Psychiatric Services, 44*(7), 666–670.

Mueser, K. T., Goodman, L. B., Trumbetta, S. L., Rosenberg, S. D., Osher, F. C., Vidaver, R., ... Foy, D. W. (1998). Trauma and posttraumatic stress disorder in severe mental illness. *Journal of Consulting Clinical Psychology, 66*(3), 493–499.

Nishith, P., Mueser, K. T., & Morse, G. A. (2015). A brief intervention for posttraumatic stress disorder in persons with a serious mental illness. *Psychiatric Rehabilitation Journal, 38*(4), 314–319.

OMH Quarterly. (1996). Abuse: Connecting the past with present symptoms. *OMH Quarterly, 2*, 13–15.

Posner, J., Eilenberg, J., Harkavy Friedman, J., & Fullilove, M. J. (2008). Quality and use of trauma histories obtained from psychiatric outpatients: A ten-year follow-up. *Psychiatric Services, 59*(3), 318–321.

Read, J., & Argyle, N. (1999). Hallucinations, delusions, and thought disorder among adult psychiatric inpatients with a history of child abuse. *Psychiatric Services, 50*(11), 1467–1472.

Read, J., & Fraser, A. (1998). Abuse histories of psychiatric inpatients: To ask or not to ask? *Psychiatric Services, 49*(3), 355–359.

Read, J., Hammersley, P., & Rudegeair, T. (2007). Why, when and how to ask about childhood abuse. *Advances in Psychiatric Treatment, 13*(2), 101–110.

Read, J., Harper, D., Tucker, I., & Kennedy, A. (2018). Do adult mental health services identify child abuse and neglect? A systematic review. *International Journal of Mental Health Nursing, 27*(1), 7–19.

Read, J., Perry, B. D., Moskowitz, A., & Connolly, J. (2001). The contribution of early traumatic events to schizophrenia in some patients: A traumagenic neurodevelopmental model. *Psychiatry: Interpersonal and Biological Processes, 64*(4), 319–345.

Read, J., van Os, J., Morrison, A. P., & Ross, C. A. (2005). Childhood trauma, psychosis and schizophrenia: A literature review with theoretical and clinical implications. *Acta Psychiatrica Scandinavica, 112*(5), 330–350.

Reiff, M., Castille, D. M., Muenzenmaier, K., & Link, B. (2012). Childhood abuse and the content of adult psychotic symptoms. *Psychological Trauma: Theory, Research, Practice, Policy, 4*(4), 356–369.

Rose, S. M., Peabody, C. G., & Stratigeas, B. (1991). Undetected abuse among intensive case management clients. *Psychiatric Services, 42*(5), 499–503.

Rosenberg, S. D., Mueser, K. T., Friedman, M. J., Gorman, P. G., Drake, R. E., Vidaver, R. M., ... Jankowski, M. K. (2001). Developing effective treatments for posttraumatic disorders among people with severe mental illness. *Psychiatric Services, 52*(11), 1453–1461.

Ross, C. A., Anderson, G., & Clark, P. (1994). Childhood abuse and the positive symptoms of schizophrenia. *J Psychiatric Services, 45*(5), 489–491.

Schneeberger, A. R., Dietl, M. F., Muenzenmaier, K. H., Huber, C. G., & Lang, U. E. (2014). Stressful childhood experiences and health outcomes in sexual minority populations: A systematic review. *Social Psychiatry and Psychiatric Epidemiology, 49*(9), 1427–1445.

Schneeberger, A. R., Muenzenmaier, K., Abrams, M., Antar, L., Leon, S. R., Ruberman, L., & Battaglia, J. (2012). Comprehensive trauma training curriculum for psychiatry residents. *Academic Psychiatry, 36*(2), 136–137.

Scott, J. G., Ross, C. A., Dorahy, M. J., Read, J., & Schäfer, I. (2019). Childhood trauma in psychotic and dissociative disorders. In A. Moskowitz, M. J. Dorahy, & I. Schäfer (eds), *Psychosis, trauma and dissociation: Evolving perspectives on severe psychopathology* (pp. 143–157). Hoboken, NJ: John Wiley & Sons.

Tucker, W. M. (2002). How to include the trauma history in the diagnosis and treatment of psychiatric inpatients. *Psychiatric Quarterly, 73*(2), 135–144.

5

DEVELOPMENT OF A TRAUMA COMMITTEE

Forming Connections

*Kristina Muenzenmaier, Gillian Stephens Langdon,
Mara Conan, Toshiko Kobayashi, and Joseph Battaglia*

Introduction

My participation in the trauma committee resulted in a major transformation in the way I worked. In the early stages of the trauma committee, the focused attention on the ways in which it was possible to open up discussion about past overwhelming experiences helped me to feel more confident in asking survivors about difficult circumstances. I also began to understand how important it was for many survivors to be able to discuss subjects that they had not been able to discuss in the past. I became more confident that by our providing a holding environment, a service user would become more trusting and would feel less hesitant talking about topics she/he had avoided in the past. I was surprised at the number of individuals who were interested in working together on a narrative about both threatening and rewarding past experiences. In addition, I realised that focusing on managing trauma related symptoms was quite effective and did not necessarily require detailed discussion of traumatic events. This was extremely important also in running trauma groups and helped to ensure that individuals did not trigger strong emotional reactions in other members.

One of the most important factors in maintaining a balanced approach to my work (in addition to engaging in rewarding and grounding activities when not at work) was my participation in the trauma committee. Committee members became a major source of support. I knew that the group of people attending the meetings shared similar assessment and treatment planning goals, and were dealing with similar intense experiences. Because we met together frequently, I

DOI: 10.4324/9781003055914-6

> experienced it as a very safe environment and knew that it I could freely express my concerns and reactions. I was confident that I would not be critically judged. It was extremely helpful to hear others talk about their own fears and feelings of confusion to unexpected and frightening reactions of trauma survivors. We often discussed the parallel process that existed in both service user and staff groups and that empathy and the development of connection was key in both.

Looking back, belonging to a smaller community within the larger framework of the facility was validating and energising. The trauma committee (TC) provided a holding environment which enabled us to engage in very meaningful though intensive work. This chapter outlines the development of the TC. The beginnings of our committee originated with our developing and implementing trauma assessments. We revised hospital policies to become trauma-sensitive and created hospital-wide trauma trainings. To address the needs of people with psychosis and childhood trauma, we developed multi-modal treatment approaches. This included a wide variety of multi-disciplinary trauma groups. Our collaborations became the foundation for improving the hospital environment by making it more trauma sensitive and by developing trauma informed treatment approaches. A critical feature of all of this was that we became a support group for each other, prioritising any committee member's overwhelming experiences during this challenging work. In a way the TC paralleled the trauma groups where group members could begin to heal in the context of safe connections.

Early Steps: Developing Trust

In the 1990s the formation of the New York State (NYS) Trauma Task Force consisting of clinicians, researchers, consumers/survivors, administrators and policy makers became an active force addressing the needs of this population. As a result of this advocacy an understanding emerged of the importance and need for this work, so that in the mid-1990s the commissioner of the New York State Office of Mental Health (NYS-OMH) recommended that each facility form a TC (see Chapter 3). Moreover, in 1995 new requirements of the Joint Commission on Accreditation of Healthcare Organizations (JCAHO) mandated that victims of abuse and neglect be identified and assessed for trauma and related symptoms in order to meet the criteria for accreditation (Carmen et al., 1996).

While initially the facility's TC started out with only a few members, the 1995 mandates triggered a more extensive recruitment of clinicians in order to be able to assess all service recipients for histories of trauma. We invited one or two clinicians (psychologists, psychiatrists, or social workers) from each unit and since we wanted to be sensitive to the needs of staff nobody was obligated to join. As noted in chapter 4 we felt the voluntary aspect was essential and avoided feelings of coercion. Over time clinicians representing different disciplines and different units joined the committee. Everybody was encouraged to speak up and voice their concerns. Together we developed a trauma assessment for the facility based on recommendations by the NYS Trauma Task Force taking into account the concerns of survivors about the potential for re-traumatisation (see Chapter 3).

In the beginning clinicians were hesitant to ask service users about experiences of childhood abuse and trauma, in particular sexual abuse. We therefore decided to develop training programmes on how to conduct a trauma assessment (see Chapter 4). We included role plays for practising the interview and also taped a mock interview in which a psychologist played an angry teenager/young adult who was acting out and reluctant to answer questions. During those training sessions we started to develop strong connections as a group, and despite the seriousness of the topic we could share a laugh about a psychologist playing a teenager wearing a baseball cap and giving the psychiatrist a hard time during the interview. Committee members were thoughtful during discussions about the interview process but also became more relaxed and started to feel that we could trust and be open with one another. We included trauma related goals and objectives in treatment plans (e.g. developing trust, safe connections, avoidance of re-traumatisation and survivors' preferences about safety protocols) and thought about what interventions might be helpful. Trauma committee members then started to consult on different units with individual therapists and treatment teams. As a result of these discussions there was a hospital-wide shift towards a focus on trauma, thereby raising awareness as well as, importantly, influencing staff's attitudes towards service users' behaviours.

Dancing Together: Developments within the Trauma Committee that Influenced Trauma Informed Interventions

In the early 2000s, the TC had become a hub of a vibrant, supportive, and diverse community of caregivers of different disciplines including psychiatry, social work, nursing, psychology and, later, creative arts therapies. As members of the trauma committee continued to meet regularly a stronger feeling of trust developed, which in turn made it easier to think creatively about new and innovative programmes. There were many factors which made this possible. TC meetings were frequent, consistent, and enriching. Attendance was voluntary and the meetings were scheduled once a week during lunch hour so as not to interfere with clinical responsibilities. With many of the participants just beginning to understand the way in which trauma influenced psychological development there was a very strong desire to learn as much as possible about different interventions.

In committee meetings we discussed trauma literature, gave feedback about workshops we had attended, and talked about our own experiences in working with survivors and in developing interventions. The pioneering work of Judith Herman (1992) greatly improved our understanding of complex post-traumatic stress disorder (see Introduction). In discussing background literature, we were able to refine our questions concerning the concepts of psychosis, dissociation and PTSD and its confusing overlap (see Chapter 1). Members were highly motivated to get feedback about ways to handle challenging situations. During our committee meetings we discussed and developed individual and group therapy approaches for trauma survivors with a particular focus on coping strategies for dealing with trauma related symptoms and behaviours. Vignettes throughout this book provide examples of trauma informed interventions.

One of the early trauma training sessions we participated in was entitled 'Risking Connection' and it strongly impacted members of the TC (Saakvitne, Gamble, Pearlman, & Lev, 2000). We also attended presentations on the 'Sanctuary Model' (Bloom, 1997), which taught us the value of a safe and interconnected community. We learnt from Harris and Anglin (1998) the importance of empowerment in healing from trauma. Moreover, in the late 1990s we presented at the yearly clinical training conferences in New York State (NYS-OMH) 'Mastering the Key Connection'. Those conferences were unique and stimulating in that they promoted a dialogue between people from a wide variety of backgrounds and included consumer-survivors, clinicians, administrators, researchers, and others who presented on various aspects of trauma informed care and related topics.

In the course of our work, we had become increasingly aware of how important it was for trauma survivors who also experienced psychotic symptoms to have their victimisation experiences acknowledged and for them to feel safe in the unfolding of the healing process. Because of that, we realised that in order to create a safe environment for survivors, we also had to have a strong sense of support and guidance for one another. Providing a safe space for each one of us, was another factor in a growing feeling of trust, and in turn increased openness. As we aimed towards a culture that was supportive and open, a member could arrive distressed and say, "I need help. I'm overwhelmed." Or: "The group was so disorganised. I don't know how to bring it together." The committee provided a holding environment where it was possible to be honest about our own struggles, vulnerabilities, and the different approaches we had in working with trauma survivors. It was analogous to survivors who could not heal in isolation but required empathic relationships for change to occur.

As we continued to collaborate, we realised there was a parallel process taking place between survivor groups and trauma committee meetings.

Moreover, our efforts to empower trauma survivors was reflected in our own process during committee meetings where we tried to verbalise our unique points of view and where we sometimes struggled to understand views and reactions that were different from our own. This endeavour helped fine tune our listening skills and served to increase our empathy to feelings and experiences of others both within the committee as well as the wider hospital system.

Core to the committee's foundation was the recognition that each member of the committee had a special viewpoint in understanding survivors, but that no one member alone was aware of the many different aspects that can be examined in understanding needs of each service user. We knew that when working in isolation there is the risk of creating, treating and reinforcing a fragmented picture including the one that survivors have of themselves. Clinicians from various disciplines and ethnic backgrounds provided different perspectives. Collaborating helped in understanding the survivor in a more complex and integrated way.

There were some situations that were particularly difficult for me. The TC was a safe place where I could go to talk when I experienced confusion and self-doubt. I very much appreciated the in-depth discussions about the meaning of survivors' actions and how to respond. I remember one day coming to the trauma committee meeting extremely distressed after one of the survivors I was working with had made a suicide attempt. She had come in for her once weekly scheduled appointment and calmly reported that earlier in the day she had swallowed a handful of pills, but then made herself throw-up. I knew that her only hospitalisation was precipitated when she cut her wrist, an action that had been considered a serious suicide attempt.

Her treating psychiatrist was available and I asked him to join the meeting. We talked with her, but she had difficulty answering questions. The decision was made to have her brought to a hospital emergency room for evaluation. The psychiatrist left to prepare the paperwork. After he walked out, she began to sob. She described how tormented she felt, but that she was terrified of returning to the hospital. I moved my chair so I was much closer to her and we sat together that way until the ambulance arrived. Questions ran through my head as we were waiting together: Should I have tried to talk to her alone before I called the psychiatrist in? How serious was her attempt? Had I missed the signs that she had become more depressed? What would her experience in the hospital be like? Had we made the right decision about the need for an emergency room psychiatric and medical evaluation? Would a hospitalisation affect our relationship and would it

---

be a set-back in the strides she had made in adopting more effective coping strategies? Would she decide to work with another therapist? But there were also different kinds of thoughts: How she had held herself together until the psychiatrist left the office; that she had trusted me enough to openly express her intense feelings; how deeply sad I felt sitting there thinking about what her life had been like. When I shared all this during the TC meeting, the empathic response of the committee members enabled me to talk about my emotional turmoil as well as considering ways of dealing with such challenges.

Facility-Wide Outreach

Within the facility, the support of the clinical administration was instrumental in the ability of the committee members to effect systemic change. The clinical director was supportive of our developing a working TC, and when time would allow, he attended our meetings and was very much involved in the discussions about trauma informed care. Throughout the years his interest and administrative support were critical to our work and the implementation of hospital-wide trauma assessments and trauma informed interventions. Staff interested in developing a trauma sensitive environment felt empowered and began to collaborate on proposing trauma sensitive policies and practices regarding restraint and seclusion, involuntary medication administration, communication patterns, night checks, and assessment of triggers for each service user.

We discussed coercive practices and revised decades old policies in order to prevent re-traumatisation. To help staff understand the reasons for change in procedures, it became clear that it was important to provide information about trauma to all hospital staff. We designed hospital-wide workshops in order to raise awareness of the issues unique to trauma survivors. This included trainings and consultations developed for nursing staff and clinicians, as well as for supervisors and administrators. Of particular importance was the recognition of how devastating traumatic experiences can be, the kinds of symptoms and behaviours that are associated with trauma, and which interactions/interventions can be helpful rather than harmful when a survivor is feeling overwhelmed.

Now both clinical and administrative staff started to reach out to committee members requesting trauma assessments when they realised a trauma history might be interfering with treatment. If there were incidents involving service users that were difficult to handle or were overwhelming such as assaultive or self-injurious behaviours, we went to the units and conducted both separate and joint meetings with service users and staff depending on the circumstances. Administrators were helpful in arranging coverage so unit staff could participate in the meetings. Staff was also released from ward duties in order to be able to attend trauma trainings and conferences. As a result, the awareness about the impact of trauma continued to grow.

Given our understanding of 'vicarious traumatisation' (Pearlman & Saakvitne, 1995), committee members stressed the importance of developing support to all staff regardless of work assignments, disciplines, and administrative levels (see Chapter 6). In addition to support for frontline staff, we also developed separate training meetings for supervisors. Learning about the impact of trauma helped in understanding not only the needs of traumatised service users but also the needs of traumatised colleagues after serious incidents. Nursing supervisors often were the first responders to frontline staff when incidents happened. While reaching out to traumatised staff they too could be overwhelmed with extremely challenging circumstances. They too needed support. Over time people became attuned to their vulnerabilities and reactions. It became clear that developing a support network for staff, as well as hospital-wide trauma trainings, were essential in the attempt to create a more trauma sensitive environment within the facility.

Continuity of care was another issue which we grappled with. We wanted to facilitate the integration of the various service delivery systems. We encouraged open communication about treatment approaches, problems encountered and overwhelming circumstances. We were aware of how challenging it could be to avoid an atmosphere of fear and blame after traumatising incidents. Since the TC meetings happened during the lunch hour, we scheduled discussions with clinicians from different services on an as needed basis. We invited staff throughout the hospital to our meetings where they could present difficult questions, challenging issues and discuss specific trauma assessments. If a service user had experienced a hospitalisation prior to turning 18, we tried to include a team member from the children's psychiatric facility in order to gain a better understanding of a survivor's experiential world as a child. We included treatment providers from outpatient services, encouraging a natural tendency to think about recovery and coordination of treatment when a survivor returned to the community. We also made ourselves available to staff in residential facilities.

Multidisciplinary Participation in Trauma Committee Leads to Multimodal Interventions

In the United States, interest in the consequences of trauma within both the general public and among clinicians working in psychiatric settings was heightened after the terrorist attacks in the United States on September 11th, 2001 (Loewy & Hara, 2002; Neria, DiGrande, & Adams, 2011). However, the paucity of studies of the effects of the terror attacks on people with psychosis was striking. The general reluctance in the mental health system to consider the effects of trauma and PTSD in individuals who were diagnosed with schizophrenia and schizo-affective disorder remained. In our facility, however, there was an increased interest by staff from various disciplines including creative arts therapies to join the trauma committee (as will be discussed in Part III).

I came to New York in 1999 to study art therapy since I had been working with people in Palestine years earlier doing origami. During that time trauma theory was not regularly incorporated into the teaching and practice of art therapy. After the terrorist attacks in the United States on September 11th, 2001 this gradually changed. I was interested in how trauma informed work could be incorporated in art therapy and how to adapt origami as a tool of treatment. Origami had not been recognised by the mainstream art therapists at that time.

When I started working at the facility, I met my supervisor, a music therapist, who emphasised that there was a weekly TC meeting that I should try to attend. In order to treat people with severe mental illness my trials and errors in both art therapy and origami paralleled my understanding of how important it is to incorporate a trauma informed approach into my clinical work. I also realised the importance of collaborating with colleagues when doing art therapy. Trauma work can be very stressful and challenging not just for service users but also service providers. I learned that a community of caregivers is an essential support. I learnt a saying – "It takes a whole village to raise a child"[1] – from one of the committee members. Indeed! This also holds true for a community of caregivers. Attending the committee meetings became a routine at work that I looked forward to.

A major thrust in the facility was to provide treatment using a group paradigm. Clearly group treatment made economic sense: it made it possible to involve more service users in treatment for more hours a week than would be possible if there was only individual therapy. But there were also other reasons why group therapy was particularly effective in the population that the facility served. Many of the trauma survivors tended to isolate themselves and found relationships with others overwhelming. In order to provide a safe environment in which healing can occur, committee members started to develop different kinds of trauma focused groups and discussed outcomes during committee meetings. Groups included: educational groups, process groups, structured cognitive behavioural therapy (CBT) groups and groups that combined CBT strategies and dynamically oriented group practices as

1   African proverb.

well as creative arts therapy groups. These groups are described in other chapters of this book.

Years before my becoming a member of the TC I was blind to the need to address trauma in a psychiatric setting. Influenced by the mainstream idea that many things that service users talk about are based on psychotic ideation, I focused on the present moment in my sessions. Considering the way I worked, I realise now that my therapeutic approach sometimes incorporated strategies that addressed difficulties that have been discussed throughout the trauma literature.

However, I remember keenly one young man who was quite provocative, often creating a situation where he was made fun of or bullied until he would lose control and threaten to begin a fight with another service user who would then hurt him. When everyone was cleaning up after a group one day, he told me that both his father and his mother beat him up when he was a child. He said it again another time. It is painful for me to remember that at the time I did nothing. I completely disregarded his words, thinking he made them up to make a scene. When, as a member of the TC, I became aware of the prevalence and effects of trauma, I remembered this survivor and thought about how I could have responded differently. In the TC I began to identify symptoms, gain knowledge of how to address symptoms, and perhaps most importantly, I had peers who supported me in dealing with my own reactions and my tendency to want to distance myself from the topic of trauma. I became actively involved in the TC when one of my interns expressed an interest in conducting a music therapy trauma group. On the same unit where she was beginning to do clinical work, a social work student had expressed the same interest. Her supervisor was the psychiatrist who was the head of the TC. We spoke together and decided it would be an informative experience for the two of them to team up and initiate a trauma group that would integrate verbal and music therapy. It would be comprised of women with trauma histories. The psychiatrist and I began to meet to coordinate the supervision, and it was not long before I became an eager member of the TC. We were excited to be pioneering this combined music-verbal therapy trauma group.

When creative arts therapists joined the trauma committee, their involvement opened many possibilities. In verbal groups it was not always easy for members to connect and express or listen to others' thoughts and feelings which could make it challenging to foster an atmosphere of group cohesion. Now, a growing emphasis in the work of the committee was to incorporate verbal and creative arts therapy techniques. This was important since many trauma survivors had difficulties in trusting and relating to others. The addition of creative arts therapists to the committee provided a multidisciplinary and multimodal approach to connect through music, movement and art. In this context, trauma survivors were given an opportunity to find their 'voice' through art, music, movement, and words, reflecting their own individual creativity and cultural identity.

While verbal trauma groups had expanded to different units, we now started the first interdisciplinary trauma group by combining the verbal modality with creative arts therapies. We recognised during the early and subsequent group work the importance of traumatic effects that can present as multi-sensory, and include auditory, visual, proprioceptive and somatic perceptions and hence the value of addressing these problems in a multimodal fashion.

An important aspect of the work of the TC involved the inclusion of trainees. Many students were highly motivated to learn about using a trauma informed approach and they joined our meetings. Educated in fields that included social work, psychiatry, creative arts therapies and psychology, the students' enthusiasm and fresh perspectives provided a significant contribution to our endeavours. Depending on the topics being discussed we provided this forum for the trainees as often as we could.

We supervised psychiatric residents in individual and family therapies, an important and at times challenging combination of interventions in the context of trauma informed treatment (see Chapter 10). We developed a trauma rotation for psychology interns and a trauma training curriculum for psychiatric residents (Schneeberger et al., 2012). In addition to didactics, the teachings included experiential learning with an emphasis on safe boundaries and the creation of a holding environment.

As we continued to work as a multidisciplinary group and learned about different approaches to healing, we organised our own trauma conferences as well.[2] We focused on specific issues related to people with serious mental illness and psychosis and discussed topics including intergenerational trauma and male sexual abuse. We also spoke about our experiences in developing multimodal and multidisciplinary approaches and in collaboration with trainees we attended and presented at national and international conferences.[3]

---

2 'The Impact of Trauma: From Individuals to Communities' (2004), 'Healing from Trauma: Individuals, Cultures and Systems' (2006), and 'From Fragmentation to Integration: Multidimensional Approaches for Working with Complex Trauma' (2009).

3 Among the organization that we presented at were: International Society for Psychological and Social Approaches to Psychosis (ISPS); International Society for Trauma and Dissociation (ISSTD); International Society for Traumatic Stress Studies (ISTSS); American Psychiatric Association (APA); APA Institute on Psychiatric Services (IPS); American

Conclusion

Establishing safety, empowerment and limiting coercive practices were some of the principles upon which we built our interventions. Over time it became apparent that the same goals that were important in our work with survivors were just as important in our work with one another. A continuous and open-ended dialogue in the context of safe connections allowed for the expression of our own fears and anxieties. With a multidisciplinary committee that embodied the elements of a trauma sensitive community each committee member's active input and participation was encouraged.

As the TC became a safe place where people could connect and share ideas there was a growing awareness of the ways in which staff from different disciplines could work together in order to develop interventions that were responsive to specific service users' needs. A major goal for the committee's interventions was the establishment of a safe and therapeutic environment in which interactions with others were encouraged. This included non-threatening and meaningful communications between survivors, survivors and group leaders, and between group leaders themselves. In this way it was possible to design a less fragmented and more integrated recovery model, that could be applied throughout the facility.

During our collaboration, we realised there was a parallel process taking place between survivor groups and trauma committee meetings. Our effort to assist each trauma survivor find their own voice was similar to our endeavour to listen and understand the reactions of other committee members. It was a group consensus that as we worked together, we became more empathic and more aware of things that committee members were concerned about and/or thought important. We came to understand that the way in which we were able to process information and support one another during our committee meetings was a major factor in continuing to work towards our goals. We were able to maintain the belief that as a committee we could develop a programme in which we could respond to the complexity of each survivor's needs and resources and at the same time validate and take into account the concerns of staff.

Association of Directors of Psychiatric Residency Training (AADRT); American Public Health Association (APHA); American Family Therapy Association (AFTA); Male Survivor; American Music Therapy Association (AMTA), Expressive Arts Therapies; American Art Therapy Association (AATA),and The First International Music Therapy and Trauma Symposium.

References

Bloom, S. L. (1997). *Creating sanctuary: Toward the evolution of sane societies.* New York: Routledge.

Carmen, E., Crane B., Dunnicliff, M., Holochuck, S., Prescott L., Rieker, P., Stefan, S., & Stromberg, N. (1996). *Massachusetts Department of Mental Health task force on the restraint and seclusion of persons who have been physically or sexually abused: Report and recommendations.* Boston, MA: Massachusetts Department of Mental Health.

Harris, M., & Anglin, J. (1998). *Trauma recovery and empowerment: A clinician's guide for working with women in groups.* New York: Free Press.

Herman, J.L. (1992). *Trauma and recovery.* New York: Basic Books.

Loewy, J. V., & Hara, A. F. (eds). (2002). *Caring for the caregiver: The use of music and music therapy in grief and trauma.* New York: American Music Therapy Association.

Neria, Y., DiGrande, L., & Adams, B. G. (2011). Posttraumatic stress disorder following the September 11, 2001, terrorist attacks: A review of the literature among highly exposed populations. *American Psychologist, 66*(6), 429–446. (doi:10.1037/a0024791)

Pearlman, L.A.& Saakvitne, K. W. (1995). *Trauma and the therapist: Countertransference and vicarious traumatization in psychotherapy with incest survivors.* New York: Norton.

Saakvitne, K. W., Gamble, S., Pearlman, L. A., & Lev, B. T. (2000). *Risking connection: A training curriculum for working with survivors of childhood abuse.* Lutherville, MD: Sidran Press.

Schneeberger, A. R., Muenzenmaier, K., Abrams, M., Antar, L., Leon, S. R., Ruberman, L., & Battaglia, J. (2012). Comprehensive trauma training curriculum for psychiatry residents. *Academic Psychiatry, 36*(2), 136–137.

6

WIDENING THE CIRCLE OF CARE

Trauma Programme for Staff

Kristina Muenzenmaier, Toshiko Kobayashi,
and Joseph Battaglia

Introduction

Recognising traumatic experiences and their effects on both service users and staff is fundamental to the creation of a trauma sensitive environment. As the trauma committee developed a trauma informed approach for service users, it became apparent that it was important to also focus on trauma experienced by staff. The building of trust, the expectation of confidentiality and the acknowledgment of the need for a safe and comfortable environment are essential for both. This chapter traces the history of the programme designed to reach out to traumatised staff in a public mental health service system. We will discuss the importance of support, and self-care in the healing process and how caring for staff impacts caring for service users.

Bills (Bills & Bloom, 1998) describes her first day as medical director of a "chronic, extremely violent, women's unit in a state hospital" (p. 350) and goes on to provide more details about the unit which she indicates was "noted to be the most difficult" in the facility (ibid.). Her description of her first day on the unit is chilling:

> As I opened the door, I looked down a long, dimly lit, drab hallway.
> I stopped at the sound of women's screams filling the air. As I stared down the long corridor, a chair flew across the hallway and crashed to the floor ...
>
> (Bills & Bloom, 1998, p. 350)

She goes on to describe the general conditions in the unit and other incidents in which a service user is violent towards self and/or others. Though the degree of violence was not typical of other units in that particular hospital her description does make clear the kinds of incidents that can leave staff

DOI: 10.4324/9781003055914-7

feeling extremely vulnerable when working in a psychiatric facility and might lead to increased emotional tension and heightened vigilance.

Trauma Programme for Staff

Background

In the late 1990s the coordinator of the Employment Assistance Program (EAP)[1] saw the need to expand services to reach out to staff within the facility. While the EAP was offering short term counselling services and/ or referrals to staff who experienced family difficulties, addictions, physical and/or mental health problems, there was a need to expand services specifically to traumatised staff. In collaboration with the trauma committee and the administration, the decision was made to develop a service that had been pioneered by several other mental health facilities. A trauma programme for staff (TPS) would provide support to traumatised employees, individuals as well as groups and clinical teams who had experienced and/or witnessed a traumatic incident related to their work environment.

The presupposition for the development of a TPS was that staff can experience emotional and physical distress including acute stress reactions, hyper-vigilance, avoidance and re-enactment behaviours and other symptoms related to the traumatic exposure. Interpersonal relationships such as connection and trust and/or emotional dysregulation resulting from traumatic experiences can influence the interactions with service users.

Over the years since, the TPS has undergone numerous changes. The different approaches and interventions depended on the needs of the traumatised employees, the programme coordinators and team members, the culture of the hospital setting, and most importantly the support of the hospital administrators. The range of services provided included responding to emergency calls, immediate consultations after incidents, individual counselling and organising group interventions as well as facility wide outreach and educational trauma trainings. While over the years we experienced some setbacks, we realised that the programme could not be sustained without an individual TPS coordinator and administrative support.

Population and Setting

There are several factors that make work in a public mental health setting challenging. Public service such as working for a psychiatric facility

---

1 The Employment Assistance Program (EAP) is a large nationwide programme that was originally developed in the 1940s to address alcohol abuse affecting work performance in employees. Over time it was expanded to also include substance abuse, family and mental health problems (Masi, 2011).

requires 'multifaceted emotional labor', meaning that emotional skills and abilities are required (Guy, Newman, & Mastracci, 2014). This 'relational work', usually not part of a job description, can be exhausting and is mostly under-acknowledged (ibid.).

Moreover, Garrett (2019) describes economic concerns in public mental health settings and the way in which funding issues directly affect the interventions that are possible. Staff/patient ratios may be lower than in private settings with shortages leading to staff feeling overwhelmed. For example, lack of adequate staffing can result in increased demands on each staff member such as higher caseloads and increased time pressure to respond to the needs of each service-user. This makes it more difficult to establish a trusting relationship with service-users. Shift work is physically demanding with additional work assignments and double shifts adding to an already stressful work environment. Increased areas of responsibility and a reduced ability to handle all services important in the process of treatment and recovery can lead to feelings of frustration. As a result, staff can become physically and emotionally exhausted and is more likely to experience *demoralisation* and *burnout* (Kristensen, Borritz, Villadsen, & Christensen, 2005).

In addition, *direct traumatisation* and workplace violence[2] add to the general stress level and may include witnessing or experiencing:

• threats of physical harm and verbal assault;
• completed or attempted physical and/or sexual assault;
• stalking;
• fatal or serious injury;
• suicide/homicide; and
• accidental exposure to blood or other potentially infectious material.

When demoralisation and burnout are compounded with traumatisation, there will be increases of absences and sick-leave due to physical injuries as well as low morale, anxiety, or depression. This in turn places more burden and work responsibility on the remaining staff leading to further burnout and stress. The likelihood of incidents increases and can result in additional traumatisation due to staff and/or patient injuries.

A further difficulty is that the majority of service users have a history of being severely traumatised. Dealing with the complexity of symptoms and behaviours exhibited by traumatised individuals is challenging. Mistrust, hostility, verbal, and physical assaults as well as self-injurious behaviours

2 The Occupational Safety and Health Agency states that workplace violence is often under reported and from 2002–2013 incidents of serious workplace violence were four times more prevalent in health care settings than in private industry. See www.osha.gov/sites/default/files/OSHA3826.pdf.

and/or suicidal attempts can be extremely stressful to staff. Responses to paranoid ideation and delusional behaviours can result in altercations and further increase violent incidents on the units (see Chapter 8). Though many of these behaviours may be due to difficulties in affect regulation and impulse control and/or to re-enactments of past trauma, they provide a challenge for staff in both inpatient and outpatient settings.

Moreover, *secondary traumatisation* occurs, for example by listening to the specific story of a traumatised client (e.g. interpersonal violence, disaster, accidents) which can lead to *secondary PTSD* (e.g. intrusive imagery, nightmares etc.), also described as compassion fatigue by Figley (1995). This needs to be differentiated from *vicarious traumatisation* (Pearlman & Saakvitne, 1995). Vicarious traumatisation as opposed to secondary PTSD is less recognised. It is not 'symptom based' but seen as the cumulative effect of emotionally connecting and working with trauma survivors over time, often with a slow onset (ibid.). Alterations of beliefs and feelings about safety in the world, self, and others and questioning of one's professional ability may occur (ibid). Vicarious traumatisation also has to be differentiated from *countertransference* (a therapist's reaction to *one* particular client). Besides general countertransference there is a special challenge when working with trauma survivors which is referred to as *traumatic countertransference* and relates to the interaction of the therapist's own history with a client's trauma history. Traumatic countertransference usually elicits strong reactions and presents various challenges that are extensively discussed by numerous trauma therapists (Herman, 1992; Pearlman & Saakvitne, 1995; Dalenberg, 2000).

While staff can feel overwhelmed by service users' intense emotions, they also can experience feelings of helplessness and even paralysis. We often observe these various reactions in trainees who have come from other placements. Fromm-Reichman (1950) points out the importance of being aware of one's own insecurities and anxieties when providing treatment. For example, accustomed to a fast-paced rotation in an emergency room or acute inpatient unit psychiatric residents arrive at a long-term psychiatric facility ready to move into action. But now their pace seems slowed down and they begin to realise that there is no pill or magic bullet to a speedy recovery for people with serious mental illness. Consequently, they might see themselves as being inadequate and incompetent which can result in emotional withdrawal and/or cynicism. Feelings of helplessness and hopelessness in trainees as well as permanent staff may lead to seeing clients as being 'chronic' and 'treatment resistant'. This lack of engagement is counter-therapeutic and reinforces disconnection.

All of the above situations can negatively impact the work environment and the interactions between service users and staff members. Moreover, a negative outlook on one's professional future and/or one's personal life may be compounded by anxiety, depression, guilt, shame, and/or substance abuse, thus limiting the day-to-day effectiveness of health care workers. The negative effects on individual employees also extend to the general staff morale on the unit. Therefore, it is imperative in supervisory and staff meetings to fully discuss aspects of parallel process and understand vicarious traumatisation in the context of working with traumatised persons. As a supervisor it is important to be aware of feelings of helplessness and demoralisation in supervisees and support the need to develop safe and trusting relationships. Supervisors also need to explore issues related to traumatic countertransference and be alert to vicarious traumatisation in supervisees and other staff members.

My internship placement at an urban psychiatric institution allowed me to learn some valuable lessons ...

When you are too tired to go on ... you go on. I was so exhausted during my internship not just because I was tired from working a full-time job, going to school full time, and interning two days per week at a psychiatric hospital, but also because in many ways the hospital was a frightening experience for me. There were long hallways and large empty rooms reminiscent of horror movies. My first day in the art therapy room a patient grabbed a scissor and attempted to attack my supervisor. Luckily the scissors were all child safety scissors.

On one of my first days, a hospital staff member in the elevator asked me if I was new. I asked her if it was that obvious. She said that she can tell when someone is new because they hover close to the walls. After a few months the hospital began to feel less scary and more routine. By the end of my year, after getting to know the service users individually, I understood better their specific needs and sensitivities and my fear lessened.

When new situations feel intimidating, perseverance provides us with an opportunity for growth. I also realised, that it is vital when doing this work to laugh at ourselves. One of my fondest memories was laughing with my supervisor on our way home on the subway. Being able to laugh was a great way to decompress after working in a stressful environment.

Goals

With staff experiencing difficulties and frustrations due to working conditions and challenging interactions with trauma survivors we realised early on when forming the trauma committee in the late 1990s that one of the important goals was to be able to build a support network for traumatised staff and be responsive to their needs. When staff do not feel protected or safe,

Table 6.1. Summary of essential ingredients for TPS.

- Confidentiality – private meeting space, confidential TPS phone line, anonymous questionnaire, locked mailbox
- TPS team diversity – recruitment across disciplines, ethnicity, gender, age etc.
- Extensive outreach regarding incidents – formal and informal to individuals, teams, units and departments (e.g. morning reports, incident report meetings, team meetings, administrative meetings, work place violence meetings, emergency calls, etc.)
- Widen the array of TPS services – immediate response, consultations, referrals, debriefings, supports (e.g. accompanying individuals, groups, team etc.)
- Teaching, trauma training, and supervision – individual, team or discipline specific, and facility-wide promoting self-care
- One of the important ideas was to take care of TPS working team as well (e.g. stress reduction programmes, creative arts therapies modalities, and annual health fair).

guilt and shame about an incident, blame of self and/or others as well as rage and anger is often directed at fellow staff, administration officials and/ or service users. In a supportive and trauma sensitive environment the aim was that after incidents staff were not blamed but understood and cared for. We saw the development of a TPS as a prerequisite for a safe and nurturing environment that also could minimise demoralisation and staff burnout. By being able to acknowledge feelings of vulnerability and victimisation we hoped that staff members could respond in an empathic manner also to the traumatic sequelae of service users.

It is so important to note that a traumatic event cannot be described with one word. In addition to the subjective experience of the traumatic incident there are multilayered processes that need to be taken into consideration when developing a TPS approach: the incident at the time of the event, how things are handled immediately after the event, medical services needed and available, relationships with supervisors and co-workers, and support systems in and outside of work environment (e.g. family). Moreover, the cultural perception of the trauma is important. How do people in the community see the traumatic event/s? How stigmatising might be the disclosure of the trauma? And how does this affect the support of the traumatised person?

All of these factors (including a person's past trauma history and coping skills) have an impact on the recovery of the traumatised person in addition to the subjective experience of the trauma itself. Moreover, it is important how follow-up is provided and how the process of returning to work is managed.

Early Beginnings

We started to develop a TPS in the late 1990s. In the beginning the coordinator of the TPS did not consistently hear about the happenings of each traumatic incident. Either administration and/or involved staff did not consider the incident severe enough to be reported to the TPS coordinator or staff might have felt uncomfortable to disclose experiences of victimisation. Traditionally the unspoken culture in medicine considered vulnerability and victimhood as a weakness. Therefore, the expectation was to 'be tough' and remain at the workplace whenever possible despite a serious incident.

Recruitment

In order to be able to assess the needs of traumatised staff, and since different disciplines have different needs, we reached out to the various departments and disciplines. Over time and with the support of the administration the coordinator was able to include volunteer staff to connect with the TPS coordinator or even participate in some TPS meetings. The various disciplines involved included nursing, social work, psychology, psychiatry, creative arts therapies, clergy, safety, maintenance, and the food service department, as well as day and night shifts. This ensured that the TPS coordinator would be better informed about incidents that happened in different locations and during off hours (e.g. during the night).

In order to assure cultural sensitivity, we tried to include staff members from different ethnic backgrounds. We hoped this would not only improve support and greater acceptance for the programme but also lead to a better understanding of the cultural perceptions about trauma and the stigma of disclosures. We also found it important to pay attention to gender roles and family dynamics across different ethnic groups.

Outreach

Information about traumatic incidents was usually made known in formal administrative meetings, nursing reports and other meetings related to workplace violence. The TPS coordinator was present in these meetings and/ or received the information from the clinical director's office. Additionally, information could be informally submitted by the affected staff themselves or by colleagues who were concerned or had witnessed an incident. Reviewing challenges to the flow of information helped us to continue to make changes. We realised the importance of providing more access for staff to relate confidential information regarding incidents. We designed a short questionnaire. Anybody could feel free to communicate their concerns in the questionnaire privately or anonymously if preferred. Questions included specifics about the incident/s, whether a follow up by the TPS coordinator is requested and if so, how they wish to be contacted. We installed securely locked mailboxes in several locations all over the facility that were conveniently located and easily accessible. Anyone who works at the facility could drop off the questionnaire and include additional comments and concerns. The TPS coordinator responded to all forms by phone or in person and would set up confidential appointments with individual people as well as reach out to staff involved in an incident. In order to introduce the questionnaire, the coordinator went to all units, to the medical clinic, to the dietary department and other service locations, met with all shifts and explained the forms, the process and the services available. Providing information about TPS services was one of the most important roles of the TPS coordinator.

Procedures

Part of the standard procedures developed by the TPS after an incident was the scheduling of a physical exam either at the worksite or with a personal physician. One of the members of the TPS tried to reach out as soon as possible to the affected staff member, often responding to the hospital-wide emergency code in order to evaluate whether a TPS service was needed. Then we would accompany the traumatised staff and find a quiet and comfortable environment to meet privately. Over the years we were able to identify a 'safe room' where the traumatised staff could take some time out, get help filling out the incident report, talk with the coordinator about the traumatic event or just rest.

In order to meet with the TPS coordinator or one of the team members during regular work hours permission had to be granted, which was also necessary when leaving the worksite after a traumatic incident and/or schedule time off. A TPS member reached out to the injured staff by telephone and/or home visits (if permitted) to offer support during the absences. Upon return we offered to accompany the traumatised staff back into the facility since it was often overwhelming to re-enter the workplace triggering flashbacks and anxiety. We also met with the Human Resources department to discuss the effects of traumatic experiences. Our goal was to increase awareness of the special needs of each traumatised staff which included the issue of reassignment to another unit.

Moreover, the TPS coordinator had regular meetings with various committees including administration in order to address systemic issues and identify changes that could be implemented in order to prevent future incidents.

This fictionalised staff box describes the procedures developed by TPS after an incident.

Suddenly the loudspeaker in the hospital announced an emergency on unit X. At the same time my telephone rang and one of the unit staff called me to let me know that Alicia, another staff member, had been hurt trying to intervene in an altercation. I quickly ran up to the unit where I found Alicia guiding service users back to the day room and the nursing staff returning to their workplaces. I approached Alicia and asked how she was doing. She replied that she was fine. She had been hit but felt OK. She was trying to get things back to normal now. I asked if I could take her to the clinic to be checked out. She replied that she was fine and there was too much to do now. I said, it's important to go to the clinic to get examined and fill out an incident report. Since she refused, I insisted: "Let's just go to a quiet place for now where you can have a cup of coffee. I'll find someone to cover here for a few minutes." She finally agreed and someone was found to cover the unit.

We walked down to the room that had been set aside for the TPS – a safe room – where there was privacy and I could offer a cup of coffee or some green tea. Alicia sat down with a sigh. "How are you doing?" I asked. "A little achy but OK." I think we should go to the clinic to check you out and to register the injury. You know how you can't really tell how hurt you are until the next day." "I just need to go back to the unit. It's important that the nursing staff know that I'm all right. We have to stay strong you know." As we spoke, she let me know that another reason was that she didn't want her family to know she was hurt. "If they know, they may prevent me from coming back to work here." Her fears reiterated comments about confidentiality that we had previously received anonymously in the locked TPS box. I was able to convince her that her privacy would be honoured. I escorted her down to the clinic where she filled out papers and was examined. After a while she told me she felt exhausted and was deciding it would be good to take the rest of the day off. We then went to see her supervisor who arranged coverage after discussing the situation.

I assessed her supports at home and let her know that I would be in touch if she did not mind my doing so. I also let her know that when she was ready to return to work, upon her request, I would meet her outside the hospital and walk in with her.

Debriefings

The goal for the traumatised individual and/or group was to process the event in a supportive and private environment. After a traumatic incident it was important to allow people on the unit to express their feelings including fear, anger, guilt and blame and move to where they felt validated and supported. The intervention was based on what the individual was comfortable with within the limits of what TPS could provide. Besides individual support and counselling a group debriefing meeting could be initiated by the TPS coordinator. However, whether to attend the meeting or not was a personal decision for each participant. This was a sensitive process and staff needed to first feel comfortable and trust the TPS coordinator. The TPS debriefings were confidential and independent from human resources or supervisory structures. They also differed from administrative debriefings which often analysed an incident by what went wrong rather than what happened.

During this learning process we initially adapted the model of Critical Incident Stress Debriefing (CISD) (Mitchell & Everly, 1997, 1999). CISD was designed for first responders, EMT personal etc. to be conducted in the initial aftermath of the incident and was thought to ameliorate the impact of a traumatic event and improve outcome and recovery of traumatised participants. TPS used the debriefings mostly in a group setting and as a minimum required two group co-leaders. All staff directly or indirectly affected by the traumatic event were invited. We adopted the recommended structure beginning with the introduction of each of the participants, the rules (e.g. importance of confidentiality) and topics for the meeting. The fact-finding phase of what happened (e.g. where were you when it happened) was followed by the sharing of one's own thoughts (cognitive) and reactions (emotional and physical). Then we discussed the effects of the incident, normalised the responses and shared self-care and helpful coping strategies. If participants consented (since the content of the meetings was strictly confidential) written recommendations could be made to the clinical director regarding improvements so that future incidents would be less likely to occur. The TPS coordinator acted as a mediator within the system if person/s involved consented. Reframing the event and talking about ways to make the environment safer was empowering and gave agency to traumatised staff members.

While CISD was supposed to be applied in the immediate aftermath of the traumatic incident, due to logistical reasons (e.g. inclusion of staff from the various shifts and sites, organisation of coverage to free up participants, staff out on sick leave) we often were not able to schedule a debriefing within the recommended time frame. However, we tried to meet with individual staff members immediately as well as for follow up when needed. It was our impression that the delay in the debriefings did not have a negative impact. In fact, it allowed staff to step away from the immediate aftermath of the trauma and have some time to process the happenings prior to the debriefings.

Our observations in terms of voluntary participation and time delay in the debriefings seemed to be supported by some of the outcome studies. In a review of the literature Rose et al. (2002) did not find CISD to be effective in preventing PTSD (even possibly worsening PTSD symptoms by re-traumatisation). In general, we felt that the debriefings strengthened clinical teams and seemed to be helpful to staff who participated on a voluntary basis. The debriefings provided an opportunity for team members to share information, listen to each other and be supportive in the aftermath of a critical incident. The group process was very important in how participants dealt with the event and the connected emotions. We also reached out to staff members individually before and after the debriefings. Follow-up studies are needed that take into consideration the various groups of participants being debriefed, their connectedness and work relationships (e.g. clinical teams vs. groups of strangers), different time frames and contexts, as well as different outcome variables besides PTSD (e.g. feelings of support, etc.) in determining the effectiveness and efficacy of the debriefings (Bisson, Brayne, Ochberg, & Everly, 2007). Later CISD was expanded to Critical Incident Stress Management (CISM) (Everly, Flannery, & Mitchell, 2000) which allowed for more flexibility and a more comprehensive approach to crisis management. More recently, as will be discussed later, psychological first aid (Freeman, Graham, & Boywer, 2000; Freeman, Flitcroft, & Weeple, 2003) has been used to provide support in the aftermath of trauma and to reduce initial distress.

Response to the Events of 9/11

We encountered a unique challenge in dealing with a violent incident that differed from the work we were used to at the facility. Below we describe the varied experiences to the events of 9/11 as opposed to trauma in the workplace.

When the planes flew into the World Trade Center on September 11th, 2001, we were all shocked. We discussed with administration how to proceed and what would be most helpful to service users and staff. We decided for TPS members to go to all units/services of the hospital and talk to staff from day, afternoon and night shifts and assess how people were feeling and what supports were needed. We were all traumatised having witnessed the incident on television and watching the flames and smoke through some of the windows. It felt extremely important to reach out to everybody. How did the incident affect service users? How did it affect staff? Many were upset, shocked and in disbelief. The smells from the burning of the towers penetrated the halls and the windows. Some worried about missing relatives and/or friends. We hoped that meeting with the various teams would help to deal with some of the distress and uncertainty. However, we were somewhat hesitant because we were overwhelmed ourselves and concerned about our own safety and the safety of our families not knowing if there would be additional attacks. But we did want to provide a safe space for staff in the face of this adversity and we did know that reaching out to staff in turn would provide a safe and non-threatening environment for the service users. We hoped that the hospital community providing support to each other would result in improved understanding and caring for both traumatised staff and service users.

Several days after 9/11 trauma committee members also went downtown to debrief employees who were told to return to their office buildings in the vicinity of the WTC with the buildings still smouldering. The air smelled toxic and returning employees were concerned about inhaling the polluted air. They were worried about the environmental safety and their physical health not just in terms of air pollution but also whether another attack might occur. They expressed frustration that their physical and mental health concerns were not being considered. Most did not want to return to their workplace but were required to do so. Parents talked about how difficult the separation from their children was during this period of unpredictability and possible danger, compounding the distress experienced.

This was also true for the mental health workers doing the debriefings. For example, one of the committee members was involved in going to two different hospital facilities to 'debrief' employees. After this experience she came back and talked to the TPS coordinator about her experience as well as her own feelings of anxiety. In addition, she shared her own fears and worries about how her sons were impacted by these overwhelming circumstances.

During this time, trauma committee members realised that we were coping with an unusual debriefing situation. In this case the persons doing the debriefings were also traumatised and had a strong emotional reaction to the traumatic event. Reliving the circumstances with each debriefing became retraumatising. We realised how different the experience was when the debriefers themselves were directly affected.

My first group after the World Trade Center disaster gathered as usual in the music therapy room in the central programming area. I had a feeling of relief at being together, that we had a place to come to that was familiar – same group members, same time. Some people shared that they could see the smoke from where the World Trade Center had been from the top floors of the building where they resided. Others, looking out of the window from where we were assembled, expressed fear that their building could also be a target since it stood out higher than others in the surrounding area. As we began to move into a musical warm up, I felt my eyes filling with tears – all these deaths! The buildings collapsing – indelibly imprinted through the repetition on the television.

"What do we need from music today?" I asked. Immediately group members replied that we should play songs of prayers for the people who had died and for the families who had lost loved ones. They understood well pain and loss and as they united in singing their prayers out into the world, the melodies and words creating a healing energy that was palpable in the room. I felt grateful to be a part of that loving embrace.

Sometimes caring comes in our joint efforts, a powerful reminder of the resilience of survivors who can sustain and support us as well.

Turning Point

After the 9/11 event awareness about PTSD was raised in the general population. The cultural perceptions of trauma changed. Now less stigma was attached to medical providers such as rescue workers, nurses and physicians who were expressing their feelings of traumatisation. In our facility TPS was more accepted as staff developed an extended awareness of the benefits.

During continued planning efforts, we felt strongly that our outreach needed to include administration and the development of facility wide educational programmes. This, we hoped, would raise awareness of the needs of traumatised staff. After we had been without a coordinator for some time, we realised the importance of such a role in responding to traumatic incidents and organising individual and group meetings. With a newly appointed coordinator we now were able to add weekly group meetings for staff support and additional gatherings with different administrative staff members. We also participated in departmental meetings and developed educational venues throughout the facility, teaching about the effects of trauma both didactically and experientially.

Staff Training

The training programme for staff was designed to be both educational and supportive. It included the development of a trauma training curriculum for staff education as well as for hospital-wide supports (e.g. annual health fair).

Didactic lectures were targeted to all staff and all services in the mental health facility. In addition to addressing education related to trauma informed care (Harris & Fallot, 2001) the trainings were designed to raise awareness about stress at the workplace and included discussions about the various kinds of staff trauma. It was important for staff to be able to recognise their own stressors while working with traumatised service users as well as to acknowledge their own traumatisation. We asked questions such as: What stressful/traumatic events have you experienced/witnessed? How did it affect others/you? How does working with traumatised service users impact staff? What are common reactions to traumatic events? Do you think any of these trauma reactions affect you/other staff in their interpersonal interactions or relationship with service users? Discussions also included the importance of personal safety and the safety of the environment. Did staff feel supported at their work setting? If not, what would be helpful? What were systems issues that need to be addressed? How can we improve TPS services? How useful is a safe recovery space for staff? We wanted staff to feel empowered and comfortable in asking for help.

We also developed discipline specific staff training workshops. By reaching out to the various disciplines we learned for example that the traumatic experiences of nursing administrators were mostly unacknowledged. While managing difficult situations throughout the facility they also had to attend to the needs of traumatised on-line staff who were in the forefront during emergencies. We came to realise that for nursing administrators support of their traumatised staff was a priority while their own needs often took a back seat in the face of adversity. The nursing administrators had to be attended to and taken care of as well.

The severity of distress and traumatisation experienced by health care workers was brought to the forefront by the global COVID pandemic. Previously not broadly acknowledged it became clear that special support had to be provided to health care professionals who were overwhelmed with stressful and challenging situations during the pandemic.

Psychological First Aid

The Psychological First Aid Program (PFA) is a model which was developed in the late 1990s in order to meet the immediate needs of traumatised individuals after natural and man-made disasters (Freeman, Graham, & Boywer, 2000; National Child Traumatic Stress Network and National Center for Post-Traumatic Stress Disorder, 2006). After 9/11, in order to be prepared for potential emergencies, mental health workers but also volunteers and lay persons who were not mental health professionals were trained to support, assess and screen traumatised people and extend 'helping hands' to deal with immediate issues. One of the main advantages was that anybody could be ready after a short training course to apply 'first aid' in mental health emergencies without having a formal mental health education (McCabe et al. 2014). The coordinator of TPS was certified as a PFA trainer in 2015 and found it helpful to introduce some of the principles of PFA in planning the trauma informed curriculum at the annual staff training.

PFA differs from CISD in that it focuses primarily on the safety of the survivors and their current needs and does not necessarily process the traumatic event(s) (Freeman, Flitcroft, & Weeple, 2003; Bisson & Lewis, 2009). Non-intrusive support and practical assistance (e.g. resources and referrals if needed) paired with teaching of coping skills and mobilisation of a so-cial support network are of essential importance. PFA has been found to be effective in the amelioration of trauma related outcomes (Everly, Phillips, Kane, & Feldman, 2006) and has been used to reach out and support indi-viduals and families traumatised by the current COVID health crisis.

Self-Care and Creative Arts Therapies

Another main topic throughout the annual mandatory staff trainings, which also included a trauma training curriculum, was related to the impor-tance of self-care: How can people take care of their personal needs? How can the stress at the work site be decreased? Does exercise help? Is your sleep affected? How about healthy eating and drinking habits? What supports can be helpful outside the work site? Each attendee received a de-stressing ball and was able to learn a simple de-stressing exercise so that they could practise it by themselves. It was a great opportunity to reach out to all staff and also inform them about the TPS.

The sombre mood of the training topic 'trauma' was eased by the sharing of personal responses of the facilitators to critical incidents at the facility. The descriptions of emotional and/or physical reactions to stressful events paved a way for those who had experienced incidents during their work sit-uation. Some felt shameful, guilty, and/or were angry at the system or them-selves. By taking part of the annual training fair the understanding was that trauma can happen to everybody, that many different kinds of reactions to a traumatic event are to be expected and that it can be helpful to acknowledge those reactions. Both trainers as well as participants shared how some of their stressful experiences had affected them and how to support each other in difficult situations.

Unique to this phase was also the introduction of the creative arts ther-apies (CATs) (e.g. art, origami, music, dance/movement) into the staff care programme. Lunch time included music, visual arts, dance movement, origami, and crafts groups led by creative arts therapists and recreational therapists. While many of the interventions of TPS were geared towards critical and violent incidents the weekly lunchtime groups were targeted towards general stress reduction and burnout in addition to dealing with traumatic and stressful experiences.

These services were provided not only to staff who worked in inpatient units but also in outpatient and residential settings, as well as across differ-ent shifts and disciplines. The most popular programmes were the 'lunch-time de-stress group' and 'afterwork yoga'. De-stress groups (which are not therapy groups) were adapted to the unique work hours of such disciplines as nursing and dietary staff, safety officers, and religious service providers. We also offered a short de-stress activity during the morning rounds, specifically the day after staff had experienced an incident. Many workers participated and seemed to really enjoy these group activities.

There were several reasons for including creative arts therapies in the staff care programme. While CATs have been applied as part of the rehabilitation services in the hospital, more and more staff had witnessed service users participating in the CATs groups. On the surface, these treatments appeared to be about fun and enjoyment, especially when individual art therapy and music therapy sessions were provided by students studying to earn master's degrees in these fields. However, staff realised the remarkable impact of these treatments as they noticed changes in service users' behaviours. Service users including those who were seen as 'treatment resistant' showed interest in attending CATs groups. The increased attendance in sessions seemed to improve behaviours (such as unpredictable and high-risk behaviours) that had prevented service users from being allowed to attend groups sessions in the first place. Participating in CATs sessions helps service users to experience a more autonomous sense of self; they are the master of each creative expression. Witnessing changes in service users, some of the staff became curious and started to participate themselves with the service users who were on one-to-one observation due to high-risk behaviours.

The CATs therapies sessions were always conducted by two or more therapists including students. Many of the art therapy students were interested in attending the trauma committee meeting and there they gained a better understanding of trauma care for the population with SMI. They also learned that trauma care does not benefit only service users but also mental health workers including themselves.

These understandings were the basis for starting a de-stress CATs group for staff. The most challenging part was the scheduling and organising one group for each of the different professions, shifts, and work locations.

Reflections

From past experiences facilitating art workshops for people working in refugee camps and settlement houses, I knew art therapy was helpful for individuals who were working in challenging and stressful situations. My background as an Asian also gave me confidence that creative and expressive opportunities are important for all. It is a common practice in Japan to provide creative activity services at the workplace, such as a tea ceremony, ikebana (flower arrangement), and calligraphy. Activities like these are designed to build a supportive working community. They serve as a de-stressing activity

---

91

where workers can begin to leave behind what happened at work. In Japanese it is commonly called 'keiko-goto'. This denotes learning from an expert, having practising time, and sharing non-competitive, non-threatening time together.

In addition, I knew from my work with service users at our facility that art therapy was a positive experience regardless of cultural background, language spoken, gender, age and life experience. Because I had recently settled in the United States, I was very aware that there might be cultural differences in the kinds of activities that were accepted within the workplace and I did wonder whether facility staff would feel comfortable with the creative arts modalities. Putting into place a trauma programme for staff when I was just beginning to get used to cultural differences was challenging for me. But I also was aware that there is no formula for trauma care that works for everyone: one size doesn't fit all. Despite my uncertainties and concerns I was able to add the use of CATs in the TPS. I persisted in this endeavour because I felt strongly about the importance of building additional supports for staff.

I was glad to hear positive feedbacks of attendees:

- "When do you have the next meeting?"
- "What will be the next topic? Percussion, origami, dance, water colour, etc.?"
- "It is great, I wanted to try these activities but it is so convenient that I can join at the workplace, and it's free!"
- "Nothing to do with my work, just relaxing!"

Conclusion

By widening the circle of care our understanding of what is vital for an environment to be safe and healing evolved. We realised that the successful implementation of a TPS depended on a commitment to a trauma informed culture in the larger facility and the full support of the administration. We also realised that we needed to not just reach out to service users but also to all employees including direct care, support, and administrative staff. On the basis of discussions in individual meetings, educational trainings and critical incident stress debriefings we came to propose formal and informal policy changes within the facility, became confident in handling challenging incidents and improved staff's understanding of the complex effects of traumatisation.

While the TPS is not providing treatment for staff, it offers advice and support to employees who work in environments in which relational and emotional demands are frequent. Severe stress reactions affect resilience and interpersonal connections and behaviours. This can result in making it difficult for staff to empathically relate to service users, an element extremely important in the recovery process. The idea of incorporating CATs activities added another modality in building support for staff. The process of implementing a TPS emphasises the vital importance of trauma informed care where the goals and principles for both staff and service users are directly connected. Safety, respect, and empowerment are the foundations for an environment in which healing can occur. All of us, providers and service users alike, are human and therefore vulnerable to stressful life experiences. These are the times when we need support and healing.

References

Bills, L. J. & Bloom, S. (1998). From chaos to sanctuary: Trauma-based treatment for women in a state mental hospital system. In B. Levin, A. Blanch, & A. Jennings (eds), *Women's mental health services: A public health perspective* (pp. 348–367). Thousand Oaks, CA: Sage Publications.

Bisson, J. I., Brayne, M., Ochberg, F. M., & Everly, G. S. (2007). Early psychosocial intervention following traumatic events. *American Journal of Psychiatry, 164(7)*, 1016–1019.

Bisson, J. I., & Lewis, C. (2009). *Systematic review of psychological first aid.* Washington, DC: World Health Organization.

Dalenberg, C. J. (2000). *Countertransference and the treatment of trauma.* Washington, DC: American Psychological Association.

Everly, G. S., Flannery, R. B., & Mitchell, J. T. (2000). Critical incident stress management (CISM): A review of the literature. *Aggression and Violent Behavior, 5(1)*, 23–40.

Everly, G. S., Phillips, S. B., Kane, D., & Feldman, D. (2006). Introduction to and overview of group psychological first aid. *Brief Treatment and Crisis Intervention, 6(2)*, 130–136.

Figley, C. R. (ed.). (1995). *Compassion fatigue: Coping with secondary traumatic stress disorder in those who treat the traumatized.* London: Brunner-Routledge.

Freeman, C., Flitcroft, A., & Weeple, P. (2003). *Psychological First Aid: A replacement for psychological debriefing.* Edinburgh: Cullen-Rivers Centre for Traumatic Stress, Royal Edinburgh Hospital.

Freeman, C., Graham, P., & Boywer, D. (2000). *Psychological First Aid: A replacement for psychological debriefing.* Edinburgh: Rivers Centre for Traumatic Stress, Royal Edinburgh Hospital.

Fromm-Reichmann, F. (1950). *Principles of intensive psychotherapy.* Chicago, IL: University of Chicago Press.

Garrett, M. (2019). *Psychotherapy for psychosis: Integrating cognitive-behavioral and psychodynamic treatment.* New York: Guilford Publications.

Guy, M. E., Newman, M. A., & Mastracci, S. H. (2014). *Emotional labor: Putting the service in public service.* New York: Routledge.

Harris, M., & Fallot, R. D. (2001). Envisioning a trauma-informed service system: A vital paradigm shift. *New Directions for Mental Health Services, 2001(89),* 3–22.

Herman, J. L. (1992). *Trauma and recovery.* New York: Basic Books.

Kristensen, T. S., Borritz, M., Villadsen, E., & Christensen, K. B. (2005). The Copenhagen Burnout Inventory: A new tool for the assessment of burnout. *Work & Stress, 19(3),* 192–207.

Masi, D.A. (2011). Employee assistance programs in the new millennium. *International Journal of Emergency Mental Health, 7(3),* 157–167.

McCabe, O. L., Everly Jr, G. S., Brown, L. M., Wendelboe, A. M., Abd Hamid, N. H., Tallchief, V. L., & Links, J. M. (2014). Psychological first aid: A consensus-derived, empirically supported, competency-based training model. *American Journal of Public Health, 104(4),* 621–628.

Mitchell, J. T. & Everly, G. S. (1997, 1999). *Critical incident stress management (CISM): An operations manual for the prevention of traumatic stress among emergency service and disaster workers,* 2nd edition. Ellicott City, MD: Chevron Publishing Corporation.

National Child Traumatic Stress Network and National Center for Post-Traumatic Stress Disorder. (2006). *Psychological first aid: Field operations guide,* 2nd edition. Los Angeles, CA: National Center for Child Traumatic Stress.

Pearlman, L. A. & Saakvitne, K. W. (1995). *Trauma and the therapist: Countertransference and vicarious traumatization in psychotherapy with incest survivors.* New York: W. W. Norton & Co.

Rose, S. C., Bisson, J., Churchill, R., & Wessely, S. (2002). Psychological debriefing for preventing post traumatic stress disorder (PTSD). *Cochrane Database of Systematic Reviews, 2002(2),* CD000560. doi:10.1002/14651858.cd000560.

Part II

TRAUMA FOCUSED INTERVENTIONS
From Fragmentation to Integration

7

EXPLORING A GROUP THERAPY APPROACH FOR HEALING FROM COMPLEX TRAUMA

*Mara Conan, Kristina Muenzenmaier,
Gillian Stephens Langdon, and Toshiko Kobayashi*

When you're in it, you can't see where you're headed or what you will create. As we move through the struggles and joys of each day, we can only catch glimpses of the trail we leave. Each day, each session, each meeting, each supervision, each conference, each reading guided our development without us seeing it clearly. We were creating our own models. We dove in with the knowledge we could glean from our past experiences, from each other in the trauma committee meetings, from trial and error and sharing, conferences we attended and readings. Neurological studies and writings began to bring us new understandings that supported the ideas we developed as we introduced a series of group approaches.

Introduction

Many of the people we were working with who were diagnosed with psychotic disorders had been impacted by compounded victimisation experiences such as childhood abuse, homelessness and adult re-victimisation. They were often isolated in their pain and fearful of making interpersonal connections. A group could become a place to develop new skills and form safe relationships. As Judith Herman (1992) states "Recovery can take place only within the context of relationships; it cannot occur in isolation" (p. 133).

During the late nineties and the first decades in the 2000s, we developed a variety of group therapy approaches for trauma survivors. Our group programme became in part a learning process as we tried different kinds of groups, met with obstacles and made changes based on what we had learned. After starting out with an educational approach we piloted a cognitive behavioural therapy (CBT) model and later added process groups. Moreover,

DOI: 10.4324/9781003055914-9   97

we came to realise the importance of creative arts therapies in reaching out to persons who are multiply traumatised and who presented, for example, with varying levels of withdrawal, muteness and/or affect dysregulation.

The major goals of all groups, regardless of modality, included first and foremost safety from physical and emotional harm and gaining confidence in negotiating current life circumstances. We believed that focusing on such factors as empowerment, the importance of privacy, ways to deal with strong emotional responses, connections among members and the development of adaptive coping skills, would strengthen survivors' sense of agency, self-esteem and confidence in relationship with others. As we developed the groups, we became aware of the effect of this challenging work on group leaders and realised the importance of focusing in trauma committee meetings on self-care of therapists. Fictionalised vignettes and staff boxes will highlight the experiences of survivors and group leaders.

Trauma Informed Care

In the 1970s and 1980s, there was a realisation of the importance of trauma and the impact it had on emotional well-being (see Chapter 1). At the time we were initiating our programmes, a heightened awareness of the relationship between sexual abuse and incest and psychological difficulties later in life started to emerge. Treatment approaches were developed that focused on psychological trauma (Courtois, 1988; Herman, 1992; van der Kolk, 1987). Moreover, there was a growing body of literature on therapeutic group interventions for women who had experienced sexual abuse and incest as children and/or rape trauma as adults. Process oriented and early CBT group approaches emerged (Alexander, Neimeyer, Follette, Moore, & Harter, 1989; Brandt, 1989; Herman & Schatzow, 1984; Courtois, 1988; Resick, Jordan, Girelli, Hutter, & Marhoefer-Dvorak, 1988). However, at the time there was little information regarding protocols for trauma treatment that included individuals with psychotic symptoms (Ford, Fallot, & Harris, 2009). With a few exceptions, existing group interventions for trauma screened out participants who were regarded as being emotionally unstable, prone to decompensation, and/or were abusing elicit substances (Alexander & Muenzenmaier, 1998).

Since the women we worked with not only reported high rates of childhood abuse, but were also likely to be revictimised in adulthood and experience periods of homelessness (Muenzenmaier, Struening, Ferber, & Meyer, 1993), we were striving for the development of interventions that could take those difficult experiences and complex realities into account. Another problem we faced was that many of the people were diagnosed with schizophrenia and schizoaffective disorders and therefore the aetiology of their illness was largely seen by psychiatrists and other clinicians as being based in biology and genetics. As a result, the prevalent treatment modalities centred mostly on pharmacotherapy. However, realising the high prevalence of childhood abuse histories, we were determined to develop interventions that would target the neglected trauma sequelae in this population.

We were influenced by Judith Herman (1992) and her elaboration of the three stages of recovery from sexual abuse trauma in her groundbreaking book *Trauma and Recovery*. The first stage is establishing safety which includes physical, emotional and interpersonal safety. When we started thinking about the development of interventions the focus on safety and a supportive, non-threatening environment in group settings was of primary importance. We knew that establishing safe connections and ensuring a safe environment would be particularly important for people who have experienced psychosis and who also have been neglected and/or sexually and physically abused while growing up. The educational trauma group model we developed was focused on the beginning stage of healing (Muenzenmaier et al., 1998).[1]

The Efficacy of Group Programmes for Individuals Who Experience Psychosis

At the time we were initiating our work there was little information about conducting trauma groups for people who experience psychosis. In discussion of group therapy treatment for individuals who experience psychosis, González de Chávez (2009) compares it to other psychotherapeutic modalities as "one of the most unknown and least systematized for its adequate use, choice and indication" (p. 251). The limited material to draw from at the time highlights the many challenges in running groups for individuals who experienced both childhood trauma as well as psychosis. Survivors may be:

- distrustful of others;
- hesitant in socialising and not comfortable speaking in a group situation;
- mentally preoccupied (e.g. experiencing intrusive memories, hearing voices and/or dissociating);
- experiencing emotional numbing as a mode of avoiding strong reactions;

---

1   As we proceeded with the implementation of the educational group, we later learned about other successful trauma groups for people with serious mental illness such as the Trauma Recovery and Empowerment Model (TREM) at Community Connections (Harris & Anglin, 1998). Other trauma group models that caught our interest, albeit for somewhat different populations, was Seeking Safety: A Treatment Manual for PTSD and Substance Abuse (Najavits, 2002), the TAMAR project working with trauma, addictions, mental health and recovery in incarcerated women (Gillece & Russell, 2001) and the Trauma Adaptive Recovery Group Education and Therapy (TARGET) for the treatment of PTSD and addiction (Ford & Russo, 2006).

- in a hypervigilant and/or paranoid state and attending to possible threatening circumstances;
- having difficulty controlling emotional reactions, resulting in self-harm or harm to others; or
- having difficulty in self-reflection and taking in other people's perspective.

Despite these circumstances González de Chávez (2009) emphasises that psychotherapy groups can be particularly effective in treating people with psychosis. He stresses the importance of the development of interpersonal relationships and the opportunity to talk together about difficulties that are common among group members.

At our facility there had been a longstanding commitment to using group paradigms and most of the trauma committee members had experience and training in running groups with individuals who experienced psychosis. We had seen how effective group programmes could be in fostering motivation to interact with others and adopt new coping strategies. Within the facility there were differences in the needs of individuals assigned to specific units whether inpatient, outpatient, short or long stay. Our task was to match specific aspects of the group (both content and structure) with the needs of the specific population we were working with.

Throughout the period we were conducting groups there was often a question in terms of how structured the group should be. We were aware that discussions about traumatic experiences could trigger strong emotional responses. We experimented with a tightly structured CBT group, but also ran more flexible groups. As we discuss group models, including creative arts therapy, we will provide detailed information about the reasons for variations in our approach.

Educational Trauma Group

The first group model *Understanding and Dealing with Sexual Abuse Trauma: An Educational Group for Women* (Muenzenmaier et al., 1998) was designed to be both informative and supportive and we hoped it could meet some of the needs of the multiply traumatised women with serious mental illness.

The trauma group was implemented in an outpatient setting. It included information about the various definitions of abuse, maladaptive coping styles and related symptomatology as well as some skills training. Additional topics discussed were feelings of helplessness, isolation, secrecy, stigma, and shame. Rather than blaming and pathologising we wanted to let survivors know that many of their thoughts, feelings and behaviours were connected to their past traumatic experiences. We felt that an educational model would empower survivors and provide the containment in which the

Table 7.1. Educational trauma group sessions.

Session 1	Contracting and Orientation to the Group
Session 2	Staying Safe Within and Outside the Group
Session 3	What is Abuse?
Session 4	Talking and Learning about Abuse
Session 5	Protecting Your Safety: Should You Disclose?
Session 6	Reactions of Others to Disclosure about Abuse
Session 7	Effects of Abuse on the Individual
Session 8	Experiencing PTSD and Dissociation
Session 9	Coping as a Child and as an Adult: Safety Issues
Session 10	Controlling Trauma-Related Experiences
Session 11	Support and Resources: Avoiding Re-victimisation
Session 12	Wrap Up

Source: Muenzenmaier et al. (1998)

group members would be able to safely connect and validate each other's feelings, including distorted beliefs resulting from self-blame, guilt and shame. The communications and connections established between group members let survivors know that they were not alone, they were not 'crazy', and, most of all, that there would be 'light at the end of the tunnel', an approach validated by the group leaders.

The manual, *Understanding and Dealing with Sexual Abuse Trauma: An Educational Group for Women* (Muenzenmaier et al., 1998), became the foundation for later group work and manuals. The box above describes the topics of each of the 12-week group sessions. The first session begins with an orientation where the goals of the group, the 'contract', the curriculum and the flow of the sessions are discussed including safety and confidentiality rules. Each of the chapters has the same structure and shares guidelines for group leaders, a handout for group members, and a small card with the 'thought for the day' for each of the participants to keep.

The structure of the sessions, the educational information provided and the safety rules are designed to help participants stay grounded in the context of emotionally overwhelming and painful experiences. The topics were selected according to what would be the least triggering and stressful and then in subsequent sessions to move to more intense and emotionally difficult topics. The last session is a 'wrap up' and includes an evaluation form where participants can provide feedback about the group.

Safety

Since safety was the first and foremost goal, the structure and content of the group sessions were designed accordingly. Safety was emphasised in each group session, in the beginning and before closure as well as throughout.

Each person was empowered to say 'no' if any remarks or topics became too triggering and stressful. The assumption was that if one group member did not feel safe the group was not considered safe. One of the ground rules was that sharing of detailed personal trauma should be avoided in the group and instead be discussed in individual sessions with the primary therapist where readiness and specific interventions appropriate for each person can be assessed. This is important since, although not always successfully, we tried to limit strong trauma related responses (e.g. affective dysregulation, dissociation, and flashbacks). We aimed for no more than eight group participants and required a minimum of two group leaders. This provided flexibility so that if one of the members got triggered, was dissociating and/or became extremely angry, one group leader could leave the room with that person if necessary. An evaluation then was made outside the group room as to what was going on and could be used to practice grounding and/or reinforce other skills that had been discussed during the group sessions. Meanwhile the other group leader was able to continue the group with the other members.

Structure and Content

The once-a-week sessions were one hour long, highly structured, and predictable. However, there was flexibility built in when major issues were brought forth by any of the group members that needed to be addressed. The sessions usually started with a review of the previous week's thought for the day and session content. A short presentation given on the weekly topic was followed by a discussion. All group members could join in the discussion but did not have to participate.

Response

Initially staff was reluctant to refer women to the trauma groups fearing worsening of symptoms and decompensation. Group leaders as well were concerned but hoped that the safety measures put into place would help to control trauma related symptomatology during the group. We were encouraged by the fact that the traumatised women were feeling empowered and seemed to experience less stigma and shame. Later we also piloted a separate group for male participants. During the process of developing these various educational trauma groups, we felt supported in personal communications with Gilchrist and Rainbow (1998), who also were part of the trauma task force in New York State (see Chapter 3). They had developed a drop-in, low intensity trauma group and felt that an entry level educational group was helpful and subsequently encouraged participants' interest in other trauma informed interventions.

Cognitive Behavioural Therapy Groups

As we moved the groups from an outpatient to an inpatient setting, we were confronted by new challenges. While the existing inpatient psychotherapy groups were process-oriented and included general support, we were interested in developing more trauma specific interventions that went beyond the educational aspects. We also needed to take into account the complex realities of the people who were hospitalised and experienced a wide array of symptoms. Major difficulties in affect regulation, dissociation, flashbacks, and psychosis were intertwined and often included aggressive and/ or self-destructive impulses that could be triggered in a group setting. In order to develop and assure a safe and holding environment we needed more structure and clear boundaries in the group setting. We did not want the trauma groups themselves to be traumatising to group members or group leaders.

While group CBT with exposure components had been shown to be efficacious in the treatment of symptoms of post-traumatic stress disorder (PTSD) (Foy et al., 2001), we were concerned that exposure would not be suitable for the multiply traumatised inpatients who also experienced psychotic symptoms. Even a two-phased approach that included skills training in affect regulation during the first 8 sessions and then added a modified exposure component during the second 8 sessions (Cloitre, Koenen, Cohen, & Han, 2002) could be destabilising for people with psychotic symptoms.

Complex PTSD (cPTSD)(see introduction) was an important component of some of the difficulties experienced by people with serious mental illness (Muenzenmaier, Spei, & Gross, 2010). We therefore decided to develop a group CBT model that would take the symptoms of cPTSD (Herman, 1992) into account. The Symptom Specific Group Therapy (SSGT) for cPTSD (Shelley, 2006) is a 12-week manualised programme and includes skills training and social support in addition to psycho-education. It provides structure and guidance for both group members and therapists. Groups last 60 minutes and generally include no more than eight participants. We also conducted gender specific groups which were manualised (Shelley, 2006). An alternative model of group CBT for PTSD – Group Education and Skills Training (GEST) (Muller, Rivera, & Muenzenmaier, 2005) – was adapted to a higher functioning outpatient population with some variations (75-minute sessions and more involved homework assignments). In Shelley's SSGT group described above, the twelve modules address cPTSD symptoms including nightmares, flashbacks, dissociation, avoidance, affective numbing, hyperarousal, impulsivity and affective lability, dangerous behaviours towards self and others, substance abuse and addictions, self-concept, bodily manifestations of trauma, and problems in relationships and trust (Shelley, 2006).

We modified the cognitive behavioural intervention to address the needs of the people with serious mental illness by clarifying concepts and using colourful visual images and stickers. This improved the understanding of the difficulties experienced ('symptoms') and illustrated the use and helpfulness of coping skills ('tools'). We practised cognitive, behavioural and social skills during the group session and gave handouts and simple assignments for the following week.

The Pre-Group consists of an introduction for all participants as well as an overview of the goals and topics for the group. Then participants are asked to cut, paste and colour their own 'stop signs' to be used in subsequent sessions. We find it is easier for the participants to hold up their stop sign rather than interrupt and speak up when they feel that the topic makes them uncomfortable. In addition to the stop signs we also include a visual distress-o-meter that is pasted on the wall to be rated by each participant both in the beginning and the end of the meetings to assess distress as well as to assure safety for each member. Each group member receives a journal to take notes when they wish to throughout the duration of the sessions.

After the pre-group session we started with the first module followed by a total of twelve for each consecutive week. All sessions are structured in a similar fashion. After the introduction that includes the summary of the prior session, the current topic is introduced. A psychoeducational presentation and the sharing of ideas about the topic are followed by skills training ('tools') on how to cope with the difficulties/symptoms, followed by practice exercises. For example, in the module which focuses on 'relationship' and 'trust', in describing trust, it is explained that "When you trust someone, you believe that they are reliable, that they tell the truth, that they will not hurt you, and that you can count on them and depend on them" (Shelley, 2006, pp. 66–67). Next, examples are provided of issues that can be explored: It takes time to really get to know someone and determine whether they are worthy of your trust; following relational trauma in childhood it can be hard to develop trust in other people; and if you believe that someone you know is not safe to be with, that relationship should be avoided. Following this discussion period there is a shift to developing skill in being assertive which involves setting boundaries and being able to "ask for what you want and say 'no' to what you don't want" (ibid., p. 69).

The structured format of the groups encourages participants to engage in a focused discussion of symptoms and coping strategies. Didactic presentations and skills training are important in the pacing of painful feelings and cognitions. This way containment of strong emotions including anger and rage can be processed more gradually during the group sessions. As the group continues and mutual trust develops the participants may be able to share some of their own feelings of vulnerability and victimisation.

The cognitive behavioural groups valued the importance of education and the normalising and reframing of 'symptoms' as coping strategies necessary for the survival of difficult circumstances. Moreover, the development of skills that were useful in dealing with trauma related difficulties and complications was of key importance. Neither of the group models included exposure treatments. While we were not able to conduct a randomised controlled trial, a preliminary small pilot study showed improvement in symptoms of PTSD, dissociation and psychosis as well as improved knowledge, including the use and helpfulness of constructive coping skills (Muenzenmaier, Battaglia, Langdon, Kobayashi, Takeda & Michaud, 2007).

In a similar population Mueser et al. (2007) implemented a cognitive behavioural intervention without an exposure component and was able to document significant improvements including trauma-related cognitions and PTSD symptoms. Moreover, an outcome study for TREM (Fallot, McHugo, Harris, & Xie, 2011) showed that psycho-education and skills training in addition to a focus on empowerment and recovery improved outcomes for participants with co-occurring severe mental illness.

Group Process

Many of the participants in the trauma committee had educational and training experiences in which group psychotherapy theory was a major focus. The ideas of Irvin Yalom who made major contributions to group process theory (Yalom & Leszcz, 2005) were helpful in guiding our work in which focus was on relationship, containment, and instilling hope and trust. Yalom's emphasis on the 'here and now', interpersonal relationships, emotional responses, and group cohesion was influential in the running of our groups. "Members of a cohesive group feel warmth and comfort in the group and a sense of belongingness; They value the group and feel in turn that they are valued, accepted and supported by other members" (ibid., p. 55). Herman & Kallivayalil (2018) state that "Caring interaction and witnessing among group members are powerful mechanisms for normalizing traumatic experience, reducing shame and isolation, and building self-compassion" (p. 8).

As we continued the cognitive behavioural trauma groups, we felt that at times the groups were too structured. Having been trained in group process and in fostering the development of group cohesion we wanted to focus more on group dynamics. By now we also felt more confident in dealing with the various topics outlined in the trauma manual as well as the difficulties that emerged in a group setting. This helped us to be more flexible in terms of responding to topics introduced by group members that were not included in the weekly module. Moreover, the importance of developing trusting connections is an essential element for healing from trauma. Our goal was to maintain a structured setting as well as an environment that would facilitate the development of interpersonal relationships. The new trauma groups we initiated, in addition to following educational and cognitive behavioural principles, placed more emphasis on group dynamics and community building. At the same time, in our early experience in process-oriented groups, it was clear that we needed to ensure that focus on details of traumatic events be avoided. The experience of feelings of safety and group cohesiveness was threatened, for example, if discussion triggered flashbacks and intense emotional reactions.

It is extremely important for survivors to believe that change in the way they negotiate life circumstances is possible. In our trauma informed groups, discussions about the different topics led to a more complex understanding of the way in which early trauma affects current behaviour, emotional reactions, and dissociative states. Using an interpersonal approach in which group members share specific psychological difficulties grounds the discussion in commonality of experience. Members realise, for example, that they are not the only ones who have experienced extreme shame and/or guilt. With increased awareness of different perspectives, members can gain insight into their own reactions and behaviours. Moreover, feeling less isolated, it is more likely that members will actively consider new skills (i.e. positive coping strategies) that others have adopted successfully.

The following is a fictionalised vignette of a trauma informed group in which there is demonstration of several of the factors we have described including: readiness for a group therapy experience, group cohesiveness, relationship among group members, group containment and commonality of experience.[2]

> *I worked with Steve for many years in individual therapy. When we started working together, he was often in a state in which his sense of reality was quite distorted. He spoke about the devil and believed that he was being punished for 'bad' things he did. Such beliefs were apparent throughout the time we worked together. During our work he developed a growing ability to focus on reality-based life circumstances that occurred both when he was a child and later as an adult. He was gradually able to express things he felt badly about including what he had done as well as the harmful actions of others towards him. He was often able to remember circumstances that had prompted his actions. Because of his developing ability to see things from a variety of perspectives and his decreased focus on fixed beliefs and delusional material, Steve was ready for a group encouraging engagement with others. I also felt that because we had worked together for years, my presence as a group leader would make it easier for him to make the transition to a group setting.*

---

2   See Yalom and Leszcz (2005) and Cabeza (2019) for discussion about therapeutic factors in groups.

Steve began attending one of the trauma groups that I ran in the outpatient clinic. Most of the group members were vulnerable and had issues with trust. However, there were also differences among members. Some were still experiencing hallucinations and delusions, some were not. There were differences in terms of ease of interacting with others. The group included both males and females and a variety of cultural backgrounds were represented. Members seemed comfortable with one another early on and group connection developed fairly quickly. Steve was very eager to talk about subjects discussed, but initially had a tendency to interrupt others and appeared to have difficulty focusing on what other people were saying. For Steve, participation in the group was an important interpersonal learning experience. Despite his eagerness to talk about himself, he gradually became better able to give others a chance to talk and he was increasingly able to focus on what others said.

There were some topics that were especially interesting to Steve and there were several occasions when ideas he brought up sparked a great deal of discussion. For example, throughout his childhood there were periods in which his mother, who was abusing drugs, was unable to care for him. At such times he was cared for by several different family members and he struggled when separated from his mother and with dealing with difficult circumstances in relatives' homes. Then, as an adult, he had been placed in a series of housing situations some of which he liked and some in which he felt victimised. In a discussion about trust, he was able to convey why certain circumstances felt comfortable and others did not. Other people readily responded by talking about their own experiences and the group was able to engage in a very meaningful discussion about qualities that effected how comfortable they were being with other people. Because Steve had often walked around the clinic talking to himself, and at times making angry statements (which were directed at the voices he experienced), other people tended to avoid interactions with him. This was not the case in the group.

Based on things that he talked about in individual sessions, it was clear that the group experience was helpful in his growing understanding of his emotional reactions. In individual sessions, I could reinforce practices talked about in the group. Having the same therapist in individual and group therapy seemed to be a very positive experience. In individual sessions, when I asked him about his thoughts about what other group members had mentioned, he talked about Anthony and what he had said about his temper. Anthony had indicated that he was really working on controlling his behaviour when he was angry. Steve readily identified with Anthony's reactive responses, was relieved that he was not the only one in the group that had trouble dealing with

anger, and thought that maybe he could try some of the things the
group talked about in terms of dealing with strong reactions.

Creative Arts Therapy Groups

Creative arts therapies had been established in the facility for many years
in music, art, dance, and drama therapies. With the advent of the trauma
committee, creative arts therapists became eager to find a new way of understanding the work they were already doing. The music therapist and art
therapist along with their interns were intrigued by the idea of developing
techniques to reach trauma survivors using the unique tools available in
each modality. Recognising that many service users were not ready for verbal therapy groups, and seeking a structured approach, they adapted the
educational (Muenzenmaier et al., 1998) and SSGT (Shelley, 2006) models
to their trauma informed group approaches. This led to a period of exploration of these group models using the unique tools of art and music. After
several years, creative arts therapists began to return to a less structured
approach that allowed for the topics to emerge more spontaneously and the
tools to be incorporated into the needs at hand.

Music Therapy

Each of the creative arts therapies function in distinct ways. Bruscia (2014)
describes four types of music experiences in music therapy: listening, im-
provising, re-creating, and composing. Although effectively used in individual work, one of the signature features of music therapy is its use in group
contexts. Music has been used throughout the ages to draw people together
to create community. One of the aspects that is particularly helpful with
individuals that experience psychosis is the ability of music to reach out
without having to make direct contact. For example, a person sitting outside
a group, perhaps responding to inner stimuli and apparently disregarding
the group, hears the music and may begin to tap their foot or look up or
even provide a single word or phrase that may be put into a song. Among
the tools in music therapy are: the ability to work on developing relationship
(Stephens, 1983), engagement of the body that van der Kolk (2014) describes
as necessary for the healing of trauma, and support for the social engagement system (Porges, 2010). The importance of these aspects in music therapy will be described more fully in Chapter 13.

After the initial attempts at the open format of the music-verbal therapy trauma groups (mentioned briefly in Chapter 5), it became clear that as
powerful as music is to express emotions, the need for musical structures is
essential when working with people who have trauma histories and experience psychosis (see Chapter 12). As we reflected on the needs of the survivors we knew we needed to titrate the emotional intensity – something that

would be manageable for the group members and for the therapists. This structure would guide both the therapists and the group members to explore creatively while providing containment for the group topics. We began to use music therapy techniques such as song writing, drumming, and guided imagery to address topics such as self-injury, re-scripting nightmares, and relationship and trust issues (see Chapter 12). The topics helped us to maintain a focus and to be clear in guiding our discussions. As an example, the following abbreviated outline of the module focused on 'relationship' and 'trust' is shared here.

As in most of the modules the group begins with a musical gathering either through an improvisation or a check-in song. Then the theme of relationship and trust is presented verbally with some prompts from the SSGT manual (Shelley, 2006). An open discussion ensues. Then the musical part is introduced.

In this example, song writing was used (see Chapter 12 for a more detailed description of this module). The act of composing a song together and integrating members individual ideas, was designed to provide an opportunity to work together, build relationships and develop a sense of community. The group members chose 'Trust' for the title of their song. A simple chord progression was provided by the music therapist to make it easier for group members to create their own melodies and words to go with this harmonic foundation. With guidance from leaders, taking cues from how comfortable each member felt with the process, as well as the containment the music provided, an integrated group song was created. The group members appeared proud of their work and comments made as the song developed suggested how positive members felt about this group activity.

Following our exploration using set topics we began to feel that sometimes we were cutting off spontaneous and vital moments by adhering to this model. We felt at times we were missing meaningful discussions or deep musical experiences and that having a fixed plan was ignoring what was most urgent for the group members at the moment. We already knew and could recognise the symptoms of trauma and we had techniques to share. We now felt we needed to let the group guide us into what were their most immediate needs.

This led us into a more flexible approach for the music-verbal therapy trauma groups. We had internalised the topics that were essential to cover and knew how to guide these both musically and verbally. We remained aware of the importance of music to frame the group, to hold the on-going concerns of group members, to regulate emotions emerging from difficult discussions, and to support playful interactions between group members. We could now enter the group space in a more receptive way. We might begin by picking up on a rhythm or melody spontaneously presented by a group member or begin with a musical warm up. Sometimes a group member burst out, "The unit is crazy today. There was a fight!" We would respond using words and/or music to find grounding, deepen a discussion, or uncover creative solutions (see Chapter 13).

Art Therapy

The initial approach to working with a group of service users in the art therapy room was to have an 'open studio' format. The open studio format was in a sense free style, with no directive except to enter and participate in 'art making'. This type of art therapy session is most effective when people are ready to work on their own and there is a well-equipped art studio. The therapist's focus during the sessions is the process of each individual artist; and the main element of structure is a group discussion, a reflection period, at the end of the session.

Choosing this type of art therapy session was designed just to encourage participants to come into the art therapy room, explore the material available and work on something that they were comfortable with. There was no judgment in terms of choice of art making and it was made clear that there would not be a focus on any artistic skill. Individuals were not used to working independently and group members made lots of requests, for example, "Draw me a flower. Do you have a note card? Can I have a snack?" Providing the individual attention needed was difficult even though there were art therapy students co-leading the groups.

Art therapy can be an individual endeavour but it also can take place in a relational group context (Malchiodi, 2003). Practising trauma informed work inspired us to consider more structured approaches. While attending the trauma committee meetings, we began to think about running groups that incorporated an educational and a SSGT approach. We decided to adapt both the SSGT manual (Shelley, 2006) and the educational manual (Muenzenmaier et al., 1998) for group art therapy sessions. It was a challenging process to figure out how to adapt a verbal therapy model to art therapy while respecting the nature of art therapy. Creative artistic expressions are seen by many as based on individual motivation and spontaneity (Kramer, 1993; Wilson, 2001). With the power of self-expression, often times, people reveal their past experiences possibly disclosing what they are not ready to express verbally (Wilson, 1998).

As we moved into this new way of working, our paradigm involved art media in combination with specific topics from the manuals. The creative endeavour was seen, in part, as a means to foster a 'holding environment', which we felt would in turn help clients to feel grounded as they explored together their thoughts and emotional reactions. Session structure and art materials also worked towards an experience of individual and group containment.

The session plan for each of the 12-week trauma groups and the format of each session was planned in detail in advance (see Chapter 14). Each week a topic (e.g. dissociation, self-soothing, and re-scripting nightmares) was introduced with an art activity (e.g. projects using paper, clay, and collage) (Kobayashi, Park, Chen, & Saito, 2007).

As the group met together over time there was a developing understanding that other members of the group shared common life hardships. A sense of connectedness began to be created. There was a focus on strengthening interpersonal skills through 'sharing time' where all were given a chance to talk about their reflections, at the same time listening to other people or choosing to be silent.

One of the goals of trauma focused art therapy is the development of trust (Schouten, van Hooren, Knipscheer, Kleber, & Hutschemaekers, 2019). A journal writing activity was incorporated for this purpose. At the end of each session, 5–10 minutes were used as a time for reflection. Every member was given their own journals which were kept in a locked drawer to maintain confidentiality. Group members were given enough time for discussions and to write or draw anything they wanted in their own journal. This was important for those group members who were hesitant to talk about their art and their art making process. Moreover, everyone became aware of the importance of being respectful of each other's privacy. The details of how group members responded to the art projects and how those projects effectively developed a supportive community will be described in Chapter 14.

Co-leadership

During the years of the trauma committee's work together, along with the development of the various group modalities there was a growing understanding of the needs and benefits of co-leadership. One of the major concerns when we began running groups, was to ensure that both leaders as well as members would feel that the group was a safe place. Since group leaders often have to deal with unexpected difficult situations and circumstances, we recommended that there be at least two group leaders present in the trauma groups. As previously, mentioned if one participant wanted and/ or needed to leave the group there was one leader available to accompany the survivor while the other could continue the group with the rest of the participants.

Moreover, co-leadership is a major factor in the development of group cohesion and the fostering of interpersonal relationships among members. It is important that the leaders have mutual respect as well as empathy for each other. Recognition of the different knowledge and resources that each leader brings to the group also helps in coordination of input. The need to observe the interplay between members, leaders, as well as members and leaders during the group session is a challenging task. As González de Chávez (2019) emphasises "Co-therapy facilitates better observation and knowledge of the details of the group dynamics and management of transferences and contra-transferences" (p. 34). We find it essential for co-leaders to meet regularly by scheduling time for pre- and post-meetings. There is a wide range of issues to be discussed including: method of addressing specific topics; what interventions foster 'trusting relationships' among members; how to handle affective dysregulation; and ways group leaders can model effective communication skills. In addition to focusing on specific interactions between the group members, it is also important for the group leaders to reflect on their own interactions.

A therapeutic factor that we have not discussed is the potential of modelling. Earlier in the chapter, we discussed how important co-leadership is in building in group safety. Co-leadership also makes it possible to teach through example rather than by didactic instruction. During the group, for example, group co-leaders can openly disagree, but can do this in a constructive and respectful manner. It is also important for group leaders to respond to group members in a way that demonstrates positive communication skills. In addition, leaders can point out when members' responses are supportive. The group leaders have to be able to discuss important concepts and adjust the discussion to the emotional and cognitive needs of the group members.

A special situation occurs when a co-leader is also an individual therapist for one or several group members. Here it is essential to distinguish between the different roles and be aware that personal information that might be overwhelming to others cannot be shared in the group setting. A stress on the need for confidentiality is also important.

When introducing other modalities such as creative arts therapies, co-leadership becomes even more complex. Artistic expressions can trigger strong emotional reactions. It is important for group leaders to discuss the potential reactivity and grounding methods for each group member. The music-verbal therapy trauma groups provide unique and challenging perspectives. Leaders of this type of group will have to learn how to alternate between words and music and determine whether verbal discussions and/ or musical interventions are preferable at specific times. As the co-leaders become more comfortable with using both music and verbal interventions during the groups, a comfortable dialogue emerges– sometimes within the group itself – negotiating which modality is best (Langdon, Margolis, & Muenzenmaier, 2018). The more verbally oriented therapist can then feel comfortable to say, "I think a song is needed here" or the music therapist saying, "Perhaps we need to talk more about this before we play music."

Conclusion

The development of trauma groups was a major focus of the trauma committee. The diversity of trauma committee members in clinical background as well as cultural differences and life experiences influenced the integration of the various trauma therapy group approaches.

There are special challenges in running groups for individuals who have experienced trauma and psychosis. In this chapter we have reviewed the evolutionary process in our endeavour to develop different kinds of trauma groups starting with an educational approach to a cognitive behavioural model to including creative arts therapies. Modifications have been made to provide safety and containment so that survivors with psychosis can participate in psychotherapy groups. The focus on symptoms and strategies without discussing details of traumatic experience is of primary importance when considering the beginning phases of recovery. Also important are the use of personal characteristics to determine the kind of trauma group that matches the needs of specific individuals, the encouragement of feelings of group cohesiveness and hope, the sharing of information that facilitates belief in the possibility of life changes, the development of positive self-esteem, and the transformation of feelings of shame into positive self-esteem.

Over the years we learned what interventions were effective and we adjusted our group modalities to the needs of the participants. It is important to emphasise that the group members played an active role in our seeing what works and what does not. Our recommendations for the future would be to document group outcomes in a systematised manner with specific research protocols and best practices.

References

Alexander, M. J. & Muenzenmaier, K. (1998). Trauma, addiction and recovery: Addressing public health epidemics among women with severe mental illness. In B. Levin, A. Blanch, & A. Jennings (eds), *Women's mental health services: A public health pespective* (pp. 215–239). Thousand Oaks, CA: Sage Publications.

Alexander, P., Neimeyer, R., Follette, V., Moore, M., & Harter, S. (1989). A comparison of group treatments of women sexually abused as children. *Journal of Consulting and Clinical Psychology, 57*, 479–483.

Brandt, L. (1989). A short-term group therapy model for treatment of adult female survivors of childhood incest. *Group, 13*, 74–82.

Bruscia, K. (2014). *Defining music therapy*, 3rd edition. University Park, IL: Barcelona Publisher.

Cabeza, I. G. (2019). Therapeutic factors in group psychotherapy for patients diagnosed with psychosis. In I. Urlić, & M. González de Chávez (eds), *Group therapy for psychoses* (pp. 20–31). New York: Routledge.

Cloitre, M., Koenen, K. C., Cohen, L. R., & Han, H. (2002). Skills training in affective and interpersonal regulation followed by exposure: a phase-based treatment for PTSD related to childhood abuse. *Journal of Consulting and Clinical Psychology, 70(5)*, 1067–1074.

Courtois, C. A. (1988). *Healing the incest wound: Adult survivors in therapy.* New York: W. W. Norton & Co.

Fallot, R. D., McHugo, G. J., Harris, M., & Xie, H. (2011). The trauma recovery and empowerment model: A quasi-experimental effectiveness study. *Journal of Dual Diagnosis, 7(1–2)*, 74–89.

Ford, J. D., Fallot, R. D., & Harris, M. (2009). Group therapy. In C. A. Courtois & J. D. Ford (eds), *Treating complex traumatic stress disorders: An evidence-based guide*, (pp. 415–440). New York: Guilford.

Ford, J. D., & Russo, E. (2006). Trauma-focused, present-centered, emotional self-regulation approach to integrated treatment for posttraumatic stress and addiction: Trauma adaptive recovery group education and therapy (TARGET). *American Journal of Psychotherapy, 60*(*4*), 335–355.

Foy, D. W., Schnurr, P. P., Weiss, D. S., Wattenberg, M. S., Glynn, S. M., Marmar, C. R., & Gusman, F. D. (2001). Group psychotherapy for PTSD. In J. P. Wilson, M. J. Friedman, & J. D. Lindy (eds), *Treating psychological trauma and PTSD* (pp. 183–201). New York: Guilford.

Gilchrist, P. & Rainbow, P. (1998). *Trauma safety drop-in group: A clinical model of group treatment for survivors of trauma.* Albany, NY: New York State Office of Mental Health Trauma Initiative Publication.

Gillece, J. B., & Russell, B. G. (2001). Maryland's programs for women offenders with mental illness and substance abuse disorders: Incarcerated and in the community. *Women, Girls & Criminal Justice, 2*(*6*), 84–89.

González de Chávez, M. (2009): Group psychotherapy and schizophrenia. In Y. O. Alanen, M. González de Chávez, A. S. Silver, B. Martindale (eds), *Psychotherapeutic approaches to schizophrenic psychoses: Past, present and future* (pp. 251–266). New York: Routledge.

González de Chávez, M. (2019). Creation of a therapy group for persons with psychotic experiences. In I. Urlić & M. González de Chávez (eds), *Group therapy for psychoses* (pp. 32–47). New York: Routledge.

Harris, M., & Anglin, J. (1998). Community Connections Trauma Work Group. *Trauma recovery and empowerment: A clinician's guide for working with women in groups.* New York: Free Press.

Herman, J. L. (1992). *Trauma and recovery.* New York: Basic Books.

Herman, J. L., & Kallivayalil, D. (2018). *Group trauma treatment in early recovery.* New York: Guilford.

Herman, J. & Schatzow, E. (1984). Time-limited group therapy for women with a history of incest. *International Journal of Group Psychotherapy, 34*(*4*), 605–616.

Kobayashi, T., Park, E. H., Chen, J. & Saito, T. (2007). *Syndrome specific group art therapy (SSGT) for complex PTSD.* Presented at the 38th American Art Therapy Association Annual Conference, Albuquerque, NM.

Kramer, E. (1993). *Art as therapy with children.* Chicago, IL: Magnolia Street Publishers.

Langdon, G. S., Margolis, F., & Muenzenmaier, K. (2018) Weaving words and music: Healing from trauma for people with serious mental illness. *Music and Medicine, 10*(*3*), 157–161.

Malchiodi, C. A. (2003). *Handbook of art therapy.* New York: Guilford Publications.

Muenzenmaier, K., Battaglia, J., Langdon, G. S, Kobayashi, T., Takeda, K., & Michaud, K. E. (2007). *Syndrome specific group therapy (SSGT) for complex PTSD: A cognitive behavioral group intervention adapted to music and art therapy.* Presented at the Male Survivor International Conference Relief, Recovery, and Restoration: Helping Men Heal from Sexual Abuse, New York.

Muenzenmaier, K., Sampson, D., Norelli, L., Alexander, K., Stephens, B., & Huckeba, H. (1998). *Understanding and dealing with sexual abuse trauma: An educational group for women*. Albany, NY: New York State Office of Mental Health Trauma Initiative Publication.

Muenzenmaier, K., Spei, K., & Gross, D. R. (2010). Complex posttraumatic stress disorder in men with serious mental illness: A reconceptualization. *American Journal of Psychotherapy, 64*, 257–268.

Muenzenmaier, K., Struening, E., Ferber, J., & Meyer, I. (1993). Childhood abuse and neglect among women outpatients with chronic mental illness. *Psychiatric Services, 44*(7), 666–670.

Mueser, K. T., Bolton, E. E., Carty, P. C., Bradley, M. J., Ahlgren, K. F., DiStaso, D. R., Gilbride, A., & Liddel, C. (2007). The trauma recovery group: A cognitive-behavioral program for PTSD in persons with severe mental illness. *Community Mental Health Journal, 43*, 281–304.

Muller, K. L., Rivera, M., & Muenzenmaier, K. (2005). *Development of an alternative model of cognitive behavioral group therapy for PTSD: Group education and skills training (GEST)*. Poster presented at the Association for Cognitive and Behavioral Therapies (ABCT), Toronto, Canada.

Najavits, L. M. (2002). *Seeking safety: A treatment manual for PTSD and substance abuse*. New York: Guilford Press.

Porges, S. (2010). Music therapy and trauma: Insights from the polyvagal theory. In K. Stewart (ed.). *Music therapy, and trauma: Bridging theory and clinical practice* (pp. 3–15). New York: Satchnote Press.

Resick, P. A., Jordan, C. G., Girelli, S. A., Hutter, C. K., & Marhoefer-Dvorak, S. (1988). A comparative outcome study of behavioral group therapy for sexual assault victims. *Behavior Therapy, 19*(3), 385–401.

Schouten, K. A., van Hooren, S., Knipscheer, J. W., Kleber, R. J., & Hutschemaekers, G. J. M. (2019). Trauma-focused art therapy in the treatment of posttraumatic stress disorder: A pilot study. *Journal of Trauma and Dissociation, 20*(1), 114–130.

Shelley, A.-M. (2006). *Men's trauma manual*. n.l.: Anne-Marie Shelley. Retrieved from www.lulu.com/en/en/shop/dr-anne-marie-shelley/mens-trauma-manual/paperback/product-1yvmnwe.html?page=1&pageSize=4.

Stephens, G. (1983). The use of improvisation for developing relatedness in the adult client. *Music Therapy Journal of the American Association for Music Therapy, 3*(1), 29–42.

van der Kolk, B. A. (1987). The psychological consequences of overwhelming life experiences. In B. A. van der Kolk (ed.), *Psychological trauma* (pp. 1–30). Washington, DC: American Psychiatric Press.

van der Kolk, B. A. (2014). *The body keeps the score: brain, mind, and body in the healing of trauma*. New York: Penguin Books.

Wilson, L. (1998). Introduction: Kramer's theoretical formation. In E. Kramer (ed.), *Childhood and art therapy* (pp. xxvii–xxxiv). Chicago, IL: Magnolia Street Publishers.

Wilson, L. (2001). Symbolism and art therapy. In J. A. Rubin (ed.), *Approaches to art therapy: Theory and technique (pp.44–62)*. New York: Brunner-Routledge.

Yalom, I. D. & Leszcz, M. (2005). *The theory and practice of group psychotherapy*, 5th edition. New York: Basic Books.

8

IMPLEMENTING A TRAUMA INFORMED APPROACH ON AN INPATIENT UNIT

Kristina Muenzenmaier, Gillian Stephens Langdon,
Toshiko Kobayashi, Mara Conan, and Joseph Battaglia

Introduction

During the 1980s inner cities in the United States became centres of an epic storm of what was often referred to as a crack/cocaine epidemic. Violence and gang fights were rampant and gun shots were a frequent occurrence. Families started to disintegrate. Many children lost one or both parents to AIDS or were taken away by child protective services due to neglectful and/or abusive parental behaviour. Others ran away from their homes and were then faced with additional challenges: some became homeless; some were placed in foster care where the cycle of abuse at times continued; some ended up in psychiatric children's facilities. It was not surprising that the inpatient psychiatric population at a public urban facility included many service users who had often moved around between several different foster homes, had a history of homelessness and exhibited symptoms and behaviours associated with complex trauma.

The following fictionalised vignette illustrates some of the kinds of interactions and challenges encountered when working with traumatised service users on the inpatient unit.

> *Antonia grew up in the inner city and was taken away from her mother after her mother's boyfriend had started to beat and sexually abuse Antonia. Both the mother and the boyfriend were addicted to crack and Antonia often spent nights alone in the apartment. Antonia did not know her biological father.*
>
> *Antonia's aggressive behaviour was first noted during the period in which she was in her first foster care placement. It was reported that she had violent outbursts and temper tantrums. She had difficulty concentrating in school and soon fell behind her classmates. Antonia was admitted to a psychiatric children's hospital, having reported that she heard voices instructing her to stab her foster care*

DOI: 10.4324/9781003055914-10

brother. She was diagnosed with schizoaffective disorder. This was the beginning of a revolving door cycle alternating between discharge and re-hospitalisation. At age 18 she was transferred from the children's facility to the adult hospital where the cycle continued.

There were many contradictions in Antonia's description of her childhood. At times she referred to her mother and foster parents as "good parents" and denied having been abused; at other times she vividly described violent sexual acts and physical cruelty. Sometimes she would sit silently and not respond when talked to. At other times she appeared full of rage and became assaultive attacking other service users and staff. As a result, she was frequently restrained and placed in seclusion, inadvertently triggering another cycle of violence and re-traumatisation. These events created chaos on the unit and were traumatic for Antonia as well as other service users and staff.

After careful observations and discussions, the trauma committee realised that Antonia's behaviours were better understood in the context of complex trauma reactions that included dissociative responses. Some of the members of the trauma committee assigned to the unit wanted to develop a relationship with her in which she could feel safe and cared for. This however was extremely difficult given the reported physical and sexual violations she had experienced first at the hands of her mother and boyfriend and then later her foster care parents, which had resulted in severely disorganised attachment patterns and a complex array of trauma related symptoms. Throughout these crisis situations we worked together with Antonia and the unit staff in order to create safety and understand what triggered her assaultive and self-injurious behaviours.

Working Towards a Safe and Cohesive Inpatient Unit

Initial Stages

In the early 2000s the hospital was comprised of different units (e.g. admissions unit, intensive treatment unit, community placement unit, etc.). These were staffed with one or two nurses for each shift, several nursing aides, and at least one psychiatrist, social worker, and psychologist as well as a rehabilitation therapist (e.g. a creative arts therapist or a recreation therapist). Each staff member had a private or shared office with the exception of the aides who sat in the nursing station in order to be able to observe the happenings on the unit.

A major responsibility of several trauma committee members was to act as consultants throughout the hospital. We were called upon to work with service users who had trauma histories and exhibited affective dysregulation and impulse control difficulties. The consultation consisted of assessing trauma histories, understanding re-enactments and developing a safety treatment plan with the team and the service recipient. Assessment and treatment plans included a description of the trauma the person had experienced; related symptoms; a statement of specific triggers leading to flashbacks and re-enactment behaviours; a safety plan for affect/behavioural management and reinforcement of positive coping skills.

The impact of doing consultations depended on the receptiveness and collaboration of the staff on the units on which we consulted. We realised that staff often felt intruded upon in their relationship with an already 'difficult to manage' service user. In addition, our outreach was mostly limited to one staff member rather than involving the whole team and follow up was often episodic.

Trauma committee members also had been running hospital-wide trauma groups that included survivors from different units. Developing specific verbal and creative arts therapy groups for trauma survivors required extra time and effort in selecting participants, getting permission from the clinical teams on the different units, scheduling time and location, and physically gathering each participant one by one to attend the groups. From the programming point of view, it would be logistically easier to conduct trauma groups on one unit.

Enacting Change: Working through Obstacles

Despite serious questions and concerns, we became convinced that a trauma unit could better address the needs of survivors. We realised that a shift in thinking would be necessary. In trauma committee meetings, we discussed the importance of gaining the trust of service users and establishing a positive relationship in order for healing to take place. We also realised that working with staff was essential in order to create a safe and holding environment (Winnicott, 1965). When considering the implementation of a 'trauma unit' creating trusting relationships as well as using a trauma informed approach in therapeutic interventions would be key factors in facilitating recovery in survivors. Sandra Bloom's book *Creating Sanctuary* (1997) served as an important guide and inspiration for our approach.

When we reviewed different proposals for implementation of a trauma unit, we were especially impressed with the Sanctuary Model (Bloom, 1997, 2000). In the early 1990s I had visited the Friends Services Hospital in Philadelphia where Sandra Bloom and her staff worked on a psychiatric inpatient unit treating adult survivors of trauma. Over a period of time, they had developed a trauma-based treatment approach within the context of a therapeutic milieu which was informed by egalitarian principles and stressed the importance of non-violence and empowerment of the whole community. This visit had left a strong imprint throughout the years and when considering the development of a trauma unit for our facility, I believed that despite all the challenges of a public psychiatry setting, a safe community and a trauma sensitive environment were achievable goals.

Members of the trauma committee were initially hesitant to organise one ward as a 'trauma unit'. However, based on doing trauma assessments throughout the hospital as well as considering the findings of the prevalence studies, we knew that many service users had experienced childhood trauma. We also understood that trauma survivors were often seen not only as being 'out of control' but also as 'treatment resistant' (Jennings, 1998) suggesting that the standard psychiatric treatment protocol did not result in much improvement. While the downside was that we would have less time to consult on other units of the hospital, now we would be able to focus our energy on one entire unit.

We looked at various units to get an idea of how we could organize a trauma unit. There was an intensive treatment unit where individuals who were considered to be dangerous to self or others were often transferred. Here the staff to patient ratio was higher than on the other units and staff were specially trained to deal with 'out of control' behaviours. Initially, the unit housed both women and men. Because many service users had experienced previous physical and sexual abuse/violence, difficulties on the unit seemed to be intensified by male/female interactions. A decision was made to create an all-female unit which then became the 'trauma unit'. The women admitted to the trauma unit often had experienced multiple psychiatric hospitalisations. They were considered to be seriously mentally ill and exhibiting psychotic symptomatology. Typical chart diagnoses included schizophrenia, schizoaffective disorder and/or a mood disorder, with or without an additional personality disorder diagnosis. Over the years and across different admissions they often had received different diagnoses. However, post-traumatic stress disorder (PTSD), dissociative disorder or Disorder of Extreme Stress, not otherwise specified (DESNOS) (APA, 1994) were rarely included. The vast majority of the women on the trauma unit were survivors of early and continuous life trauma (see Chapter 3) resulting in behaviours and symptoms that could often be seen as consistent with complex PTSD (Herman, 1992; Van der Kolk et al., 2005; Courtois &

Ford, 2009) and dissociation (Kluft, 1987; Moskowitz et al., 2009). Difficulties in affect regulation and impulse control had led to frequent use of emergency medications and seclusion and restraint procedures. With this new unit, treatment could now also be addressed in a trauma context rather than being limited to a diagnostic framework of psychotic disorders such as schizophrenia and schizoaffective disorders.

It soon became apparent that the idea of an all-female trauma unit was not embraced by everybody. Concerns about serious management difficulties and increased risk of violence towards self and others made recruitment to work on this unit a challenge. Nursing staff who were often the first responders during an incident were more likely to get hurt and be subject to investigations if violence occurred. This could result in transfers of staff to other units or even suspensions. Despite the known and expected challenges many staff did apply to work on the unit and were committed to the task at hand.

Growing Awareness of the Complexities

One of our goals was to empower staff in the development of the unit and the decision-making process. The initial steps included meetings with the unit staff to present some of our thoughts and goals. We made it clear that we wanted to get input from all staff on how to go about developing a trauma informed unit. Though we also wanted to include survivors in the planning process, we delayed that task until we had developed relationships with staff and a culture of collaboration had evolved among the members of the treatment team. Our aim was to create an inclusive environment in which every staff member independent of discipline felt comfortable voicing concerns and contributing to discussions. We hoped that a professional culture of inclusiveness and interdisciplinary connectivity would empower all staff and also contribute to the empowerment of service users. Regularly scheduled meetings and educational trainings would include discussions of clinical and systems issues as well as our interactions with service users and each other.

In early meetings in which we discussed the structuring of the unit we made clear one of our key beliefs was that the medical model failed to recognise the way in which service users were impacted by overwhelming life experiences.[1] By focusing on diagnosis, (e.g. schizophrenia, schizoaffective disorder, affective disorders), we had been failing to develop trauma based interventions for people with psychosis and trauma histories. While psychopharmacological treatment was often helpful, we found that people who received

---

1   A detailed discussion on how the assumptions in a trauma-based model differ from those in a medical model is provided by Bills & Bloom (1998).

higher dosing of psychotropic medications reported more co-occurring categories of stressful childhood experiences than those who received lower dosing (Schneeberger et al., 2014; Anda et al., 2007). Moreover, treatment approaches based on separate diagnostic categories served to recreate the fragmented pictures survivors had of themselves. Therefore, we felt that it was essential to develop an integrated approach that included trauma informed care and was empowering to the survivors (Muenzenmaier et al., 2010).

As we started to develop the unit in 2006, the complexities involved became more apparent. There were constant emergency calls. Seclusion and assault rates were high, so were incidents of self-injurious behaviours, putting both service users and staff at risk of injuries. More staff seemed to be calling in sick and the ones who were present expressed feelings that they did not get enough support. In addition, rotation of staff to different units presented difficulties in providing consistency in our approach to service users. We felt exasperated; the unit was overwhelming to both service users and staff, and we had clearly underestimated the challenges. Similarly, when Bills attempted to develop a trauma-based unit in a state psychiatric hospital system she wrote: "Violence was normative behaviour. On the average, there were 100 reported violent episodes per month, which included violence to self, others, and accidents" (Bills & Bloom, 1998, p. 351).

We had to address these frustrations, and realised that administrative support would be essential in working towards changing the attitudes towards trauma survivors within the facility. Training, support, and empowerment of staff would be a pivotal part of this process. We also started to look at and work with the hospital administration on ways that we could implement hospital-wide systemic changes for trauma informed care (Harris & Fallot, 2001). Developing trauma informed practices included changes in hospital policies and release from clinical duties to attend trauma related training. Often the clinical director of the hospital modelled trauma sensitive interventions when crises occurred. He supported the ongoing work of the trauma committee and helped us stay informed about challenging situations throughout the facility.

Developing Trusting and Inclusive Relationships

Despite the disruptions, we believed that trusting and inclusive relationships among staff were key to developing a safe and structured environment for the whole community. We continued to strive for regular meetings with all staff including meetings with evening and night shift staff. The goal was to develop and maintain ongoing communications within and between shifts as well as among the various disciplines so that everybody was familiar with the interventions helpful for each of the service users.

We also discovered that finding a comfortable space to hold our meetings was more difficult than we had expected. We started out in the nursing station; a room surrounded by windows looking onto the unit. This allowed the nursing staff to participate while fulfilling their responsibilities for observing happenings on the unit. The nursing station was a small, narrow rectangular room in the middle of the unit in which there was not enough room for everybody to sit. The room was enclosed by big plexiglass windows so that staff could easily oversee the hallway and the day room where most of the service users gathered. For our staff meetings we all tried to squeeze inside, sitting and standing, in order to discuss clinical issues. From the outside service users could observe us as well. It appeared that some were even able to read our lips. Service users would walk up and down in the hallway gazing at us from outside the window. Some tried to get our attention by gesticulating, banging on the windows, or interrupting the meeting by opening the door. Fighting would erupt and we would have to stop the meeting to intervene. While we knew that there was potential for violence and boundary violations on the unit, we did not expect this level of disruption. The nursing station was clearly not the right place for our clinical meetings. We felt as if we were sitting in a cage and it was as uncomfortable for us as it was for the service users. However, we now understood how service users must have felt being constantly observed.

On the other hand, with the newly created unit we were able to develop ongoing relationships with staff as well as service users and their families. In team meetings we could discuss trauma informed interventions for each service user and work together with staff in highlighting re-enactments and re-traumatisation practices. We now would be able to maintain consistency in the interventions targeting trauma specific behaviours. It was quite rewarding when we began to see positive changes on the unit.

Staff Training as an Integral Part in Developing the Unit

Besides educational goals regarding trauma relevant information we felt it was of primary importance for all of us to learn and understand the barriers and prejudices we faced as individuals and as team members on the unit. We strove for inclusiveness in training. We wanted everybody on the unit to participate in the development of a trauma sensitive environment from nursing, psychology, psychiatry, social work, creative arts therapies, nutritional counselling to administrative staff such as team leaders. The trainings also served to encourage connections among staff members.

The educational goals included providing trauma relevant information to questions such as: How prevalent is a trauma history in the population we serve? What are the effects of trauma, in particular childhood trauma? How do we recognise PTSD in people with psychosis? Are some of the symptoms and behaviours we observe related to trauma exposure? What biases do we have about the women we work with? How safe/unsafe do the women survivors feel on the unit? How do we respond to their behaviours (e.g. losing control) and their feelings (e.g. becoming afraid)? How safe do we as staff feel on the unit? What and how does this impact our interventions? Does it affect how we deal with control issues and procedures such as restraint or seclusion? How aware are we that inpatient psychiatric environments and practices can be traumatising to both service users and staff (e.g. use of emergency medication, restraint and seclusion practices, nightly checks, etc.) (Jennings, 1998).

In order to achieve inclusiveness, we proposed, in addition to the regular scheduled daily rounds and weekly clinical and staff meetings, formal training sessions for all staff regardless of educational backgrounds, disciplines and shifts. This was particularly important since not all shifts could attend team meetings. With special permission from administration, once a month all disciplines were able to participate in trainings. Night and evening shift staff were paid overtime if they were able to attend. In addition, trauma committee members met with the morning, evening and night staff to discuss survivor's trauma histories and treatment plans as well as identification of triggers and coping skills.

The trainings used multidisciplinary approaches. For example, creative arts therapists educated staff in the uses and importance of creative arts therapies when addressing issues of trauma and extreme emotionally dysregulated states (Kobayashi et al., 2009). What might appear as playful diversions could be understood as carefully thought-out interventions. Hands-on-experiences during in-service trainings helped staff to recognise the power of art, origami, music, drama, and dance/movement therapy. Creating community, expressing feelings, and gaining a sense of empowerment through creative arts therapies were key components in the healing from trauma.

The starting point for the training sessions was safety. Bloom (1997) emphasises several facets of safety including physical safety, psychological safety, social safety, and moral safety. Physical safety in a psychiatric inpatient setting was of particular concern. Restraining and lowering a person who is agitated is traumatising to the person being subdued. The experience of restraints and seclusion often is reminiscent of past traumatic experiences, both by re-enacting past violence as well as by being left with feelings of isolation. Moreover, such an incident also is traumatising to others witnessing the event. This includes other service users as well as staff.[2]

But there is so much more to safety than not experiencing sexual, physical and/or verbal violence. For example, nightly checks by nursing staff, done to assure safety in the bedrooms can be re-traumatising to survivors and trigger flashbacks to past traumatic experiences. In trainings we have frequently used an excellent table developed by Jennings (1998, pp. 335–337) in

---

2   Chapter 6 will discuss the development of the Trauma Program for Staff (TPS).

which she compares how early traumatic experiences are re-enacted within an institutional psychiatric setting leading to further victimisation of survivors. In order to interrupt the cycle of violence staff needs to become aware of triggers and traumatic re-enactments and enter into a dialogue with the survivor. Moreover, they can assist service users to recognise and negotiate challenging environments and collaborate in the development of positive coping skills. This includes understanding how to avoid re-victimisation experiences and how to be safe inside but also outside the hospital (e.g. when on community passes, not responding to sexual propositions). Moreover, the whole community needs to be safe. This also includes staff. If staff do not feel safe on the unit, how can service users feel safe? We wanted staff to be able to express their own fears, both for themselves and for the women they are responsible for, without worries of being judged. We also wanted to understand our own barriers and prejudices and how they might impact our work with survivors.

Therefore, we designed role plays which were some of the more popular trainings. We chose challenging situations that had happened on the unit during the preceding weeks which we re-enacted. Staff were assigned different roles outside their disciplines and professional tasks: A day shift staff member played a night shift staff member feeling left out of the communication; a staff member who had secluded a service user played the individual becoming agitated and reacting to staff's interventions; a member of the nursing staff played the psychiatrist being inattentive to the needs of the nursing staff; a psychologist played a nursing staff member responsible for one-on-one observation of a self-injurious service user, etc. The role reversals were as much fun as they were eye opening. Amazement, laughter but also anger and frustration were brought to the fore. Team members became aware of their own preconceived notions as well as their emotional reactions. This included: ideas about culture, race, and gender; ideas about behaviours that might not have been previously recognised or understood; feelings about being controlled and maintaining control; understandings of fear-based behaviours and triggers; ways to deal with emotion dysregulation and re-enactments; and feelings of hopelessness and disempowerment. The role plays elevated our understanding of implicit and explicit biases and increased awareness of our emotional reactions. The experience fostered collaboration among team members and we felt that it was one of the pillars for the development of a solid team approach.

Stress was placed on inclusive decision making and the need to carefully listen to one another. Control issues were particularly important to focus on since they were a barrier to empowerment. The hierarchical structure of the medical model led inherently to issues of control. Moreover, the fear of violence and the need for boundaries could reinforce stricter limit setting and control. We practiced how to defuse crisis situations and work together in a circle of support, at times encircling the survivor in a protective way. By feeling more comfortable in our roles and the decision-making process and becoming aware of our own vulnerabilities (e.g. our own victimisation experiences) we hoped to improve our understanding of the survivors, as well as to feel more confident in ourselves when coping with challenging circumstances.

Issues with specific service users, as well as unit systems problems, could also be targeted in clinical trainings. Moreover, we supervised various staff members on an individual basis and could focus specifically on trauma related issues (e.g. complex PTSD, self-destructive, aggressive, and acting out behaviours) by including these formulations in treatment planning.

The music therapist describes her experience in running a music therapy in-service.

In order to help staff members express feelings about working on the unit and at the same time to help promote a sense of community, we planned a music therapy experience for the staff. I wondered how staff would react. Because I had conducted music therapy groups (including trauma groups) throughout the hospital and supervised music therapy students, many of the staff knew me. However, I was not a member of the trauma unit.

I entered the room where the staff was seated. The group was larger than I had expected and I felt nervous. I thought, "Who am I to 'help' staff here?" But I was already there holding my guitar with a cart of instruments so I started singing "Hello" using a simple accompaniment and strum on the guitar. Continuing to sing, I added "Tell us how you're feeling?" From the back of the room I heard the words, "Fed up!" As I embraced these intense words adjusting the guitar strum to be more forceful and my voice to create emphasis, the group started to laugh. Others began sharing, "angry", "tired", "hopeful", as the guitar and voice supported the affect for each of these feelings.

As the session continued, we shared rhythms using the percussion and melodic percussion instruments as well as movement, ending with a familiar song from one of the trauma groups. It was clear through the common rhythms and the sharing of meaningful words that the sense of community was growing. The group had been open to my beginning intervention and had responded to my embrace of difficult emotions. The song allowed for 'negative' feelings to be expressed and shared without extensive verbal discussion. The song itself wove into a group song which led to a feeling of openness and camaraderie, a step on the road to building community.

Creating a Safe Space Leads to a Stronger Sense of Community

As we have indicated, a very important factor in being able to implement a trauma informed approach has to do with the investment that staff members have in the unit which is at least partially related to how safe they feel. During the period in which we were struggling to find a place for our staff meetings, a new clinician, a creative arts therapist, was transferred to the unit. Her efforts played a major role in the initiation of unit changes.

The art therapy room had become a comfortable community space in which service users felt empowered to express themselves. The fact that they felt relaxed and safe helped to make it easier to focus on projects they were working on. As interactions took place, it provided an opportunity to focus on communication styles and the importance of discussing things in a respectful manner. Because of the pleasant atmosphere there and our continued search for a meeting room that would accommodate all staff, we proposed that meetings be moved from the nursing station to the art therapy room. The art therapist, however, was reluctant to open up her room for staff meetings since she saw the art therapy room first and foremost as a safe room for service users (Killick, 2017). She wanted to establish an open-door policy and a safe environment where service users could feel free to enter at any time during the daytime and felt that staff meetings could be a hindrance in this endeavour.

After ongoing discussions, the art therapist finally agreed and opened the room to staff as well. She developed a culture of respect and warmth toward whomever entered her room, staff and service users alike. Service recipients learned to respect staff meetings and there were less disruptions. Staff seemed to feel calmer and more centred. We now were able to sit as a team for the length of our meetings without interruptions. Team members developed trusting connections with each other. While initially we only focused on clinical issues (such as trauma, trauma related symptoms, and triggers), now, we started to discuss our relationships with the survivors and with each other. We became more open and were able to share our own feelings and difficulties. Staff started to bring food to the unit meetings. As we began feeding each other the meetings became nurturing for us physically and emotionally. An understanding that all staff members, no matter what their discipline, had important roles in the team became widely accepted.

The art therapy room became a main centre for the unit and a safe place for the whole community. When the door was closed, while never locked, people respected the boundary. The ward had a schedule for activity programmes to be held at certain times during the day. Now, instead of the nursing station, the psychiatrist used the room to talk about medication and medication side effects. The psychologist and nursing staff started to run groups in this space instead of the visitor's room. Now staff members helped out, co-led groups, and generally were more inclined to participate in various ward activities.

There were other notable changes on the unit. Team members started to spend more time together in the nursing station. This made it possible to also informally discuss observations about interactions and behaviours among community members as well as concerns and differences of opinion among staff outside of the regular scheduled meetings. Staff developed a better understanding of the value of trauma informed care including specific interventions such as verbal, music, and art therapies.

Our ability to restructure the unit was enhanced by the encouragement, guidance and support of the facility administration. The clinical director of the hospital understood the experience staff were going through and was aware of the supports we needed. He had often participated in trauma committee meetings and was knowledgeable not only of the high prevalence of childhood trauma but also how to work with the traumatised women.

There were many foundations that had to be established in order to start an effective art therapy programme on the unit. I felt that in order to be supported by staff, it was important to convey that the art therapy programme was a therapeutic practice and not simply a recreational activity. In order for staff to understand the nature of my work it would be important to discuss the therapeutic aspects of art therapy.

When I first opened the art therapy room, initially no one came. I turned to nursing staff for help and they announced that the art therapy room was open. I also went inside the dayroom and invited people one by one; many of them were sleeping and ignored me or said "no thank you". However, as I continued to greet people every morning and before I left in the evening a few people started to exchange nods, then greeted me in response. Gradually relationships began to be formed and simultaneously my concerns about establishing a meaningful programme disappeared.

It didn't take a long time before people started entering the art therapy room. Some service users were very curious about what was going on inside and first peeked through the window before they were ready to enter the room. Some people knocked on the window to attract attention. When people started coming to the door, some of them curiously pointed out a karaoke machine. They asked if they could use the attractively displayed art materials and I responded, "Of course, all of them are for you." With that invitation, one by one, they decided to enter the room. Once some people entered the room, others followed. They started to ask about folding specific origami (paper folding) objects. Gradually, I introduced simple and playful origami models that they could create independently. (The use of origami as a tool for trauma care will be discussed in detail in Chapters 14 and 15.) I played music on the karaoke machine that service users requested. I also made arrangements to get CDs based on the cultural background of the people on the unit. (e.g. Greek songs, hip hop songs, soul music, Latino music, and popular songs in different languages). I was impressed when recipients requested Japanese songs. I felt that this demonstrated sensitivity, awareness of the other, and respect for my culture.

By reaching out to service users, staff and administration, our efforts to establish a feeling of community on the unit began meeting with success. The importance of establishing a therapeutic community was a concept introduced early in the facility's development. Therapeutic community meetings were seen as an essential forum for understanding the concerns of the community and arriving at possible ways to resolve problematic issues by identifying unit issues and encouraging all community members to express their feelings and viewpoints. The historical origins and concepts of a therapeutic community as a healing and corrective experience are extensively discussed by Bloom (1997). Moreover, its specific application to trauma-based inpatient care is further elaborated on by Bills and Bloom (1998). In the early stages of the trauma unit, there were three weekly therapeutic community meetings that often included only one staff member. We were highly motivated to establish a more inclusive meeting. The expectation on the unit was that not only would all service recipients attend these meetings but also all staff including those who had leadership roles in directing the unit (e.g. psychiatrists, team leaders). We wanted service users to take responsibility for running the meeting and establish a patient government that would discuss and take responsibility for important unit issues. A fully participant community would serve to counteract a hierarchical power structure. We wanted to build a unit in which every service user and every staff member was taken seriously and played an important role. Therapeutic community meetings were an essential part in this process and a decision was made to increase the frequency from three to five days a week. Running the meeting was empowering to service users and the full participation of staff made clear that staff was taking unit issues seriously. It was helpful that each meeting was structured in the same way (i.e. the rules of the meeting and schedule of the day were reviewed, and then community issues were discussed) and became an established routine. Because all members of the community were encouraged to be respectful and attentive during discussions, and because of the consistency in the structure, over time the meetings ran more smoothly, provided a safe holding environment, and fostered change on the unit.

The development of the creative arts therapies programme also was a major factor in instilling a feeling of community. For example, when the hospital administration wanted each unit to create a mural, everyone was invited to participate in this project. Service users and staff including all disciplines (e.g. psychiatry, social work, psychology, and nursing) worked on the mural together in the art therapy room. Each individual created a doll that was a self-representation. The dolls were cut out in a human shape using cardboard and decorated with fabrics, yarns, watercolour, origami paper, and other available materials. When the mural was completed, it was hung up on a big wall in the hallway of the unit for everybody to see.[3]

Consolidation: Integration of Programming

The above implemented changes led to an increased sense of safety for the whole community and a belief that staff was genuinely able to provide support. We were able to successfully implement multimodal and multidisciplinary interventions. Individual and group modalities included verbal, music, and art therapies in addition to medication management and skills training programmes. Staff began to refer service users to specific groups based on individual needs and interests. The development of important relationships (both among staff and service users) led to less volatile responses during stressful situations. There was less hesitation in approaching staff when support was needed and survivors became increasingly interested in participating in specific trauma informed interventions. We reached out to family members and included them in therapeutic programmes whenever possible. For example, the unit psychologist held family therapy sessions in which family issues could be discussed in a safe environment. Issues addressed could include intra-familial trauma, domestic violence, substance abuse, environmental safety, struggles with poverty and resilience, among others (see also Chapter 10).

---

3   The book cover design replicates a similar group project created by people involved in the creation of this book.

By the second year of working on the unit, I was able to see a clear change. The general feeling was more positive and I no longer felt tension when I opened the front door of the unit. It also appeared that the nursing staff truly appreciated the therapeutic value of art therapy. Most importantly, I felt that staff now was aware that when service users participated in art therapy sessions, they were focused and productive and able to control problematic behaviours. I was also pleased with the role that art therapy activities played in the building of community and equal participation. Objects that service users created, such as origami models and drawings became thoughtful gifts and were received positively. Service users and staff participated in decorating the unit to celebrate different events, prepared art exhibits, and regardless of discipline and background were invited to submit their pieces.

Fictionalised Vignette Continued

Returning to the vignette of Antonia's story at the beginning of this chapter, we describe the multidisciplinary and multimodal integration of the programming and how Antonia moved from a state of anger and isolation to one in which she fully participated in unit programmes, established relationships, and was ultimately discharged to the community.

Initially it was extremely difficult for Antonia to feel safe and cared for and to connect with others. Therefore, our first goal was to work with Antonia to develop one-on-one relationships with staff members. The treatment team worked closely with her to develop a connection and identify therapeutic interventions that took into account Antonia's resources and limitations. Involvement in activities with other service users was also difficult for Antonia. The introduction to the different group programmes was a gradual process. In staff meetings, we discussed her readiness for therapeutic interventions including individual creative arts therapy and specific group therapies. Staff agreed that it was important for Antonia to gain insight on ways to control her strong emotional responses. This would involve learning how to self-monitor and recognise triggers that resulted in rageful outbursts. The next step would be to develop skills to help her in grounding and calming herself.

Every day, the therapist greets her with a "Good morning," and at night says, "See you tomorrow." For many weeks Antonia just glares at her. One day when the therapist says goodbye, Antonia asks if she is coming back tomorrow. "Yes. I'll see you tomorrow", the therapist answers. Antonia is silent and stares.

This brief communication is seen by staff as perhaps a sign that Antonia is becoming more responsive to others. The rest of the staff is also intent on establishing a relationship with Antonia and often approach her to say hello. Slowly she starts to respond to questions.

Around this time Antonia obtains a set of headphones and the staff notice that music seems to calm her as she paces around the unit. One day Antonia asks the therapist, for batteries. She replies, "No, but would you like to listen to music on the karaoke machine?" Antonia comes in and stands by the karaoke machine and takes the microphone the therapist hands her. Almost inaudibly she sings along with the song, "No one who really cares …". As the weeks progress, she enters the activity room requesting to hear this song.

A new music-verbal therapy trauma group is being formed by members of the trauma committee. This group utilises words and music to help survivors understand trauma-related symptoms and gain tools for coping (see Chapter 12*). The clinical team decides that music-verbal therapy might be a good modality to include in her treatment programme. Perhaps she might come to this group.*

Antonia enters the group room. She stands in a corner glaring at the group members who are singing the opening welcome song and starting to discuss one of the topics about trauma symptoms and strategies for self-care. Abruptly she storms out of the room. A couple of days later she returns for the next group meeting. One day she sits next to the music therapist at the keyboard. She pounds the piano keys randomly but soon appears to be creating a rhythm. Everyone looks surprised but quickly catches hold of this rhythm and supports her. However, this musical cohesion doesn't happen again; she continues to appear hostile in the group sometimes impulsively beating on a drum or picking out random notes on the keyboard. Although group members attempt to play along with her, she appears to have no connection to the playing of the other group members. When discussing the group, the leaders wonder if she is benefitting from the group. Even though she isn't speaking she appears on some level to be listening. As a result, Antonia is invited to attend the next group series of sessions.

Over time Antonia becomes more responsive to staff and service users on the unit. She now attends art therapy sessions regularly. In one group she is standing by the karaoke machine. She is watching intently as one of the group members draws people's names in outlined bubble letters. Antonia asks her to make her one. She sits and colours in her name.

At some point Antonia is able to indicate to her individual therapist that watching violence on TV is frightening to her and that it triggers bad memories. As a team we discuss Antonia's triggers and begin to observe precursors to her assaultive incidents. She seems to stare off into space and begin to tremble. Eventually Antonia lets one of the nursing staff know that walking around the unit with someone helps her calm down. The nurse encourages her to name a particular staff member on each shift with whom she feels safe. These staff members agree to try to be available to walk with her if she says she is feeling unsafe.

Working in this way makes an important change for Antonia. Perhaps she feels more empowered and is beginning to believe that staff members care and are trying to work with her. Staff also feels empowered and, rather than responding to a violent incident, now they can develop and work on a safety plan together. Instead of having to respond to random, unpredictable violence, they now have some tools to work with and the unit begins to feel safer. This work has revealed a piece of the puzzle that helps lead to Antonia's healing.

In the creative arts therapy meetings and in staff meetings the art therapist and the music therapist discuss the possibility of Antonia attending individual music therapy sessions off the ward. Antonia's violent episodes have decreased so the team agrees that if Antonia is comfortable, she can meet the music therapist who will work with her in a room where there are a selection of instruments including a piano – a good place for individual music therapy. The art therapist introduces them and Antonia agrees.

Antonia is delighted that the music therapist can play her favourite song and she can sing along. As their work together continues, sometimes Antonia refuses to attend but afterwards asks the art therapist whether she is coming tomorrow. The art therapist encourages Antonia, writing the name of the music therapist, date and time on a piece of paper for Antonia to keep. Antonia often loses the paper and returns to her to write out a new one.

After several months, Antonia becomes more comfortable in individual music therapy. She begins to sit at the piano with the music therapist. In one session she vocally improvises over the therapist's flowing accompaniment on the piano. As Antonia continues to vocalise she begins to release a flood of words unfolding the traumatic story of her abuse. Later in supervision the music therapist reports having felt lost in the music and overwhelmed with Antonia's story. In trauma meetings, the need for musical boundaries is discussed – the need for more structure and for the music therapist to use her own voice to catch one of Antonia's phrases to create a refrain – a place Antonia can return to – a musical life raft - that allows Antonia to come back to the present and become aware of the therapist's presence.

The music therapist continues to work with Antonia, supporting her improvisations while musically grounding her at the same time. In one session she becomes more and more attuned to the therapist and her rhythm becomes more decisive. As the therapist slows down her playing slightly Antonia follows this change. She appears to be present in the here and now and is no longer talking to herself. For the first time she makes eye contact with the therapist. At the end of their improvisation Antonia smiles broadly and claps her hands. Instead of talking in a disorganised way and referring to delusional relationships she looks up and asks what's next?

Antonia begins to ask about the music therapist's world. The therapist appears to be becoming a real person to her and maybe a role model. From someone who was either silent or rageful she is beginning to find her own voice and establish connections with others.

Antonia's case is discussed in the various venues for staff discussion: the trauma committee, rounds on the unit, and in the creative arts therapies meetings where we try to assess what would be the best treatment for her. Over time, trust is built with the entire community. In trauma groups Antonia eventually serves as a helper to other survivors experiencing difficulties and is able to share strategies for handling difficult situations. After many months on the unit, the ward staff now starts discussing a possible discharge with Antonia.

After living in the community for about a year Antonia is re-hospitalised for a brief period. Although there is a difficult journey ahead, it is clear that Antonia's sense of self and agency remains strong.

Conclusion

As a result of this intensive work not just with trauma survivors, but also with staff, the focus shifted from discussions of violence and assaults, to victimisation and re-victimisation behaviours; and from restraints, control, and power struggles, to understanding of re-enactments. This change in turn had a ripple effect on the traumatised women who started to feel safer and became less prone to self-destructive and assaultive behaviours. Gradually clinical meetings went more smoothly and the unit became more trauma sensitive. The number of violent incidents such as assaults and self-abusive behaviours decreased over a period of three years. As a result, staff felt safer, had a more positive attitude about working on the unit, and felt empowered to express their concerns and fears. Different viewpoints and emotional reactions were more readily discussed resulting in a greater acceptance of listening and responding to each other and to service users. We were very much invested in adopting an approach so that team members would not fear retaliation or feel judged.

As the ward environment changed over time, we became increasingly confident. Looking at problems as systems issues was extremely helpful and administrators became supportive in the implementation of a trauma informed approach. We also knew how important it was that all staff felt empowered to actively participate in unit planning. We saw ourselves as facilitators rather than directors whose role was to give staff and service users norms and rules to be followed. However, at times when we felt that discussions were becoming divisive and could result in undermining the work towards our goals, we took a more directive stance.

The importance of connecting and developing safety in relationships is fundamental in the healing process. Based on what we learned in our readings and discussion of the trauma literature we came to believe that the creation of a safe and holding environment was the foundation for recovery in any unit. The step-by-step building of trusting and empowering relationships between service users, between staff and service users, and between staff members as illustrated in the chapter is the basis for developing a safe community in which traumatised individuals can begin to trust others, establish connections, and develop a sense of agency. It became clear that the most important principles we had emphasised in the trauma committee meetings materialised and crystallised in the trauma unit. The fictionalised vignette described above provides an example of the integration of different perspectives and interdisciplinary collaborations. The attempt to integrate the various treatment modalities fostered collaboration within treatment team members so that we were able to overcome discontinuity in treatment which often mirrored the fragmentation of the survivor.

Finding connections and searching for meaning in fragmented thoughts and feelings, survivors are often able to piece together the missing aspects of their personal narrative. Shared hope and belief in recovery in addition to the development of a more integrated sense of self provide the background in which hospitalised service users who experience psychosis, can risk to negotiate and overcome countless obstacles and difficult life circumstances.

References

Anda, R. F., Brown, D. W., Felitti, V. J., Bremner, J. D., Dube, S. R., & Giles, W. H. (2007). Adverse childhood experiences and prescribed psychotropic medications in adults. *American Journal of Preventive Medicine, 32(5)*, 389–394.

APA. (1994). *Diagnostic and statistical manual (DSM-IV)*. Washington, DC: American Psychiatric Association.

Bills, L. J. & Bloom, S. (1998). From chaos to sanctuary: Trauma-based treatment for women in a state mental hospital system. In B. Levin, A. Blanch, & A. Jennings (eds), *Women's mental health services: A public health perspective.* (pp. 348–367). Thousand Oaks, CA: Sage Publications.

Bloom, S. L. (1997). *Creating sanctuary: Towards the evolution of sane communities.* New York: Routledge.

Bloom, S. L. (2000). Creating sanctuary: Healing from systematic abuses of power. *Therapeutic Communities: The International Journal for Therapeutic and Supportive Organizations, 21(2)*, 67–92.

Courtois, C. A., & Ford, J. D. (eds). (2009). *Treating complex traumatic stress disorders: An evidence-based guide.* New York: Guilford Press.

Harris, M., & Fallot, R. D. (eds). (2001). *New directions for mental health services: Using trauma theory to design service systems.* Hoboken, NJ: Jossey-Bass/Wiley.

Herman, J. (1992). *Trauma and recovery: The aftermath of violence-from domestic abuse to political terror.* New York: Basic Books.

Jennings, A. (1998). On being invisible in the mental health system. In B. Levin, A. Blanch, & A. Jennings (eds), *Women's mental health services: A public health perspective* (pp. 326–347). Thousand Oaks, CA: Sage Publications.

Killick, K. (2017). *Art therapy for psychosis: Theory and practice.* London: Taylor & Francis.

Kluft, R. P. (1987). First-rank symptoms as a diagnostic clue to multiple personality disorder. *American Journal of Psychiatry, 144,* 293–298.

Kobayashi, T., Langdon, G., Muenzenmaier, K., & Rhodes, D. (2009). *Integration through creative arts therapies with survivors of chronic, pervasive trauma in an inpatient psychiatric setting.* Presented at the 2009 International Society for the Study of Trauma and Dissociation (ISSTD) Annual Conference, Washington, DC.

Moskowitz, A., Read, J., Farrelly, S., Rudegeair, T., & Williams, O. (2009). Are psychotic symptoms traumatic in origin and dissociative in kind? In P. Dell & J. O'Neill (eds), *Dissociation and the dissociative disorders: DSM-V and beyond.* (pp. 521–533). New York: Routledge.

Muenzenmaier, K., Battaglia, J., Conan, M., Kobayashi, T., Langdon, G., Margolis, F., & Spei, E. (2010). *Is treatment for psychosis possible in a public mental health system?* Presented at the Eleventh Annual Meeting of the International Society for Schizophrenias and other Psychoses (ISPS-US), Stockbridge, MA.

Schneeberger, A.R., Muenzenmaier, K., Castille, D., Battaglia, J., & Link, B. (2014). Use of psychotropic medication groups in people with severe mental illness and stressful childhood experiences. *Journal of Trauma & Dissociation, 15(4),* 494–511.

Van der Kolk, B. A., Roth, S., Pelcovitz, D., Sunday, S., & Spinazzola, J. (2005). Disorders of extreme stress: The empirical foundation of a complex adaptation to trauma. *Journal of Traumatic Stress, 18(5),* 389–399.

Winnicott, D. W. (1965). *The maturational processes and the facilitating environment: Studies in the theory of emotional development.* New York: International Universities Press.

9

TRAUMA INFORMED CARE IN OUTPATIENT CLINICS

Mara Conan, Gillian Stephens Langdon,
Toshiko Kobayashi, and Kristina Muenzenmaier

Introduction

The goal of this chapter is to demonstrate the way in which a growing under-standing of a trauma informed perspective altered the way facility outpa-tient therapists worked with trauma survivors during the first two decades of the twenty-first century. Fictionalised vignettes demonstrate the way in which this knowledge informed interventions in both individual and group treatments. Efforts to coordinate services both within the facility and via networking with other agencies are summarised and the impact of creative arts therapy are described.

I began working in the outpatient department in the mid-1980s and prior to this worked in the inpatient service.[1] When the trauma committee was formed in the late 1990s, it included outpatient and inpatient therapists. It became clear to me, after joining the committee and reviewing the preva-lence rates of trauma experienced by service users at the facility, that it was important that psychiatric assessment and treatment include a focus on the effects of traumatic circumstances.

But I had ambivalent feelings when I was asked to join the trauma com-mittee. I knew that many of the service users I worked with had experi-enced trauma in childhood as well as in adulthood. Almost all had been hospitalised and as a therapist I was concerned that a focus on emotionally charged experiences could be disturbing, re-traumatising and could trigger decompensation. The majority had been diagnosed as having a form of schizophrenia and at times had periods in which they experienced psychotic symptoms (e.g. delusional and/or paranoid thought and auditory halluci-nations) that made it difficult to negotiate challenging circumstances while living in the community. They often felt overwhelmed and scared, and expe-rienced difficulty managing emotional reactions when frustrated and angry.

---

1 When the first person pronoun is used it refers to reflections and experiences of one of the authors of the chapter.

    DOI: 10.4324/9781003055914-11

Some exhibited impulsive behaviour and could become agitated and/or violent towards themselves or others. The ability and willingness to participate in explorative verbal discussions varied depending on each individual.

When I had moved from the inpatient to outpatient service, it took a while to get used to the idea that the people I worked with had much less support than when they were hospitalised. Many were living in their own apartments; though some were living in supervised residences, they were not monitored and supported in a way that is typical on an inpatient unit. They were more independent and could come and go as they wished. While it was the case that some service users had additional supports (e.g. supportive family/friends and involvement in community work and activity programmes), others did not. Though many came to the clinic once a week, some were seen as infrequently as once every four weeks.

As a therapist, I tended to be very careful about the issues that were focused on in sessions and I closely monitored emotional reactions. Since many of the individuals I worked with had histories of physical violence and/ or suicidal ideation, I experienced a great deal of anxiety when they were not doing well. It was hard for me to adjust to a non-linear way of recovery, in particular when clients became so overwhelmed that they could not cope without a great deal of support and at times needed to be re-hospitalised. It has been extremely helpful for me to learn about the impact of trauma and the resulting needs of the individuals I was working with. This included the growing literature on therapeutic practices with trauma survivors (Herman, 1992; Bloom, 1997; Harris & Anglin, 1998; Karon & Van den Bos, 1981; Ogden, Pain, & Fisher, 2006; Saakvitne, Gamble, Pearlman, & Lev, 2000; van der Kolk, McFarlane, & van der Hart, 1996) which provided guidance for my work.

The trauma committee's support was essential in developing confidence in doing this challenging work. I was able to talk about the many difficult circumstances I encountered (see Chapter 5 for more detailed information about staff support). Training sessions both in committee meetings, as well as in workshops and conferences, helped me to acquire a new set of skills enabling me to use a trauma informed approach in my ongoing work with survivors. It became quite clear that the emphasis on the biological/ genetic basis of schizophrenia prevented consideration of the role traumatic experiences and dissociative processes play in the development of problematic and 'treatment resistant' symptomatology.

Trauma Training for Staff

In order to familiarise clinic staff with concepts related to trauma informed care, trauma committee members working in the outpatient department developed a trauma curriculum which focused on the way in which many of the service users were impacted by past trauma. During the first decade of the twenty-first century, as staff at the clinic became more familiar with a trauma informed approach, their responsiveness and support played an important role in the development of a trauma programme for outpatients.

The structure of the clinic facilitated the focus on issues related to trauma. There were weekly rounds, staff meetings and conferences attended by all staff including social workers, nurses, mental health therapy aides, psychologists, psychiatrists and trainees from various disciplines. We instituted seminars on trauma informed care and trauma committee members held a series of training sessions which included discussion about: research that showed the prevalence of traumatic experience among individuals diagnosed with severe mental illness; symptoms associated with trauma (e.g. re-enactments of traumatic relationships and difficulty in managing emotional reactions); concepts related to a trauma informed approach (e.g. triggering and coping strategies); assessment tools that included assessments of post-traumatic stress disorder (PTSD) and dissociative symptoms; and therapeutic approaches adapted for the clinic population. The last part of the training included a presentation of the social, psychiatric and trauma history of a person enrolled at the clinic. The goal was to formulate a trauma assessment and a treatment plan that was based on an understanding of the way in which traumatic circumstances and coping strategies had impacted the survivor's current functioning.

Trauma Informed Individual Psychotherapy

To provide a sense of the way I worked with trauma survivors, I will present a fictionalised case, 'Gina', not based on an actual service user, but on circumstances and symptomatology which were often apparent in the outpatient population we were serving. When I began to work with Gina, I had a limited background in terms of the relationship between trauma and psychological processes. I had closely read through Gina's medical record including both inpatient and outpatient charts. As an inpatient she had been given several different chart diagnoses including paranoid schizophrenia and schizoaffective disorder. Emphasis was on descriptions of her symptoms as well as her response to medication. As I became more familiar with trauma literature and began to have a better grasp of dissociative responses, I began to integrate her history, current behaviour and psychological needs differently. This growing understanding and the ability to make sense of behaviour that was somewhat confusing led to changes in my therapeutic approach. It also affected my own confidence in working with her.

Gina was 25 years old when we began to work together. She had a younger brother, and she had lived with her mother and stepfather until she was 20 at which time she moved to her own apartment. Her stepfather could become easily enraged when drunk. At such times he became threatening and started to scream at anyone who was around. Gina was terrified of her stepfather, and would quickly disappear. Gina's mother indicated that although Gina had occasionally been beaten by her husband it was her youngest son who bore the brunt of his anger. She disclosed that she too had been physically attacked by him.

Gina did well in school, and was able to get a job as a secretary after high school. She continued to see her friends after she graduated. She had several intimate but problematic relationships with men who were abusing drugs and who could become verbally abusive.

Gina's first psychiatric hospitalisation was in her early twenties. Medical records indicate that at the time she was hospitalised she was paranoid and experiencing auditory hallucinations. It was reported that she would often walk around the unit appearing fearful, repeatedly telling people to leave her alone. When asked what she was experiencing, she had difficulty describing her concerns in an organised fashion. I began to work with Gina following her second hospitalisation. During both hospitalisations she was prescribed anti-psychotic medication (fluphenazine in the first admission and haloperidol in the second), and her symptoms quickly resolved.

Once back in the community Gina consistently attended outpatient day programmes and clinical appointments. She was able to work with her psychiatrist in terms of changes in medication. Her physical health was good, but she often complained about severe pain in her neck and shoulders. She was not experiencing auditory hallucinations or delusional thinking. Her dress and neatly combed and parted hair suggested that she took pride in her appearance. She was able to budget money, pay her bills, shop for food and clean her apartment. In clinic sessions we often focused on practical issues and we worked together considering steps involved in carrying out her plans. She got to know many people at the clinic and would chat with both service users and staff.

However, there were also times during our sessions when the easy flow of conversation suddenly changed. For example, one day appearing calm at the beginning of the session, she mentioned that when she had left her building, she saw her landlady. She then started to become unsettled and tense as the session went on while talking about a time when she was almost evicted from another apartment. She kept talking in a pressured manner without any breaks in her speech and jumped back and forth from one topic to another. It became extremely difficult for us to engage in a meaningful conversation. At such times it was hard to discern whether she was holding back information, had lapses in memory or was unable to focus on what we were talking about.

There were also periods, often brought on by a stressful event, in which there was a marked change in Gina's functioning. When she *came into the clinic, she appeared somewhat dishevelled. Her clothes were wrinkled and her hair uncombed. She was late in paying her bills and had difficulty handling daily routines and responsibilities in an organised fashion. She was less cautious in her interactions with other people, sometimes entering into situations which were potentially unsafe. In a session during one of these periods I found myself lost in her long run-on sentences. She jumped from one time period to another and throughout suggested that she did nothing wrong and that she did not feel safe. When I asked questions to get a better sense of what she was thinking about she continued what seemed to be disconnected thoughts and I could not get a clear picture of what she was describing. During such periods we put several supports into place. For example, I became concerned when she missed an appointment and I couldn't reach her by phone. A clinic staff member and I went to her apartment and found her anxious and having some difficulty carrying on a conversation. We found a safe and comfortable place to talk, had something to eat and as she settled, we listened to her story.*

A Trauma Perspective: Reassessing 'Gina'

Considering Gina's difficulties, both when hospitalised and at the outpatient clinic, an assessment was made based on a mental status evaluation that emphasised impulsivity, dishevelled appearance, evasive attitude, paranoia, pressured speech, poor insight, disorganised thought, loosening of associations, and auditory hallucinations. When re-examined using a trauma informed approach described by van der Kolk et al. (1996) a very different understanding of the underlying factors associated with her thoughts, behaviour and emotional reactions emerged.

Re-experiencing Accompanied by Increased Emotional Reactivity

"Remembrance and intrusions of the trauma are expressed in many different ways: as flashbacks, affective states, somatic sensations, nightmares, interpersonal reenactments (including transference repetitions), character styles, and pervasive life themes" (van der Kolk et al., 1996, p. 421).

The manner in which Gina appeared to jump from one time period to another and the intensity of reaction to these different events suggested an internal intrusion based on traumatic circumstances from the past. The tendency to declare her innocence became a recurring theme and it is possible that at these times she was responding to auditory hallucinations. Entering into troubling social relationships may have been a re-enactment of early relationship patterns.

Cognitive Difficulties

When survivors are "easily triggered into hyperarousal by trauma-related stimuli, and beset with difficulties in paying attention, they may display symptoms of attention-deficit/hyperactivity disorder" (van der Kolk et al., 1996, p. 422).

Throughout the period Gina was seen at the clinic, there were extreme fluctuations in her ability to handle cognitive tasks. This may very well have been based on increased agitation related to triggered trauma associated memories. At times, she was quite organised in handling follow-up requirements of housing and social service agencies. On the other hand, there were periods in which she was unable to structure herself. At those times her thought pattern became disorganised and it was difficult for her to consider different perspectives or follow instructions.

Memory Fragmentation

Dissociative tendencies are often associated with childhood trauma. "Patients who have learned to dissociate in response to trauma are likely to continue to utilize dissociative defenses when exposed to new stresses" (van der Kolk et al., 1996, p. 423).

As indicated above, at times it was difficult for Gina to give a clear picture of past events, this being especially true of situations that were stressful to her. Memories appeared fragmented and not integrated in a meaningful way. When alluding to specific circumstances, she would often leave out contextual information and it was as if she was alone in her own world and had lost awareness that she was engaged in a discussion with another person. I wondered whether this was a dissociative state that was reminiscent of what she had experienced as a child when trying to escape from the family chaos that surrounded her. It is possible that specific topics being discussed in sessions triggered such a reaction.

Bodily Responses to Stress

"Many traumatized patients suffer from alexithymia - an inability to translate somatic sensations into basic feelings, such as anger, happiness, or fear" (van der Kolk et al., 1996, p. 423).

It was not unusual for Gina to focus on the discomfort felt because of her stiff neck and shoulders. However, it was not typical for her to talk about emotional reactions. She seemed to not be aware of the possible relationship between the tightness of her body and her feelings of fear and anxiety.

Trauma Informed Therapeutic Approach

In the discussion that follows I will focus on several key issues that influenced the way in which I worked with Gina.

Vulnerability vs Feeling Safe

Despite often coming across as quite resourceful and highly motivated to accomplish goals, Gina experienced periods when she clearly felt fearful and vulnerable. In working with her, I was aware of how important it was to help her to experience safety and trust. Growing up, her exposure to a chaotic and threatening household, coupled with the lack of anyone who could provide protection, resulted in dissociative tendencies which served as a way to block out what was going on around her. An important focus in treatment was how to evaluate the relative safety or danger of situations involving other people. In discussing relationships, we talked about trust, and we considered the people in her life who she felt comfortable and safe being with. We considered the qualities that made her feel she could trust them and what made her feel that she should avoid a relationship. We talked about situations that could be unsafe. Because Gina often felt that she was being judged in a negative way, the process of learning how to protect herself needed to be normalised as something that had to be learned. It was fortunate that Gina and I were able to work together for an extended period. With time, my growing attunement in terms of when things could be said and how best to frame them, and Gina's growing trust in me helped to make therapeutic interventions more effective.

Emotional Reactivity vs Managing Feelings

Saakvitne et al. (2000) have focused on the process of learning to manage feelings. They describe the importance of a survivor being able to "recognize, tolerate, modulate, and integrate his/her own feelings" (p. 60). It seemed very important for Gina to come across as independent and competent and getting a sense of her feelings was generally only possible when witnessing her fearful reactions. One of the goals of treatment was to heighten her awareness of the different feeling states she experienced. One way this was approached was considering her physical reactions (Ogden et al., 2006), explaining that it was very common for bodily discomfort to serve as a clue to an emotional reaction. For example, given her neck and shoulder sensitivity, I would inquire whether she sometimes noticed that parts of her body seemed to tighten up. Helpful as well was a general discussion about the way the past can influence the present. Triggering was discussed as a common occurrence that most people experienced. She was gradually able to think about the way in which certain circumstances were particularly frustrating or hurtful. With discussion aimed at normalising some of her reactions (e.g. "most people get frustrated when ...") it became easier for her to talk about unnerving situations.

During her childhood there was no one available to help Gina to understand and modulate her emotional responses. As a result, she had difficulty noticing the gradual increase in the intensity of her reactions. In therapy it was important to focus on ways to register the strength of these responses. We focused on skills that were helpful in calming emotions (e.g. grounding and relaxation exercises) and how she could use these tools when she realised she was becoming hyper-aroused. I encouraged Gina to talk about things she liked to do and things that helped her to feel more relaxed. She liked to draw and staff provided her with art pads and pencils to keep readily available at home. She also enjoyed listening to music and she liked the idea of keeping certain CDs near her CD player so she could easily play them. We talked about different music to play depending on her mood.

Shame vs Feelings of Self-worth

Based on Gina's tendency, when in an anxious state, to repeatedly indicate that she had not done anything wrong, as well as my impression that a genuine sense of her positive attributes was lacking, I wondered if Gina's feelings of shame and inadequacy were related to the fear, vulnerability and immobility she experienced when her father was physically and verbally abusive.

Because it was important for Gina to experience her competency, I was intent on encouraging discussion which highlighted her resources. Often when she mentioned something she wanted to do, we talked about her plans, encouraging a step-by-step approach. We emphasised success centring on the obstacles she overcame when dealing with very difficult situations. Sometimes I would compare her achievement to the way in which she handled situations when she was employed, pointing to the way she was building on skills that she had developed earlier in her life.

143

Intact Memory and Thought Process vs Fragmented Memory and Disorganised Thought

Gina did not readily talk about her psychiatric hospitalisations. It is possible that she did not remember some of what had happened both when she needed hospitalisation as well as when she was a child. As previously suggested, it was important to take a very measured approach in exploring past traumatic circumstances. But I also knew that by listening to Gina's specific concerns, and noting her emotional reactions in her preoccupied state, I was witness to the extreme fear that she was experiencing. For me this was a window into Gina's inner experience and was an important step in gaining a sense of the nature of her early experience. I suspected that as a youngster her needs were often unattended to and her feelings were not acknowledged. Her best protection from the chaos of her household was to escape into her own world. Although I felt shut out during periods in which she was in a highly emotional state and felt helpless in terms of supporting her, I knew that because Gina could not verbalise what was happening it was important that she tell her story the best way she could.

Treatment Summary

An important element in working with Gina involved increasing the awareness of her strengths as well as identifying the factors that were a challenge in reaching her goals. Support was essential in her developing ability to notice, understand and modulate her emotional reactions. Though we never got to the point of talking in depth about her childhood experiences, through the period we worked together her memory became less fragmented (e.g. being able to more clearly report on her current experiences) and her abilities to integrate ideas and utilise a more thoughtful approach in handling problematic circumstances increased. It is noteworthy that during the years we worked together, Gina remained living independently, did not require re-hospitalisation and was able to work towards meaningful goals.

Group Psychotherapy[2]

Throughout the years at the clinic starting in the mid-1980s, I ran therapy groups, often with co-therapists. Soon after I joined the trauma committee in the late 1990s, I decided to run a group using material which took into account the needs of trauma survivors. I had the same concerns as I did when

---

2 A very different kind of outpatient trauma sensitive group was developed by Ekaterina Spei. She integrated a trauma informed therapy group with a cognitive remediation programme (see Spei, Muenzenmaier, Conan & Battaglia, 2014).

doing trauma assessments and meeting with survivors in individual therapy. I worried that participants who might have been triggered during the group by upsetting memories would be alone with unresolved feelings when they returned to the community. This was taken into account in structuring the group and in choosing session topics.

In selecting topics for the group, I was influenced by a variety of trauma informed approaches (Gilchrist & Rainbow, 1998; Harris & Anglin, 1998; Muenzenmaier et al., 1998; Najavits, 2002; Saakvitne et al., 2000) and other group manuals available at the time (Linehan, 1993). I was also influenced by work of theorists who have focused on therapeutic factors associated with process groups (Yalom & Leszcz, 2005). I modified the way in which concepts were explained and altered the suggested handouts based on the specific topics and detailed information I wanted to emphasise.

One of the requirements for being in the group was the ability to accept the structure and rules of the group. Participants in the group were told that the group would focus on the struggles associated with overwhelming life experiences and the concept of 'trauma' was explained. It was made clear that although we would be talking about topics that were related to traumatic circumstances, the emphasis would be on how to establish safety, handle emotional reactions and manage relationships rather than discussing the details of specific traumatic events. The group met for eight weekly sessions and included focus on the following topics: Participating in groups; feeling safe; safe environments; self-soothing; stress triggers; warning signs; discomfort talking to other people; and using sound judgment in developing trusting relationships. There were checklist handouts for each group. (For example, the self-soothing handout had a list of different activities that might be helpful when anxious). It was emphasised that the group was in part a skills training group and that members would be building on the resources that they had already developed as they handled independent living.

In general, group topics in later sessions built on previously introduced information and ideas discussed in earlier meetings were often reiterated in later groups. Initially, there was a tendency for members to not respond to what other people said, but instead to present their own, often unrelated, thoughts. With encouragement and questions about what had just been said, members' skills in listening improved. Using the checklists was somewhat helpful in stimulating conversation, although it was often necessary for the leader to select items on the list to discuss when members didn't pick items on their own. At times it was necessary to redirect discussion if someone was monopolising the group. This was done by picking up on what was just said and asking if someone wanted to say more about the topic. In order to prevent confrontational responses, it was made clear that it was helpful to be sensitive to people's reactions to criticism and to be thoughtful and respectful in verbal responses.

In addition to conveying information about trauma, I tried to foster an environment that was likely to enhance participants' feeling of safety in the group. When the opportunity arose, commonality of experiences and feelings were pointed out. At the same time the way in which two people could have a very different reaction to a specific difficult circumstance was also noted. It was emphasised that specific emotional reactions, behaviour and thoughts were often related to prior life experiences.

Building Community: Coordination of Care

It is not unusual for outpatient trauma survivors to alternate between periods in which they are successful in handling challenges of living relatively independently with intervals when they feel more vulnerable. Though at times seemingly lost in their own world, many have developed resources that enable them to negotiate challenging circumstances in the community. It was extremely important, however, to have supports in place when survivors experienced stressful circumstances followed, for example, by episodes of dissociation or psychotic decompensation. Coordination of care efforts with other facility departments and community agencies made a major difference when service users were struggling. This was especially important during periods immediately following discharge from the hospital. Survivors' continued contact with inpatient therapists were at times helpful in developing increased belief in constancy of relationships. In this section several of the services provided will be described and fictionalised vignettes involving trauma survivors will be presented.

It should be emphasised that in addition to the supports that are described below, there were other factors which were extremely important in providing outpatient trauma informed care. This approach would not have been possible if it was not recognised and encouraged by the hospital administration and clinical departments.

Transitioning into the Community

The transition from an inpatient unit to the community was an important step in the recovery process. Networking efforts on the part of clinicians with other facility staff, agencies, family members as well as residential programmes were essential in the coordination of care. Discussions in the trauma committee meetings included the challenges survivors encountered in the community and how to provide continuity of trauma informed care. To ensure that survivors once discharged could continue trauma focused treatment, we emphasised referrals to outpatient therapists familiar with a trauma informed approach. We held case conferences which included inpatient and outpatient staff and put special practices in place. For example, after consultation with the treatment team a survivor could choose to continue attending inpatient trauma informed groups after discharge or if still on the inpatient unit could choose to attend groups in an outpatient clinic. In addition, trainees from various disciplines could decide to continue to work with the survivors they had worked with on the inpatient unit after their discharge to the outpatient service. The following fictionalised vignette is an example of one of the ways in which transitioning was supported.

As a child Ramona had been placed in foster care because of parental neglect and physical abuse. At age 18 she began experiencing auditory hallucinations and suicidal ideation. She was hospitalised for six months and gradually began to respond to treatment. When her therapist started to discuss discharge plans with her, she was excited by the prospect.

She worked together with her therapist reviewing the steps involved in transitioning into the community and in finding a living arrangement she would be most comfortable in. During her hospitalisation Ramona had worked with her therapist on issues related to her traumatic childhood and also participated in a trauma informed therapy group. When planning her discharge, she indicated that she wanted to continue to work on issues related to trauma. A referral to an outpatient clinician, also a member of the trauma committee, would ensure frequent meetings between in and outpatient staff. Discussions about Ramona's concerns and emotional reactions as well as therapeutic approaches that she was responsive to could then serve as a guide to the way in which Ramona and her therapist could work together.

However, as the time for discharge approached, Ramona was reluctant to talk about concrete details of her plan with her inpatient therapist. One day during the trauma group she began to talk about how much she would miss the group when she left the hospital and how it would be hard to leave her friends and the staff she had grown close to on her unit. During the trauma committee meeting members discussed the pros and cons of her continuing to attend the inpatient trauma group even as an outpatient. It was decided, with administrative approval, that during the transition she could return and group members welcomed her continued presence. Ramona's participation was not only helpful for her but also for the other group members as she shared her experiences of returning to the community and of her new living arrangement. In outpatient individual therapy, Ramona and her therapist discussed the challenges she was dealing with now that she was living in the community. She also shared what it was like for her to continue to be with her inpatient friends and group leaders and how she felt leaving them for her new residence. Ramona's weekly return for group provided a very positive transitional and grounding experience.

Creative Arts Therapies:[3] Bridging the Gap

During the 1970s creative arts therapies were widely offered in outpatient clinics. In one clinic as you walked in there was a large room that lent itself to large meetings and groups. The dance therapist ran a group there that involved everyone: psychiatrists, social workers, therapy aides, housekeepers, and service users in a vast chain linking the whole community in movement. Many groundbreaking programmes were initiated: dance/movement therapy with mothers who were recently discharged along with their children; art therapy groups incorporating a whole class of interns that became the foundation of extensive internship programmes; and later music therapy groups helping in the transition of inpatients into the community (Langdon, Pearson, Stastny, & Thorning, 1989).

By the time the trauma committee was forming in the late 1990s, these programmes had ended due to budget cuts and the reorganisation of the hospital. Yet there continued to be many recipients at the clinics who, despite being able to live in the community, had difficulties in situations involving verbal interaction and managing emotional reactions. Verbal group therapy could be a challenge for these individuals. When creative arts therapists, who by now spent little time in outpatient clinics, began to attend the trauma committee meetings, they began discussions about working with trauma survivors in the outpatient clinics. There were several considerations in doing this including: the kinds of treatment that creative arts therapists could provide in the clinic; criteria for selecting service users to participate; the way to coordinate communication between inpatient and outpatient clinicians; and providing creative arts therapists with a consistent time and space for their programmes.

Some of the important lessons learned were: how to integrate the inpatient and outpatient programmes; ways to coordinate programmes without the ongoing presence of an outpatient creative arts therapist; the significance of training staff about creative arts therapy and trauma informed care; and the importance of providing a secure, safe, and comfortable therapeutic space for conducting groups.

The time available to creative arts therapists was quite limited so it did not allow for attendance in outpatient meetings and it could be difficult to obtain referrals for a trauma group. The contact between creative arts therapies and outpatient therapists in the trauma committee helped to bridge this gap. At times outpatient therapists acted as liaisons between the creative art therapists and the clinic. In situations in which this was not possible, it was more difficult for the inpatient therapists to provide consistent treatment with specific service users. Often the connections creative arts therapists made in the outpatient clinic were unplanned and unpredictable

---

3 See Section 3 in book for further descriptions of creative arts therapies.

but at times there was important work that was accomplished as can be seen in the following vignette.

Music Therapy

Alma was drawn to play the piano when I met her in the inpatient service and she had expressed an interest in individual music therapy. In our first session we sat at the piano. She chose the bass register and I had the higher register. I let her lead the improvisation and I followed. The chords she played became dissonant. I mirrored this in the upper register. The feeling I had was intense. It felt like we were creating a very emotional and important sound. She stopped suddenly and said, "I don't want to play anymore." She was unable to verbalise what had happened and what caused her to stop. After this incident she refused to come to individual music therapy.

This was one of the early sessions that caused me to realise the specific needs of trauma survivors; that the tendency to express fully without boundaries could be harmful rather than therapeutic. Much as I might experience my own feeling of connection and release in the midst of what might be beautifully expressive music, I learned that it is not necessarily beneficial because of the experiences survivors have endured. Many weeks later, Alma disclosed that when playing together she felt like her hands were not her own or that they were on fire. Reluctantly and painfully, she recounted the sexual abuse she had suffered at the hands of her music teacher when she was a 10-year-old girl.

Alma had a longing to play music but could never follow through. She had bursts of virtuosic playing. At those times it looked like her hands were flying over the keyboard – free. As an audience often feels in listening to great music, I wanted to fly with her. I didn't want her to stop. But always, bars came down – a prison. Sometimes she would come to a music therapy group but never continued. When she was discharged, I had no connection with her.

One day she appeared at the outpatient clinic where I worked two mornings a week with a music therapy intern. Alma seemed pleased to find people she knew and was interested in attending individual music therapy sessions with the intern as she was between programmes, waiting to be placed. Since the intern and I were regular attendees of the trauma committee we approached this session very differently than I had earlier. We reviewed Alma's opting out of individual music therapy sessions. We became aware of the possibility of Alma being triggered and experiencing flashbacks. We emphasised the need for boundaries. While one on one in music therapy could be a positive expressive experience, it could also be one that easily triggered her to dissociate and relive the abusive relationship from the past. The sessions would need to be held with great care.

Alma attended music therapy consistently for about 10 sessions. Throughout, there was a dialogue between Alma and the intern, carefully negotiating which instruments to play. Sometimes they played the same instrument, at other times the intern played the drum while Alma played the piano. They explored verbally what each experience was like. At times Alma seemed to space out and refer to her therapist as a family member. They worked on grounding through breathing exercises. The intern would help Alma feel the floor under her feet, look around the room to identify familiar objects and return her awareness to the present. She would ask Alma what she needed to feel safe. Was there music that would feel soothing? Would she like to drink a glass of water? Her delight in playing music was a support in her developing trust and willingness to build on grounding herself as well as enabling her to identify those moments when she was in her own world and seemed to be dissociating. Her improvisations became more exploratory. She even suggested at times having instrumental conversations, the experience of which reinforced the sense of boundaries. She became more clear about what she wanted to express and listened carefully to the response of the intern to determine what she played next. The regularity of her attendance suggested how important the sessions were to her. It was our hope that she would take this experience of boundary work with her into her future relationships and that music therapy and the trauma informed work would support her in her journey to resolve her complex and ambivalent relationship with music.

Art Therapy

In the second decade of the twenty-first century with guidance from the trauma committee, several art therapy trauma groups were initiated in the outpatient clinics based on requests from both clinicians and service users. Many service users requested art therapy or origami groups, having had positive experiences in the inpatient programme. Interns reported that they were often approached with greetings of, "I miss your group!" With the guidance and supervision of the senior art therapist, art therapy interns who attended the trauma committee meetings began working in the outpatient clinic. They tailored material from the educational and cognitive behavioural manuals described in Chapter 7 in order to develop trauma focus in art therapy groups. The details of one of the outpatient groups will be discussed in Chapter 15. The group evolved in order to meet both the needs of the outpatients and the programme structure of the outpatient clinic. It was difficult to put into place a 'closed' group (i.e. consisting of same participants each week) which is the ideal setting for a trauma focused group.

However, in time a core group of six to seven participants became regular members with a few other people joining each week. The group focused on the group members' individual issues, including handling everyday life circumstances, interpersonal relationships, and learning about specific triggers that led to dissociative states.

Clinic Team as Community: A Systems Approach

In the outpatient department, the staff was focused on the needs of individual service users. There was an emphasis on regularly scheduled meetings and the importance of working together as a team. In rounds, conferences and staff meetings, individual service users were discussed to gain a better understanding of dynamics and problematic coping strategies. One of the goals during these discussions was to develop a treatment plan which could help the service user adopt more constructive behavioural strategies.

Many of the survivors we treated at the clinic had psychological difficulties related to early relationships. It was not unusual, for instance, for an abusive figure to have been a family member, often a parent or parent figure. There had been instances in which the non-abusive parent failed to intervene and protect the child. Such situations were confusing to a child who was not able to predict what to expect from people whose availability was inconsistent and who were at times terrifying to be around.

The possibility of survivors recovering from these experiences does not simply involve therapeutic interventions (Bills & Bloom, 1998; Harris & Fallot, 2001). It is extremely important that the therapeutic environment of a mental health facility be one that offers containment and safety. If that is accomplished service users can grow to trust staff members and other participants in clinic programmes. An expanding expectation of being listened to and respected is extremely important in the development of positive self-esteem, a sense of agency and hope for the future.

On occasion there were circumstances in which it was helpful to arrange a meeting in which two team members met together with a trauma survivor. The approach was often exploratory and the emphasis was on service users being able to talk about circumstances they were struggling with. Even if there were 'problems' being discussed (e.g. inconsistency in taking medication), this approach made possible discussion about service users specific concerns (e.g. feeling over-medicated and in turn more vulnerable). Considering and exploring the trauma history instead of labelling a person's behaviour as 'non-compliant' and 'treatment resistant', can open up discussion of survivors' fears and mistrust of others. At the end of such a meeting, one survivor who had parents who abused drugs and often left him home alone, said that it felt like having a mother and father who were both concerned enough to talk with him and calm enough to overcome their disagreements with one another.

Networking with Community Agencies

An important source of support for vulnerable individuals attending the clinic was provided by case management agencies serving the facility area. Case managers were assigned to work individually with clinic service users many of whom were survivors of trauma. They routinely made home visits and made sure service users were able to attend all of their medical and social service appointments. Communication between case managers and clinicians was frequent and at times details were discussed that would be helpful in understanding how to best work with the survivor. Occasionally the case manager, clinician and service user all met together. There were also times, especially if clinic appointments were being missed in which joint home visits were made (which included family members if available). Service users were encouraged to talk about their concerns and participate in treatment planning. These visits were often instrumental in the service user's decision to continue treatment. Very often when appointments are missed, it is because of negative feelings about the clinic that are difficult to express and may have to do with overwhelming past experiences. Home visits give service users an opportunity to talk about emotional reactions in their own homes.

Many people who attended the clinic were living in community residences and many were also involved in work and activity programmes. In most cases, service users felt comfortable and agreed to communications between clinic staff and community agencies. An example of networking with staff from a community residence follows. It describes a situation in which a service user who had been separated from an abusive mother and placed with a family member, was having difficulty managing emotional reactions.

One of the counsellors from the residence that Deborah lived in called me to say he was quite concerned about the way in which Deborah failed to follow residence rules (e.g. calling in when late for curfew). Often at such times Deborah would refuse to talk to residence staff. In individual psychotherapy, Deborah would sometimes talk about her relationship with her mother who was extremely strict and used to beat her with a strap when she felt she had done something wrong. In individual therapy sessions Deborah told me that the best way she could handle anger and not lash out was to avoid any interaction that involved discussion of the anger inducing issue. She was able to recognise that her refusal to talk to residence staff, though helpful in containing anger, was problematic in other ways. Deborah had a positive reaction to the suggestion of talking together with residence staff. Prior to getting together I was able to talk with Deborah's counsellor about her difficulties controlling her anger and the work we were doing in therapy sessions around issue of increased control. We also discussed ways of ensuring a positive experience for her during our joint meeting. In addition, I was able to talk with Deborah in session about the concerns she had about what the staff would say.

The meeting with the residence staff and Deborah included helping her to recognise her many resources (e.g. how well she got along with other people in the residence) as well as her negative reaction to having to follow residence rules. Deborah did not appear to find the discussion threatening and was able to comfortably participate. As we talked, I got a better sense of what triggered Deborah's anger (e.g. her impression that no one cared about what she had to say and her desire to see herself as not dependent on others). This helped to open up new avenues of exploration in our therapy sessions. Residence staff reported that in the weeks following the meeting Deborah was more willing to talk to staff about the rules of the residence. At times tension again escalated and the residence counsellor and I met again with Deborah.

Conclusion

My ability to work with outpatient survivors using a trauma informed approach was greatly enhanced by my participation in the trauma committee. I became more attuned to indications of trauma while reading medical records and more sensitive to symptoms indicative of trauma. I was intent on integrating knowledge from psychodynamic and developmental theory with my understandings of the impact of trauma. The weekly committee meetings were an important forum for discussion of this and other ideas. Participation in the committee also helped me to more openly talk about the overwhelming emotional reactions I sometimes experienced during a session with a survivor. It was reassuring when other members acknowledged being impacted in similar ways, and their feedback on processing these feelings was very helpful.

Looking back at the years I spent in the outpatient department working with trauma survivors, I have thought about how important it was to provide a setting in which individuals could acquire and sustain skills and a sense of agency that enabled them to safely and independently navigate the daily circumstances they encountered. It was important as well for me to be attuned to survivors strengths and resources as well as their fears and challenges. As Courtois and Ford (2016, p. 124) have indicated, "safety is most likely to be attained not when the therapist rescues but when he or she assists the client in developing a realistic awareness and appraisal of potential dangers and a sense of both responsibility and options for maintaining personal safety".

References

Bills, L. J. & Bloom, S. L. (1998). From chaos to sanctuary: Trauma-based treatment for women in a state hospital system. In B. L. Levin, A. K. Blanch, & A. Jennings (eds), *Women's mental health services: A public health perspective.* (pp. 348–367). Thousand Oaks, CA: Sage Publications.

Bloom, S. L. (1997). *Creating sanctuary: Toward the evolution of sane communities.* New York: Routledge.

Courtois, C. A. & Ford, J. D. (2016) *Treatment of complex trauma: A sequenced, relationship-based approach.* New York: Guilford Press.

Gilchrist, P. A. & Rainbow, P. L. (1998). *The trauma safety drop-in group: A clinical model of group treatment for survivors of trauma.* Albany, NY: New York State Office of Mental Health Trauma Initiative Publication.

Harris, M., & Anglin, J. (1998). Community Connections Trauma Work Group. *Trauma recovery and empowerment: A clinician's guide for working with women in groups.* New York, NY: Free Press.

Harris, M. & Fallot, R. D. (2001). Envisioning a trauma-informed service system: A vital paradigm shift. In M. Harris & R. D. Fallot (eds), *Using trauma theory to design service systems* (pp. 3–22). San Francisco, CA: Jossey-Bass.

Herman, J. L. (1992). *Trauma and recovery.* New York: Basic Books.

Karon, B. P. & Van den Bos, G. R. (1981). *Psychotherapy of schizophrenia: The treatment of choice.* New York: Jason Aronson.

Langdon, G. S., Pearson, J., Stastny, P., & Thorning, H. (1989). The integration of music therapy into a treatment approach in the transition of adult psychiatric patients from institution to community. *Music Therapy, 8(1),* 92–107.

Linehan, M. (1993). *Skills training manual for treating borderline personality disorder.* New York: Guilford Press.

Muenzenmaier, K., Sampson, D. E., Norelli, L., Alexander, K. A., Stephens, B., & Huckeba, H. (1998). *Understanding and dealing with sexual abuse trauma: An educational group for women.* Albany, NY: New York State Office of Mental Health.

Najavits, L. M. (2002). *Seeking safety: A treatment manual for PTSD and substance abuse.* New York: Guilford Press.

Ogden, P., Pain, C. & Fisher, J. (2006). A sensorimotor approach to the treatment of trauma and dissociation. *Psychiatric Clinics of North America, 29(1),* 263–279.

Saakvitne, K. W, Gamble, S. J., Pearlman, L. A., & Tabor, B. T. (2000). *Risking connection: A training curriculum for working with survivors of childhood abuse.* Baltimore, MD: Sidran Press.

Spei, E., Muenzenmaier, K., Conan, M., & Battaglia, J. (2014). Trauma informed cognitive remediation. *International Journal of Group Psychotherapy, 64(3),* 381–389.

van der Kolk, B. A., McFarlane, A. C., & van der Hart, O. (1996). A general approach to treatment of posttraumatic stress disorder. In B. A. van der Kolk, A. C. McFarlane, & L. Weisaeth (eds), *Traumatic stress: The effects of overwhelming experience on mind, body, and society* (pp. 417–440). New York: Guilford Press.

Yalom, I. D. & Leszcz, M. (2005). *The theory and practice of group psychotherapy,* 5th edition. New York: Basic Books.

10

FAMILY THERAPY MODEL FOR TREATING TRAUMA IN SERIOUS MENTAL ILLNESS

Madeleine Seifter Abrams and Kristina Muenzenmaier

Why We Created the Model

The prevailing view about including families in the treatment of individuals has always been that family work is less valued and is generally assigned to social workers who are also less valued in the field of psychiatry. When I first began working with families, I had to struggle against the stigma in order to incorporate families. Having seen many families, I was aware of the level of trauma they faced both from the illness of their family member and from traumatic experiences both within the family, often intergenerationally, and from the systems of care with which they interacted. Families were shamed and blamed. Witnessing the attachment between service users and families, regardless of what had happened and in spite of what had happened, was a humbling experience. Working with families that have dealt with serious mental illness, trauma, and the psychosocial factors of poverty, cultural differences, immigration, racism, gender discrimination, lack of resources and other forms of discrimination in a system that often does not care calls upon the use of multiple strategies. Most important is the relationship and genuine interest in the experiences of the family. The therapist must be flexible and open to the needs of the family. I have had the good fortune to get to know the strengths and resilience of families and how well they have navigated almost impossible situations. I have heard stories of their joys and have heard details of their traumatic experiences while eating a meal from their culture that they have cooked for us in their homes, while visiting places in their community, while accompanying them to appointments, while meeting with them in the hospital.

This model derives from years of working with trauma in families. While both authors had worked as therapists and supervisors in individual and family therapy, we felt that interventions with trauma

DOI: 10.4324/9781003055914-12

were parallel though separate, and could benefit from the integration of both modalities. Our work together in integrating individual with family therapy drove us to create this model. It is conceived as a guide for therapists and supervisors who are confronted with the difficulties that present themselves when working with trauma that occurs within the family system. The work is difficult and creates much avoidance and countertransference. Our hope is that this model will provide a way of thinking about this difficult task.

Introduction

In this chapter, we will outline a family model for working with trauma-tised families and individuals in the context of serious mental illness. Included are those situations in which mental illness itself is traumatic and/or in which ongoing trauma from childhood experiences may have contributed to serious mental illness (SMI). While individual treatments and psychopharmacological approaches are important interventions, it is essential to include family interventions in the process of recovery and healing whenever possible. Education, reconnection of family members to each other, and resolution and/ or coming to terms with the reality of the situation are among the goals of family therapy. Even when it appears that reconnection may not be possible because of the severity of the traumatic experiences, we have found that in many cases a rapprochement can occur and, in fact, can lead to healing of the individual and the family. The treatment model for working with traumatised families in the context of SMI includes four phases: (1) the building of a trusting relationship, (2) intervention, (3) integration, and (4) consolidation. A fictionalised clinical vignette will be utilised to demonstrate the model.

Serious Mental Illness and Families

The value of family involvement in the recovery process from SMI has been well established (Marsh & Lefley, 2009; McFarlane, 1983; Torrey, 1995). As more families have been included in the treatment process, they have come to have more of a voice, and contemporary models view the family as central to the recovery process (Lefley, 2009).

The importance of family interventions as part of trauma treatment has also been gaining recognition (Johnson, 2002; Sheinberg & True, 2008). When the individual or the family or both experience additional traumatic events, the relationship between family members is even more complex and likely affects recovery. A major contributing factor is that people with serious mental illness have often been stigmatised and marginalised (Torrey, 1997). This marginalisation extends to people with trauma histories in particular when stressful experiences occur in childhood and include sexual abuse and/or ongoing family stressors (Finkelhor & Browne, 1985, 1986). Thus, when working with traumatised persons, the issues are complicated and multiple barriers to including families present themselves. Awareness of the significance of compounded traumas is essential for a therapist working with a family coping with the impact of SMI and trauma.

Serious mental illness has a profound impact on the entire family system. Roles and expectations are altered, symptoms and behaviours can be confusing and frightening, and the stress on the family and the individual becomes magnified. SMI disturbs the equilibrium of the family. However, the family is also suffering and needs education and support as well (Martindale, 2017).

It has often been the case that when help is being sought for an unwell family member, the family itself is refused help, blamed, intimidated, or ignored (Backlar, 1995). Because of the stigma of SMI, families as well as the unwell individual feel shame and become isolated (Wong et al., 2009). In families in which a violent incident has happened in the context of the illness, especially those in which an earlier unspoken and unresolved traumatic experience has occurred, trust has been violated within the family and/ or between the family members and the outside world. It is, therefore, difficult to engage these families. Moreover, secrecy and silence often characterise the communication pattern in families coping with traumatic experiences, thus compounding the trauma (Hinshaw, 2017).

Trauma in Families Coping with Serious Mental Illness

In our clinical work, we have noted that SMI is in itself a traumatic experience for the individual and the family for several reasons. The onset of the illness often occurs at the phase of the family life cycle when parents prepare to launch adolescents toward their own independent life; instead, families are pushed toward the ill child becoming more dependent and the parents needing to be more involved. The hopes and expectations for the individual's future tend to be lost or severely damaged (Carter, Carter, & McGoldrick, 1989; McDaniel, Hepworth, & Doherty, 2009; Lavis et al., 2015).

Stressful childhood experiences are essential considerations when formulating an assessment and treatment plan for someone diagnosed with SMI (Goodman, Rosenberg, Mueser, & Drake, 1997; Muenzenmaier, Spei, & Gross, 2010; Rosenberg, Lu, Mueser, Jankowski, & Cournos, 2007). The consequences of migration, poverty, stigmatisation, intergenerational transmission, sexism, racism, discrimination, childhood abuse and neglect have a profound effect on long-range mental health of individuals and families (Abrams, 1999; Anda et al., 2006; Schneeberger, Dietl, Muenzenmaier, Huber, & Lang, 2014; Sluzki, 1979). Trauma can lead to disconnection between family members. Depending on the nature of the trauma and the dynamics of the family, a wall of silence and shame may develop. Sometimes families are already fragmented and the trauma intensifies the problem. The above situations as well as the impact of the mental illness itself contribute to isolation of individuals and of families.

The relationship between trauma survivors with SMI and their families can be complicated. This is particularly true when trauma has occurred within the family. We have seen many trauma survivors that are angry with their families. Sometimes, in fact, they refuse to involve their families at all and the work of the therapist is to gently encourage contact when it would be acceptable to the person. Helping the individual to come to terms with unresolved family issues can be useful whether or not trauma survivors are able or willing to actually have the family be present. Bowenian theory (Bowen & Kerr, 1988) states that cut-offs from family leave people stuck and their development stunted, leading to long-term consequences. While it is optimal to involve family members in the resolution of conflict, in some cases, family members are not available while in others, the individual feels that the family is too toxic or they are afraid of opening frightening memories or the family members may be deceased. In these situations, helping the individual to work through family issues is essential. Use of interventions such as creating rituals or writing exercises, among others, may be ways of doing family therapy with an individual. In others, where the family members are available, gradually working with the individual to allow for the contact can be highly productive.

A further complication is intergenerational transmission of trauma. Traumatic events including related feelings and/or behaviours are often transmitted unconsciously and symptoms may appear long after the original event (Abrams, 1999). While the actual trauma may not have been discussed or even be in conscious awareness, the long-term impact can be devastating. Often, secret trauma creates "stuck" families. Double stigma and shame about trauma and mental illness are hallmarks of the situations mentioned above. Therefore, treatment and healing are more complicated when both trauma and mental illness are present. It is highly significant that opening and working through past trauma can prevent problems in future generations.

It must be noted that there are circumstances in which it is impossible to involve the family. For example, if the service user forbids our contact with the family, we respect their right to refuse. In addition, there are times when the family is unavailable for one reason or another. In these situations, we may help the individual to explore family issues without the presence of the actual family members.

Because of the complex challenges that come with treating trauma, SMI and families, we have developed the Family Intervention for Trauma Treatment (FITT) model (Abrams & Muenzenmaier, 2002) for the purpose of promoting individual and family development. The model takes into account all of the challenges outlined above.

The purpose of a phase specific model has to do with the significance of developing a safe and trusting relationship first with family members before introducing difficult and painful experiences that have been traumatising to the involved individuals and to the family as a whole. Further, it is important to recognise that therapists working with traumatised individuals and families need also to feel safe in dealing with painful and distressing material. The model helps to guide therapists to address complex issues in a more gradual and predictable manner. It is important to note that therapists and treatment teams have counter-transference reactions to families and individuals involved in situations in which traumatic events have occurred. Supervisory guidance is essential when dealing with these complexities.

The stepwise fashion allows for the evolution of a gradual process.

Phase-Oriented Family Trauma Treatment Model

Phase I: Engagement – The Development of Trust and Safety

Families and individuals who have experienced trauma and serious mental illness suffer the effects of stigma and marginalisation associated both with trauma and mental illness. Fragmentation of the systems of care and negative attitudes toward families lead to compounded effects of isolation and disconnection. As a consequence, frequently professionals may be viewed with scepticism, anger, and/or mistrust. Therefore, attention to engagement is critical if there is to be a solid alliance and collaboration in care. The following are steps toward engagement.

First, it is important to *meet with all available family members*. It must be noted that frequently, it is only initially possible to meet with one or two family members. Therefore, starting with what the family members are able to manage is essential. Relationship building can best occur in the frame of introducing non-toxic issues. Those coping with trauma and mental illness are often isolated from members of their own families. Family members may have feelings of guilt and remorse or may be themselves suffering from the effects of both trauma and serious mental illness. Silence characterises families in which these issues occur. Providing a forum for discussion is critical to beginning the process of healing and acceptance. In order to foster an environment of safety and trust, *answering questions* and *providing information for knowledge and empowerment* is critical. In many situations people have been left alone to try to navigate complex systems. Therefore, *assisting with concrete requests when possible, such as helping families to access resources*, can foster the building of an alliance. Concrete assistance is particularly important in building trust since many families are dealing with limitations in their basic resources.

Many families come to initial meetings with fear and resentment due to negative past experiences with systems of care. Therefore, *asking about prior experiences with the mental health system* allows people to express their distress and to be heard and understood. However, *do not probe for more information than the family is prepared to give.* This discussion is the beginning of a dialogue and when trust is better established, more information will emerge.

In whatever is discussed, *take an open, non-blaming position.* Essential to trust is the belief that information can be discussed openly without judgment. Maintaining neutrality can be challenging for the therapist in many situations and it requires attention to countertransference reactions. Thus, when more difficult issues begin to emerge, people will feel safe. Although it may seem obvious, *validating experiences and providing support* are central to building an alliance. Often, people have had painful experiences which have never been validated, contributing to a sense of hopelessness and disempowerment. Most of all, *be consistent.* Many situations have included an inability to predict what will happen next, and being able to count on stability goes a long way.

Phase II: Intervention – Beginning the Dialogue

In accordance with principles of resilience and working with family strengths, as people develop comfort with each other, discussion should first centre on areas of strength and competence rather than immediately reaching for problems. The focus on a resilience model is essential, since individuals and families dealing with traumatic experiences are likely to be focused on problems and to experience shame. It is important not to retraumatise people and also to create an atmosphere of safety and trust. Thus, initial dialogue emphasises getting to know the family and their resources. In this phase the therapist can assess the family's ability to problem solve as well as come to understand important relationships and the social network. Gradually, more difficult issues can begin to be introduced as the family is ready.

It is important to first *discuss non-toxic issues* as a means of developing comfort in communication and getting to know the family. Families are more than the sum of their problems. They are people with stories and strengths and resilience. When families are encouraged to *recall pleasant memories and anecdotes and life experiences,* they feel empowered. Family memories of all kinds can be deeply meaningful. The therapist is also able to learn about the family's internal and external resources that will be available for them as they begin to solve problems. *Greater comfort within the relationship* is a critical goal of this phase. Once the alliance is better established and a safe space has been created, it will be possible to introduce more difficult topics. At every step, it is important to *assess how much discussion of issues* of relationships and traumatic experiences can be tolerated by all involved parties. It is also important to note that victim and perpetrator can only face each other in direct discussion if safety is well-established. The perpetrator has to be able to accept and feel remorse for their actions and the victim needs to feel that they will not be revictimised even by the discussion.

Phase III: Reintegration – Working Through

In this phase the family is given alternative ways of interacting rather than continuing prior patterns of coping or problem solving. The family is encouraged to practise strategies at home and discuss their effectiveness with the therapist. Family competence is praised and strengthened. During this process, the family learns how to tolerate discussions connected to traumatic experiences. Stressors will be addressed first by discussing the effects of trauma on the family system as well as on each individual. If possible, this is the stage in which not just the effects of the traumatic experience/s on the individual and/or the family system but topic of the trauma itself can be processed. While the actual trauma may be raised, caution is taken as to how much the details of the traumatic experience is part of the discussion. It is important not to retraumatise people. Rather, the goal is to manage the details of the story. More useful than a detailing of the experience is for family members to be able to share the impact with each other.

In Phase III, sessions are used to assist the family in *finding new ways of interacting*. Families with a history of trauma frequently communicate indirectly, avoid difficult topics, and have secrets. Both silence and shame are hallmarks of families coping with serious mental illness and trauma. Facilitating the family's development of a greater range of feelings is an important goal of this phase. Since anger may be experienced as a dangerous emotion, the family can be *educated about ways to regulate emotions* when opening conflictual areas of discussion. Greater emotional equilibrium will lead to positive emotional expressions as well as the negative.

In sessions, the family members can practise talking about anger and problem solving within a safe environment. This conversation occurs by discussing a particular topic that makes someone angry or is unresolved in the session and the therapists can guide the family to speak to each other in a way that is heard and understood. Such areas as separation and control issues can be addressed. The family should then be encouraged to practice utilising the problem solving and communication skills when the mediator is not present and give feedback in successive sessions. Successes should be praised and, when needed, suggestions for improved interactions be given.

Phase IV: Consolidation – Developing a New Model for Relationships

In this phase, the family is able to reconnect in a more constructive manner. Past experiences have been placed in perspective and family members have developed new ways to interact. Families and individuals are able to look toward the future. Since the individual and family therapists are in communication with each other with the permission of the individual, the family therapist will communicate to the individual therapist what has occurred in the family sessions. Having improved communication not just between the individual and family therapist but also within the family can facilitate opening the individual to process their own victimisation experiences. This may happen first in individual therapy and then might extend to family members as well. Individuals have the capacity to work on their own issues without the burden of blame and guilt. Family members are able to be supportive of each other and understand the impact that trauma has had on each person.

The final phase consists of helping the family to feel secure about *discussing issues on their own and navigating their relationships with each other.* Since the family has discussed past experiences, they can have *the perspective to focus on the present and future.* They are able to have *more realistic expectations of each other.* In some cases, in which the trauma occurred within the family and was connected to the serious mental illness, *forgiveness may be given.* As the family comes to peace with what has occurred, it is not unusual for the individual, supported by family, to *begin to work on the unresolved past trauma.*

The following is a fictionalised description of the family and individual treatment of a young woman who was diagnosed with SMI and who had a history of trauma. The collaboration of both family and individual therapists occurred over several years.

Carmen had been diagnosed with paranoid schizophrenia when we began working with her. She had been hospitalised in a psychiatric setting for numerous years after her mother discovered she had sexually molested her younger sibling. On admission, she was described as exhibiting delusions of grandeur and paranoid ideation and was hearing voices. Her mother had left their home country to join her husband in order to find employment abroad when Carmen was ten years old. Carmen remained in the family home with her extended family and it was during that time that she had been sexually abused by an older cousin. She had never disclosed the abuse to anybody.

When Carmen was an adolescent, she came to the US to live with her parents. The parents had given birth to another child. The readjustment to the family and the new culture at a vulnerable age was difficult. Carmen started to abuse illicit substances. In her late teens she began to develop paranoid ideation which was not severe enough to draw attention or lead the family to seek treatment. It was during this time that Carmen began to sexually molest her younger sibling for a period of several months. During this time, she also reported to be hearing voices. She was diagnosed with paranoid schizophrenia and admitted to a psychiatric hospital. During her lengthy hospitalisation both parents remained supportive of Carmen and visited with her regularly with the hope of Carmen returning to the community.

Engagement

We consider working with families to be a priority in recovery from mental illness and trauma whenever possible. Carmen initially resisted having meetings with her family since, home visits having begun, she felt there was nothing further to discuss. Our position was that the time of beginning reintegration into the community is the most important time for family meetings to occur. Carmen grew increasingly resentful. She said that her parents worked and were tired and she did not want to burden them to come in for meetings. While family involvement is encouraged, the service user has the right to refuse contact with the family. After much discussion, Carmen decided that it would be useful to her treatment objectives that she involve her family, and we met first with Mrs. S. Mr. S. had a more difficult work schedule and thus was unable to attend initial meetings. Mrs. S. reported that she had sought treatment for Carmen's sibling, that things were going well, and that the entire family was comfortable with Carmen's visits. She noted that she had some concerns, but that she was reluctant to open things up because everyone was doing all right for now, at least superficially. She did not want to hinder this progress. We hoped to meet with the entire family because we felt that now that Carmen was visiting home, it would be important to know how everyone was handling being together again. However, it was clear that we would first need to build an alliance Mrs. S. and Carmen before attempting to deal with more difficult material. We helped the family with concrete arrangements and facilitating holiday visits and met with Mrs. S. at a convenient time for her.

Beginning the Dialogue – Intervention

One session marked a turning point in the alliance. Carmen was sullen during the family session. In the midst of the session, dinner was served and the smell of food was pervasive. With our encouragement, both mother and daughter reminisced about family meals back home and described the cooking and smells in the kitchen. A discussion of special foods ensued, which led to a discussion of holiday celebrations. The therapists were brought into the family's culture. Carmen became animated and mother and daughter shared numerous family stories from their life. This session began to transform the therapy from a guarded, distant relationship to a more collaborative and trusting experience.

Having the basis for beginning to discuss more difficult material, we continued the process of developing trust by having meetings with the parents alone as well as together. The meetings were now more acceptable to Carmen. Mrs. S. told us about how members of the family were currently functioning. She said that her other child was doing well in school and having had therapy, was feeling more resolved about what had happened. Gradually, the mother agreed to a joint session with the two siblings to discuss what had happened. We held several meetings with the three of them. When we met with mother and sibling first before including Carmen, it was clear that much work had already occurred and that the sibling was doing well, was interested in working things out together, and that Carmen's visits to the home were welcome. The atmosphere when they were all in the room together felt comfortable. We were also able to have a few meetings with Carmen and both parents. Her father was supportive, although he acknowledged that he had gone through a difficult time accepting that one of his children had harmed the other. At this point, he understood about the illness and was more able to support Carmen. The atmosphere was warm in the room with the family members.

Working Through

During this phase, while we continued family meetings, Carmen continued to have regular visits to the family home. Carmen was eager to return to the community. By this time, Mrs. S. was sharing her feelings openly with us and, feeling less guilty, was able to be more assertive with her daughter. While Carmen was engaged in family therapy, individual therapy was occurring simultaneously. It was during this time and after several years of treatment that Carmen disclosed in individual therapy for the first time, that, after her parents had left the country, she had been sexually abused by an older cousin. She had never before told anyone about this experience. Therefore, it was particularly significant that she was able to begin to talk about it. She recalled how upsetting it was and how unprotected she had felt. After many months in her individual work with her therapist, Carmen was able to share her traumatic experience with her mother in family therapy. This reinforced and brought to the open the extreme guilt the mother felt when leaving her daughter to come to the US to seek employment. Carmen talked about her guilt and shame she had experienced as a result of her perpetrating the sexual abuse. Mrs. S. also was able to talk to Carmen about feeling guilty that she had left and not been able to protect her. Both mourned her traumatic past together. Carmen was able to tell her parents that, although she had been angry and had felt abandoned, she now understood why her mother had come to the US. She also was able to share that an additional reason she was angry was that she had been sexually abused after the parents had left and that she had felt lonely, victimised and vulnerable.

Consolidation

An important part of this phase was our encouragement of the family to discuss at home the issues that were being brought up in sessions. Mr. S., who had not been able to attend some of our meetings because of his work schedule, was included in these discussions. They gradually became more comfortable in sharing their concerns and would report back about their progress. Through this process, they learned improved ways of communicating with each other about whatever issues arose including relationship matters. The family relationships became more solid and more layered. Each understood the others' experiences and feelings and they were able to talk about these.

Carmen's relationship with her parents had deepened. This set the stage for enhancing Carmen's transition to the community. During this phase, Carmen began to feel more empowered and competent and began to think about living arrangements following discharge. Finally, as she neared discharge, extended family members attended some sessions in order to broaden the support network for Carmen as she returned to the community. Following discharge, we had several follow-up meetings with the family to ensure a smooth transition to the community. Even later, from time to time, the family would call to ask a question or report progress.

Discussion

The model outlined above is designed to provide guidance to therapists who may be daunted by the complexity of helping families to cope with both serious mental illness and trauma. In the first phase, both the family and the therapist begin to feel engaged and develop a connection to each other. When, in the second phase, the family's story and resources begin to emerge, both the therapist and the family in a parallel way, begin to feel empathy and understanding of each other. The third phase is empowering and instils hope. Finally, change and new connections are solidified.

Regardless of what has happened, people are tied to their families in powerful ways. Families who are coping with the impact of serious mental illness and trauma are in pain, feel overwhelmed, hopeless, helpless, angry, rageful or can be in denial and may experience the emergence of unresolved past issues of their own. Therapists engaged with these families may experience similar emotions. As a result, work with these families can be challenging and the treatment personnel may feel overwhelmed, in particular if a family member was a perpetrator. In order to protect the individual, staff may avoid contact with the family. However, because of the strong attachment bond, the individual often continues to be involved with the family without the input or awareness of the treatment staff. If a therapist refuses to engage a family due to a judgment about the family, he/she may miss an important opportunity to understand and intervene in family relationships.

No matter what the experience of the individual with the family, in most cases the need for a relationship with family members remains strong since the family is embedded on a psychic level even if not physically present. Trauma may have occurred within the family or the entire family may have been traumatised over generations by social conditions, immigration, racism, wars or genocides, illnesses or many other contextual situations out of the control of the individuals now coping with the ongoing impact. External people, events, culture, and the social context influence both individuals and families. People live within a context and whenever possible, for healing to occur the family can be helpful and needs to be included in the recovery process.

The parallel process mentioned above extends to and is replicated by systems of care with which the individual and family interact during the course of a protracted recovery period. The systems of care may be disconnected and isolated from each other and from the family just as the members of the family become isolated and disconnected from each other. It is not unusual for a family to be blamed and/or ignored by service providers. Unfortunately, the mental health care system often perpetuates the problem by fragmentation of treatment objectives and resources. Thus, special attention needs to be paid to addressing the needs of individuals, families, and systems of care in order to foster resolution and, whenever possible, reconnection.

References

Abrams, M. S. (1999). Intergenerational transmission of trauma: Recent contributions from the literature of family systems approaches to treatment. *American Journal of Psychotherapy, 53(2)*, 225–231.

Abrams, M. S., & Muenzenmaier, K. (2002). *Phase-oriented model for working with the families of trauma survivors in a state psychiatric center.* Paper presented at the 19th International Conference of the International Society for the Study of Dissociation (ISSD) (Joint Session with ISTSS), Baltimore, MD.

Anda, R. F., Felitti, V. J., Bremner, J. D., Walker, J. D., Whitfield, C., Perry, B. D., … Giles, W. H. (2006). The enduring effects of abuse and related adverse experiences in childhood. *European Archives of Psychiatry and Clinical Neuroscience, 256(3)*, 174–186.

Backlar, P. (1995). *The family face of schizophrenia: True stories of mental illness with practical advice from America's leading experts.* Putnam, NY: Jeremy P. Tarcher.

Bowen, M., & Kerr, M. E. (1988). *Family evaluation.* New York: W. W. Norton & Company.

Carter, B., Carter, E. A., & McGoldrick, M. (1989). *The changing family life cycle: A framework for family therapy.* New York: Allyn and Bacon.

Finkelhor, D., & Browne, A. (1985). The traumatic impact of child sexual abuse: A conceptualization. *American Journal of orthopsychiatry, 55(4)*, 530–541.

Finkelhor, D., & Browne, A. (1986). Initial and long-term effects: A conceptual framework. In D. Finkelhor & Associates (eds), *A sourcebook on child sexual abuse* (pp. 180–198). Newbury Park, CA: Sage.

Goodman, L. A., Rosenberg, S. D., Mueser, K. T., & Drake, R. E. (1997). Physical and sexual assault history in women with serious mental illness: prevalence, correlates, treatment, and future research directions. *Schizophrenia Bulletin, 23(4)*, 685–696.

Hinshaw, S. (2017). *Another kind of madness: A journey through the stigma and hope of mental illness.* New York: St. Martin's Press.

Johnson, S. M. (2002). *Emotionally focused couple therapy with trauma survivors: Strengthening attachment bonds.* New York: Guilford Press Publications.

Lavis, A., Lester, H., Everard, L., Freemantle, N., Amos, T., Fowler, D., ... & Birchwood, M. (2015). Layers of listening: qualitative analysis of the impact of early intervention services for first-episode psychosis on carers' experiences. *The British Journal of Psychiatry, 207(2)*, 135–142.

Lefley, H. P. (2009). *Family psychoeducation for serious mental illness.* Oxford: Oxford University Press.

Marsh, D. T., & Lefley, H. P. (2009). Serious mental illness: Family experiences, needs, and interventions. In J. Bray & M. Stanton (eds), *The Wiley-Blackwell handbook of family psychology* (pp. 742–754). Hoboken, NJ: Wiley Blackwell.

Martindale, B. (2017). A psychoanalytic contribution to understanding the lack of professional involvement in psychotherapeutic work with families where there is psychosis. *British Journal of Psychotherapy, 33(2)*, 224–238.

McDaniel, S. H., Hepworth, J., & Doherty, W. J. (eds). (2009). *The shared experience of illness.* New York: Basic Books.

McFarlane, W. R. (1983). *Family therapy in schizophrenia.* New York: Guilford Press.

Muenzenmaier, K., Spei, E., & Gross, D. R. (2010). Complex posttraumatic stress disorder in men with serious mental illness: a reconceptualization. *American Journal of Psychotherapy, 64(3)*, 257–268.

Rosenberg, S. D., Lu, W., Mueser, K. T., Jankowski, M. K., & Cournos, F. (2007). Correlates of adverse childhood events among adults with schizophrenia spectrum disorders. *Psychiatric Services, 58(2)*, 245–253.

Schneeberger, A. R., Dietl, M. F., Muenzenmaier, K. H., Huber, C. G., & Lang, U. E. (2014). Stressful childhood experiences and health outcomes in sexual minority populations: a systematic review. *Social Psychiatry and Psychiatric Epidemiology, 49(9)*, 1427–1445.

Sheinberg, M., & True, F. (2008). Treating family relational trauma: A recursive process using a decision dialogue. *Family Process, 47(2)*, 173–195.

Sluzki, C. E. (1979). Migration and family conflict. *Family Process, 18(4)*, 379–390.

Torrey, E. F. (1995). *Surviving schizophrenia: A manual for families, patients, and providers*, 3rd edition. New York: HarperCollins.

Torrey, E. F. (1997). *Out of the shadows: Confronting America's mental illness crisis.* New York: John Wiley.

Wong, C., Davidson, L., Anglin, D., Link, B., Gerson, R., Malaspina, D., ... Corcoran, C. (2009). Stigma in families of individuals in early stages of psychotic illness: family stigma and early psychosis. *Early Intervention in Psychiatry, 3(2)*, 108–115.

11

TOWARDS AN LGBTQI+ AFFIRMATIVE AND TRAUMA INFORMED APPROACH IN PEOPLE WITH PSYCHOSIS

Andres R. Schneeberger

Introduction

People who suffer from trauma and psychosis are among the most vulnerable members of our society (Mueser, Rosenberg, Goodman, & Trumbetta, 2002). Vulnerability in this context refers to an increased likelihood of being attacked or harmed, on a physical, emotional, or spiritual level. Service users, within the community or the mental health care system, in homelessness, in prison, and in other settings, often find themselves in an environment that increases the chance of being maltreated and injured. Trauma informed work as described in this book, focuses on how to address these vulnerabilities by striving to provide the person with a safe environment and address consequences of trauma and psychosis from a diversity of different and integrated treatment modalities. It is paramount to provide a safe environment for service users to embark on their journey of recovery. In this chapter, I will focus on the difficulties in providing a safe space for people who have experienced trauma and psychosis but at the same time also belong to an additional minority population. While minorities are often defined by ethnic background, language, or religion, I would like to move the attention to gender identity and sexual orientation as central factors related to the minority status of a human being and discuss these in the context of trauma and psychosis.

In recent years, there has been a great deal of attention paid to the marginalised populations. This chapter will focus on LGBTQI+ (lesbian, gay, bisexual, trans, queer, intersex, and others) populations. It goes without saying that there are many minorities and marginalised populations who all continuously experience the consequences of discrimination and stigmatisation. Exclusion, aggression, and violence can affect humans because of their sex, race, gender identity, sexual orientation, socioeconomic status and other factors that might differentiate them from a dominant group within society. Many examples in this book have emphasised the traumatic

 DOI: 10.4324/9781003055914-13

experiences of women. Women all over the world experience continuously the consequences of belonging to a minority based on power differentials. While the discussion regarding the effects of the minority status of women in general is of upmost importance, I will concentrate my efforts on a sub-group of women as well as men who identify of being part of the LGBTQI+ community.

This first fictionalised vignette tries to exemplify the struggles that LGBTQI+ people face by looking at different structural levels including their family of origin, their school, and work environment and lastly also the health care system. The person I describe, I will call her Maribel, is a fictionalised creation but represents women that I encountered in an inpatient setting where I worked as an individual therapist as well as a group leader.

Maribel, a 42-year-old woman with a history of childhood sexual abuse and psychosis, refused to participate in group therapy, stating that she did not want to talk in front of other people about her personal issues. In individual sessions with me, she repeatedly stated that it would be enough for her to talk with staff and discuss her problems. Initially the treatment team conceptualised her refusal to talk in groups as social anxiety, possibly connected to some paranoid thoughts. Every now and then she had mentioned that she felt observed on the wards and that she preferred to stay to herself. Maribel would avoid most service users, except an older woman who she would sit with for lunch and dinner. At times she would react rather violently when other service users would approach her. After adjusting her medications and trying to explore together her concerns about being with other people, Maribel's reluctance to participate in group meetings remained. We abandoned the discussion and focused on other aspects of her treatment relating to problems she was experiencing in her life. After a few weeks, to my surprise, Maribel brought up the matter of participating in the women's group. The older woman who she was friends with had told her about the group. I encouraged her to participate on a trial basis. The day arrived and she joined the group for the first time. From that moment on, Maribel continued to be part of the group but for several weeks did not utter a word, instead listened attentively to what other people said and watched the group therapists react. She eventually started to speak up and told me later that it took a great deal of courage. In the beginning, she would just comment on other people's statements. More and more Maribel started talking about her own experiences. She decided to talk about some of the violence she had experienced at home and the other group members reacted supportively, and in fact, her account encouraged other service users to share their family stories.

As a teenager Maribel and her mother moved from a Caribbean island to a major city in the US where her aunt lived. She was sad to be leaving the island, as she was leaving behind her grandmother. But she was relieved because she knew she would be far away from the man who had been abusing her. The city, where her aunt lived, turned out to be a difficult place to live. She had a hard time learning English, going to school, finding new friends. She began to recognise that she felt attracted to women but felt ashamed of herself. It was not the image she wished for herself. It all felt very overwhelming. It was then that she found a group of people on her block that she would hang out with. They smoked marijuana and so, at the age of 13, Maribel tried cannabis. It was like a miracle to her. The anxiety, memories and self-doubt would disappear. She started smoking regularly. To pay for marijuana, she would steal money and eventually started to resell the marijuana to finance her needs. At times people on the street would make fun of her and call her a lesbian. She suffered from being outed in this way. Around age 17, Maribel started to withdraw socially and started to feel that people wanted to harm her. A year later, after hearing voices telling her to cut her wrists, she was hospitalised for the first time in her life. The odyssey of many inpatient and outpatient treatments began, while at the same time she started to explore her own sexuality. It was all very confusing to her. She was attracted to women and remembered falling in love a few times, but at the same time experienced a deep-seated thought that this was not right.

Maribel appeared to be beginning to feel safe in the group on the unit. In individual sessions, Maribel would tell me her experiences during the group therapy. I encouraged her to continue this journey. However, she was reluctant to share anything about her sexual orientation and her traumatic sexual experiences. Only in the individual setting was she able to open up to me and share that her sexual orientation has always been a burden for her. She was attracted to women but at the same time, she did not like that aspect about herself. On some level, she had always wished to have a family and children but was not able to see herself raising children with another woman. She herself felt being less of a person because she did not fit into her image of how a family was supposed to be. Maribel was afraid that people knowing about her sexual orientation would expose her to more traumatic experiences, as it had been the case in the past. We continued exploring topics of relationships, trust, and safety. After another member of the group had found the courage to talk about her own sexual traumas, Maribel was able to share some of her traumatic experiences as well. Nevertheless, she continued to be scared of talking about being a lesbian woman.

Maribel's reluctance to reveal her sexual orientation was based on the fear of rejection. She had learned that disclosing her sexual orientation had led to more discrimination and confrontation with her traumatic memories. This vignette exemplifies how internal and external factors are intertwined and affect the person. Minority status is determined by specific external factors that determine whether a person belongs to a certain group based on a characteristic. In contrast, the minority identity represents the internalised identification with the minority status (Mccrone, 2018). The minority status of a person can significantly affect this person's health based on psychological and physiological mechanisms. The minority-stress model provides a framework to understand the complex interactions and pathways leading to increased morbidity (Meyer, 2003). The stressors that people belonging to a minority experience are divided into two categories: distal stressors related to the minority status and proximal stressors linked to the minority identity. The minority-stress model describes the impact of distal stressors such as prejudice, discrimination, and violence as well as proximal stressors, such as expectation of rejection, concealment, and emotional stress on the mental and physical well-being of minorities. Meyer's minority stress model describes how minority status, such as sexual orientation or gender identity, influences objective stressors such as discrimination (distal) but also affects minority identities that in return can influence stressors from within the individual (proximal) (Meyer, 2003). In combination with general environmental factors and stressors, it cumulates and affects the allostasis[1] of an individual, leading to diverse allosteric states and response patterns of the individual. Depending on existing resilience factors, such as coping strategies, social support and community resources the allosteric load will influence the physical and mental health of the person. This theoretical background emphasises the importance of improving the support and safety of, and the therapeutic approaches in working with, survivors of abuse who suffer from psychosis and identify as part of the LGBTQI+ community (Corliss, Cochran, & Mays, 2002). Unfortunately, the current political climate in many parts of this world is encouraging stigmatisation and discrimination of these vulnerable populations and hence increasing their distal stressors.

Trauma Histories of LGBTQI+ People

Children who do not conform to traditional gender roles are also at particular risk of becoming victims of violence and discrimination (Plöderl & Fartacek, 2009). The coming out process, which often occurs in

---

1   The concept of allostasis refers to the regulation requiring anticipation of the needs and preparing to satisfy them before they arise.

adolescence or young adulthood, also increases the risk of discrimination both in the private and then in the professional environment. In particular, transgender people experience a significant increase in discriminatory and stigmatising experiences during the coming out.

Overall LGBTQI+ populations are more vulnerable to victimisation experiences throughout their lives (Rothman, Exner, & Baughman, 2011). In our systematic review (Schneeberger et al., 2014) we found that in LGBTQI+ populations 32.2% of women and 22% of men reported childhood sexual abuse, while 46% of women and 45% of men presented a history of childhood physical abuse. Compared with heterosexual women, both bisexual women and lesbians experience more contact sexual violence. Compared with heterosexual men, both bisexual and gay men experienced more contact sexual violence and noncontact unwanted sexual violence, and gay men experience more stalking (Chen, Walters, Gilbert, & Patel, 2020). Stressful childhood experiences, including childhood abuse and dysfunctional household environment, show high prevalence rates in LGBTQI+ populations. The following fictionalised vignette is a practical depiction of the difficulties this population face.

Jeremy started to experience mental health issues at the age of 10 and was getting into fights at school and not being able to adjust to the classroom setting. He received outpatient counselling for approximately one year at the age of 14, at the request of his mother. During that time, Jeremy reports, he had had several arguments with his mother. He realised his homosexual orientation when he developed crushes on other boys at age 12. He already knew that he was not supposed to feel this way and was afraid that his parents would be angry and disapproving. His father would threaten him with a belt if he did not behave according to his rules. Jeremy's father used to discipline all the siblings physically. Jeremy would often respond by breaking things or attempting to assault his father. While he disclosed the physical abuse, he did not at first speak about the sexual abuse he had experienced when he was a child. After being in treatment for months, he disclosed that his uncle, who visited him frequently, had abused him on multiple occasions. Jeremy did not reveal this information to anyone for several years. He grew up pretending to be straight, forced himself to have relationships with girls and often tried to act in a very masculine way. He would go to the gym to work out and gain muscle mass. It was also at that time when he first started using anabolic steroids to increase his mass even further.

After leaving home and finishing high school, Jeremy was able to find a training opportunity and a subsequent job offer at an airline company as a flight attendant. He was beyond excited to be hired and to be able to do a job that he liked and that gave him the opportunity to see the world. As an adult, he never came out to his parents, but embraced his sexual orientation when he was flying. His job gave him the opportunity to live his true self and not have to hide. The work environment was very open towards his sexual orientation and the fact that he was travelling to different places and other countries gave him the anonymity he wanted and the possibility to be who he was without his family or his neighbourhood knowing.

After working for six years as a flight attendant, Jeremy was laid off. The only explanation he received was that his performance was not at the level that was expected of him. Jeremy could not understand this reason because he had been promoted in the past and his annual assessment never showed any major deficiencies. He got into a fight with his superior, insulted her, and threatened her. The loss of his job, his lifestyle, and his identity led to a massive resentment. His experience of freedom came crushing down the moment he lost his job. He was completely blocked, unable to look for another job. He withdrew, constantly ruminating about the injustice that he had experienced. He started to smoke marijuana and consume other substances such as cocaine and crystal meth on the weekends, often in combination with sexual encounters with men.

Jeremy was 30 years old when he was transferred to the psychiatric facility. He had been developing paranoia and was very preoccupied with people around him as he was afraid that they had bad intentions and would want to harm him. He had been taken to the emergency department several times because he was found talking to himself on the street and acting erratically in public. At the emergency department, he became aggressive towards staff and tried to attack a nurse. Over the past months, he had been losing weight because he believed there were people out there trying to poison him. It was not clear whether the psychotic symptoms were just caused by his substance abuse or the clinical presentation of some other underlying problem. After receiving antipsychotic medication Jeremy calmed down significantly but the preoccupations did not stop. He would react very violently in minor conflict situations with other patients. On other occasions, he would just withdraw and look out of the window without reacting to his environment. Throughout the therapy, it became clear that the symptoms of erratic behaviour that presented as psychosis were dissociative phenomena. He would experience a sense of being detached from himself and having a perception that people and things around him were distorted and unreal. These symptoms would mostly be triggered by aggression in his environment, for example another patient getting loud and upset. After several months of therapy, Jeremy was able to connect his traumatic experiences to current reactions. Subjectively perceived injustices would trigger him as they reminded him of his father's erratic behaviour and ensuing physical abuse.

This fictionalised vignette illustrates the phenomenon, described in other chapters of this book, that childhood abuse presents itself in many different and multiple forms. As in Jeremy's story, physical abuse, sexual abuse, and emotional abuse present comorbidly. Jeremy's struggle incorporates the proximal stressors based on the internalised fears of being discriminated against and his complex trauma experiences leading to alterations in his capacity to regulate his affect and impulses, eventually also impacting the way he handled his problems at work. It shows the different layers that affect survivors of trauma, and in the case of LGBTQI+ people adding an additional layer of possible discrimination due to their sexual orientation and gender identity.

Gender Identity, Sexual Orientation, and Severe Mental Illness

Gender and sexuality encompass many facets of human existence, including biological, physical, erotic, emotional, social, and spiritual aspects (Greenberg, Bruess, & Oswalt, 2014). The way people express and experience themselves goes beyond pure sexual attraction or reproductive functioning. Gender identity, gender expression and sexual orientation are crucial aspect of how humans experience themselves. The facets that determine a person beyond their biological sex are dimensional and flexible. A person's gender identity does not determine their sexual orientation, which in turn does not determine their gender role. The term LGBTQI+ tries to encompass this variety of human expression. As my work with survivors of trauma evolved, it became evident in my clinical work that gender and sexual minority groups are especially vulnerable to being the victims of stressful childhood experiences. While gay men and to a lesser extend lesbian women have seen an improvement regarding their acceptance in Western societies, trans men and especially trans women are still the target of stigmatisation, discrimination, and violence (Casey et al., 2019). People with severe mental illness who belong to a minority regarding their gender identity or sexual orientation may experience multiple kinds of discrimination and neglect, not only within their families and social environments, but also on a systemic level including the healthcare systems. For an LGBTQI+ child growing up in a predominantly patriarchal and heteronormative society, being different not only puts them at risk of discrimination but also of increased violence, abuse, and neglect (Schneeberger et al., 2014). The following fictionalised vignette aims to exemplify how LGBTQI+ children and adolescents are at risk of becoming the victims of multiple and cumulative traumatisation. I use the fictionalised example of Sara, a transgender woman, representing the history and experiences of many transgender women in the US.

Sara H. was born into a working class family. At birth, she was considered male and named Samuel. She grew up with her mother, grandmother as well as her four siblings in a small house. Her father was absent and her mother had to work in order to support the family. Her mother dated a few men, and often these men would stay at their place. The grandmother was a very stern and strict woman; she would spank the children when they did not obey her. Sara was often the target of her disciplinary actions as she was a very lively child. At the same time, she was also effeminate and her grandmother would not tolerate her acting like a girl or even dressing like a girl or playing with dolls. In addition, she would often be the target of teasing and aggression from other kids in the neighbourhood. Her mother would come home in the evenings and be too tired to react and defend her. Going to school was very difficult for Sara. Not only was she again the target of aggression and violence, but she also had a hard time concentrating due to her inattentiveness and hyperactivity. The conflicts at home continued and escalated. At the age of 16, she decided to leave home and move to a major city on the East coast. She did not know anyone there, but she had seen different shows on TV and the open and luxurious life appealed to her. After saving some money for the bus, she left without telling anyone about her whereabouts. She arrived at Port Authority bus station with only a few belongings and without knowing where to go. The first few nights she slept on the street and met other homeless people. Quickly her dream dissipated and was replaced by the harsh reality of the city streets. It was then when she agreed for the first time to accept money in return for masturbating a man. Her inability to find a job led to a continuing engagement in sexual activities with older men for money. To deal with the disgust she was feeling, another transgender woman she had met on the street gave her some Oxycontin (a prescription opioid pain medication). Sara felt a big relief and started consuming the pills regularly when meeting men for sexual encounters.

At the outpatient clinic, I would see young survivors who were mostly homeless, unemployed, often using psychotropic substances and who had very difficult and traumatic histories. Most young people would need the evaluation to apply for supported housing or enter a regular psychiatric treatment, in some cases even an inpatient stay.

I met Sara on a Friday evening. The social worker referred her to me and mentioned that she had just arrived and that she was behaving strangely. She seemed reluctant to talk to me. After I offered her a glass of water, she agreed to talk and very quickly opened up. At the age of 12, she had realised that she liked boys but kept the secret to herself. Her mother had several boyfriends, and when she was 10 years old, one of them had approached her and forced her to touch his penis. She never spoke about it, but at that time swore to herself to escape. It took a few years for Sara to come up with a plan and money and at age 16, she finally took the bus to the city. It was her dream to live as a woman like the women in the television series. During the assessment, her speech seemed pressured and she expressed thoughts that she was being persecuted on the streets. She continued saying that she was aware of the organisation I was working for as she had information that the FBI was involved in covering up the traces of a plot to get rid of all black transgender women.

This short vignette illustrates how complex the histories of survivors of trauma can be if they also struggle with an environment that does not recognise their gender identity. Already at a young age, they might be confronted with massive social problems, often caused by being abandoned by their families and other social systems, including school and education as well as the health care system. The attitude towards the LGBTQI+ population depends on many other factors. Transphobia and homophobia are complex phenomena that cannot be explained by a unidimensional construct of negative attitudes. For example, Herek (1984) postulates different categories, the first one representing a form of homophobia based on experiences with homosexual people. The second category describing a defensive attitude that arises from the projection of one's own fears and conflicts into homosexual people. Lastly, the author formulates the symbolic category based on abstract ideological concepts, where homosexuality threatens one's own integrity or one's own social group from the point of view of the discriminator. In order to illustrate the complexity of issues of homophobia, I will focus on homophobia in men. Using the example of homosexual men, Diefendorf and Bridges (2020) indicated that gendered sexual prejudice changes in ways, which allow the relationship between masculinity and homophobia to endure. Taywaditep (2002) presents two forms of anti-feminine attitudes: (1) a prevalent male ideology or belonging to a system of values, which understands masculinity as advantageous and superior over femininity and women; and (2) a masculine attitude highlighting masculinity in relation to self-image and self-concept. In particular, it turns out that the homophobia is less directed against the male aspects of the person but much more against the femininity of the victims. Studies show that homophobia is associated with increased levels of masculinity, thus postulating that these males are generally threatened by female characteristics in both gay men and women (Parrott, Adams, & Zeichner, 2002). Among other things, this phenomenon explains why transphobia and homophobia are strongly related (Nagoshi et al., 2008). In other words, aggression is mediated by the fear of being feminine rather than the fear of not being male.

LGBTQI+ and Psychosis – Double the Stigma and Discrimination

We have to differentiate the locus of discrimination as it occurs at different levels in the lives of gender and sexuality nonconforming people. Discrimination and exclusion often occur in an interpersonal context. Discrimination in the family comes first; rejection in the family environment of transgender people is a frequent manifestation and has grave consequences (Klein & Golub, 2016).

Survivors of trauma have a hard time talking about their trauma histories and due to those frequent interpersonal experiences, they show alterations in relations with others. For LGBTQI+ people this is often complicated by the inherent possibility of prejudice due to their sexual orientation or gender identity in relation to the trauma. Their experience with distal stressors due to discrimination and stigma has taught them to be careful with their environment to avoid aggression and violence. On the other hand, these vignettes show the internalised aspects of homophobia and the proximal stressors caused by this phenomenon. This double stigmatisation – relating to his sexual orientation, gender identity and the internalised homophobia or transphobia might lead to an emotional withdrawal and potentially hindering the therapeutic alliance that would be the basis for a trauma specific treatment. The person reflexively may assume that the psychiatrist or psychotherapist is cis-gendered heterosexual and has no knowledge of the life circumstances of LGBTQI+ people or worse, disapproves of them. Hence, the difficulties that sexual minorities with severe mental illness encounter due to those stressors can lead to suboptimal treatment and subsequently to chronic illness or worsening of the psychiatric disorders.

Towards a Trauma Specific Treatment for LGBTQI+ Persons

In the early 1990s, the focus of trauma specific treatment was on building trauma informed treatment settings and increasing staff awareness for trauma histories among service user. The issues of sexual orientation and gender identity were not considered in the treatment planning process. However, in the facility where I worked a change occurred when a men's group was created that focused on specific male issues. The group dynamic changed and men were able to share their trauma history, leading to an increased openness and cohesion of the group. The group set the stage for other men to reveal not only traumatic experiences but also intimate experiences related to sexuality and gender. This positive experience shows how important it is to provide an open and safe environment for LGBTQI+ service users with severe mental illness and traumatic histories. Surveys have shown that nearly 30% of transgender persons have had negative discriminatory experiences with psychiatrists and psychologists and 45% were dissatisfied with their treatment (European Union, 2014). Likewise, comparative studies showed that homosexual and bisexual clients were significantly more dissatisfied with their psychiatric-psychotherapeutic treatments than those in a general population (Avery, Hellman, & Sudderth, 2001).

LGBTQI+ affirmative treatment needs to address a variety of factors. On one hand, an increased awareness of diagnostic, psychodynamic and therapeutic stigmatisation is needed. On the other hand, the affirmative position has to be communicated to provide a safe environment (Garcia Nuñez & Schneeberger, 2018). Diagnostic stigmatisation refers to the diagnostic characterisation of minority sexual orientations and gender identity. Early diagnostic classifications of the World Health Organization (WHO) and the *Diagnostic and Statistical Manual of Mental Disorders* (DSM) pathologised homosexuality and hence strongly contributed to the social discrimination of gender and sexual minorities (Drescher, 2015). The short fictionalised description of Maribel in group therapy mentioned in the beginning of the chapter exemplifies how difficult it is for LGBTQI+ persons to open up in this setting because of dual stigmatisation of being mentally ill and afraid to experience homophobia and discrimination.

The development of the individual and group therapies illustrate some important points. While all survivors of trauma need a safe therapeutic environment, it is paramount to focus on the topic of safety for the subgroup of LGBTQI+ service users. The same unit can be a very safe place for one person but at the same time unsafe for a gender non-conforming person. Distal stressors can be present as stigmatisation and discrimination by fellow consumers and treatment staff. Most therapists, psychologists, psychiatrists, and other mental health worker are not necessarily informed about the needs of LGBTQI+ people. However, this non-malevolent ignorance might lead to stigma and discrimination. 'Unreflected' remarks about gender identity, gender roles, gender expression, sexual partners, masculinity or femininity, and family constructs might increase the uncertainty whether the therapeutic space is safe or not. This difficulty does not mean that only mental health professionals within the same group can support LGBTQI+ consumers, it demands an openness regarding the subject matter and the willingness to broaden the therapeutic horizon. Providing a safe space for staff to talk about gender issues, including discussion and a heightening of awareness of the effects of 'unreflected' remarks and the importance of thinking about trauma in minority groups, has been very helpful.

Trauma informed therapeutic approaches with LGBTQI+ people require a special focus on the topic of safety. LGBTQI+ persons often have had experiences of aggression and violence related to their different sexual orientation or gender identity. These experiences lead to hesitation not only regarding coming out about their sexual orientation and gender identity but also about traumatic histories. Hence, in the treatment of LBGTQIA+ people, it is important to assess whether this status acts as an additional stressor. The cumulative effects of traumatic experiences relates to increased psychopathology (Muenzenmaier et al., 2015), emphasising the importance of seeing issues related to sexual orientation gender identity as a significant stressor. It is therefore very important to ensure safety, stable relationships and trust in the treatment.

Conclusion

LGBTQI+ People with severe mental illness and trauma histories are one of the most vulnerable populations. Historically, the treatment of people with severe mental illness has ignored topics such as sexuality, sexual orientation, and gender identity. It appears crucial to address these topics in LGBTQI+ people but also in sexual non-minority populations as it affects the possible treatment outcome. As we understand gender identity and sexual orientation across a spectrum, it is important to extend these topics also to cis gender individuals who have experienced trauma and psychosis. A LGBTQI+ affirmative – in broader terms gender and sexuality affirmative – treatment and trauma informed approach is crucial and can build the safety and trusting relationships needed to successfully help these populations.

References

Avery, A. M., Hellman, R. E., & Sudderth, L. K. (2001). Satisfaction with mental health services among sexual minorities with major mental illness. *American Journal of Public Health, 91(6)*, 990.

Casey, L. S., Reisner, S. L., Findling, M. G., Blendon, R. J., Benson, J. M., Sayde, J. M., & Miller, C. (2019). Discrimination in the United States: Experiences of lesbian, gay, bisexual, transgender, and queer Americans. *Health Services Research, 54*, 1454–1466.

Chen, J., Walters, M. L., Gilbert, L. K., & Patel, N. (2020). Sexual violence, stalking, and intimate partner violence by sexual orientation, United States. *Psychology of Violence, 10(1)*, 110.

Corliss, H. L., Cochran, S. D., & Mays, V. M. (2002). Reports of parental maltreatment during childhood in a United States population-based survey of homosexual, bisexual, and heterosexual adults. *Child Abuse & Neglect, 26(11)*, 1165–1178.

Diefendorf, S., & Bridges, T. (2020). On the enduring relationship between masculinity and homophobia. *Sexualities, 23(7)*, 1264–1284.

Drescher, J. (2015). Out of DSM: Depathologizing homosexuality. *Journal of Behavioral Sciences, 5(4)*, 565–575.

European Union. (2014). *Being trans in the European Union comparative analysis of EU LGBT survey data*. Brussels: Publications Office of the European Union.

Garcia Nuñez, D., & Schneeberger, A. R. (2018). Trauma unter dem Regenbogen: Stigmatisierung von Gender-und sexuellen Minderheiten. In M. Büttner (ed.), *Trauma unter dem Regenbogen: Stigmatisierung von Gender-und sexuellen Minderheiten* (pp. 167–195). Stuttgart, Germany: Schattauer.

Greenberg, J. S., Bruess, C. E., & Oswalt, S. B. (2014). *Exploring the dimensions of human sexuality*. Burlington, MA: Jones & Bartlett Learning.

Herek, G. M. (1984). Beyond 'homophobia': A social psychological perspective on attitudes toward lesbians and gay men. *Journal of Homosexuality*, *10(1–2)*, 1–21.

Klein, A., & Golub, S. A. (2016). Family rejection as a predictor of suicide attempts and substance misuse among transgender and gender nonconforming adults. *LGBT Health*, *3(3)*, 193–199.

Mccrone, S. (2018). LGBT healthcare disparities, discrimination, and societal stigma: The mental and physical health risks related to sexual and/or gender minority status. *American Journal of Medical Research*, *5(1)*, 91–96.

Meyer, I. H. (2003). Prejudice, social stress, and mental health in lesbian, gay, and bisexual populations: Conceptual issues and research evidence. *Psychological Bulletin*, *129(5)*, 674.

Muenzenmaier, K. H., Seixas, A. A., Schneeberger, A. R., Castille, D. M., Battaglia, J., & Link, B. G. (2015). Cumulative effects of stressful childhood experiences on delusions and hallucinations. *Journal of Trauma & Dissociation*, *16(4)*, 442–462.

Mueser, K. T., Rosenberg, S. D., Goodman, L. A., & Trumbetta, S. L. (2002). Trauma, PTSD, and the course of severe mental illness: An interactive model. *Schizophrenia Research*, *53(1–2)*, 123–143.

Nagoshi, J. L., Adams, K. A., Terrell, H. K., Hill, E. D., Brzuzy, S., & Nagoshi, C. T. (2008). Gender differences in correlates of homophobia and transphobia. *Sex Roles*, *59(7–8)*, 521–531.

Parrott, D. J., Adams, H. E., & Zeichner, A. (2002). Homophobia: Personality and attitudinal correlates. *Personality and Individual Differences*, *32(7)*, 1269–1278.

Plöderl, M., & Fartacek, R. (2009). Childhood gender nonconformity and harassment as predictors of suicidality among gay, lesbian, bisexual, and heterosexual Austrians. *Archives of Sexual Behavior*, *38(3)*, 400–410.

Rothman, E. F., Exner, D., & Baughman, A. L. (2011). The prevalence of sexual assault against people who identify as gay, lesbian, or bisexual in the United States: A systematic review. *Trauma, Violence, & Abuse*, *12(2)*, 55–66.

Schneeberger, A. R., Dietl, M. F., Muenzenmaier, K. H., Huber, C. G., & Lang, U. E. (2014). Stressful childhood experiences and health outcomes in sexual minority populations: A systematic review. *Social Psychiatry and Psychiatric Epidemiology*, *49(9)*, 1427–1445.

Taywaditep, K. J. (2002). Marginalization among the marginalized: Gay men's anti-effeminacy attitudes. *Journal of Homosexuality*, *42(1)*, 1–28.

Part III

COLLABORATION WITH CREATIVE ARTS THERAPIES OPENS UP NEW DOORS IN TRAUMA TREATMENT

12

MUSIC THERAPY

Exploring a Structured Trauma Informed
Group Therapy Model

*Gillian Stephens Langdon, Gina Kijek,
and Stacie Aamon Yeldell*

Introduction

The practice of music for healing appears in ancient writings among peoples all over the world as well as in pre-literate societies. In an ancient prestigious Chinese medicine textbook "it was written that before the use of herbs or acupuncture, people in China applied musical compositions to heal ... [In fact] the Chinese character for medicine ... [is] a combination of [the character for] music and herbs" (Cui, Agyeman, & Knox, 2016 p. 67). The Bible (I Samuel 16:23, King James version) tells of David playing the harp to heal Saul. Plato describes the connection of music, body, and soul. (Pelosi, 2010, p. 198). As expressed by Nordoff and Robbins:

> Music is a universal experience in the sense that all can share in it; its fundamental elements of melody, harmony, and rhythm appeal to, and engage their related psychic functions in each one of us ... It can lead or accompany the psyche through all conditions of inner experience, whether these be superficial and relatively commonplace or profound and deeply personal.
>
> (Nordoff & Robbins, 2004, p. 14)

In the nineteenth century, music began to be brought to asylums for the mentally ill in Europe and in the United States through music listening, music performance, and music instruction:

> [In New York City] prominent soloists and ensembles ... took part in sessions which were carried out at Blackwell's Island (now Roosevelt Island) an infamous, overcrowded facility designed to care for impoverished women with emotional and/or behavioural disturbances ... This attempt at using live music to relieve suffering

DOI: 10.4324/9781003055914-15

of women with psychiatric illnesses is important because it is likely the first example in U.S. history of music therapy used in a large institution.

(Davis & Hadley, 2015, p. 21)

In France, Philippe Pinel and his followers placed "much hope...in the power of music to calm the restless, and to stimulate the apathetic through mood and behaviour regulation." (Lecourt, 1993, p. 223). Music therapy as a discipline became more developed after World Wars I and II with soldiers returning from the war with physical and emotional trauma:

[C]ommunity musicians of all types, both amateur and professional, went to veterans' hospitals around the country to play for the thousands of veterans suffering both physical and emotional trauma from the wars. The veterans' notable physical and emotional responses to music led the doctors and nurses to request the hiring of musicians by the hospitals. It was soon evident that the hospital musicians needed some prior training before entering the facility and so the demand grew for a college curriculum.

(American Music Therapy Association, 2021)

Training programmes were developed at Michigan State College and the University of Kansas in the United States in the 1940s and are now available worldwide. In the 1950s and 1960s music therapy associations were formed in the United States and in England. Certification boards have been created to support the standards of music therapy practice with board certification (MT-BC) established in the United States in 1983 and licensure for Creative Arts Therapies (LCAT) in New York State in 2005.

Until the 1990s, trauma histories in people with psychosis had mostly been neglected in adult long term psychiatric facilities (see Chapter 3). In music therapy, a few discussions of music therapy and trauma existed (Wigram & De Backer, 1999). In 2002 Sutton's book *Music, Music Therapy and Trauma: International Perspectives* was released with the majority of the cases discussed relating to trauma, however it had only a few references to psychosis and trauma. In 2008 a symposium was organised in New York City and an edited publication by the same name was released, *Music Therapy and Trauma: Bridging Theory and Clinical Practice* (Stewart, 2010). This drew together much of the current thinking regarding music therapy and trauma and included work with people experiencing psychosis (Borczon, Jampel & Langdon, 2010). More recently additional writings have been published which address music therapy and its usefulness for people who exhibit trauma symptoms and psychosis (Cadesky, 2022; Langdon, 2022).

In this chapter we present some of the ways that music therapy helps build community, provides a holding environment for difficult discussions, and deepens the experience of healing using the topics of the Symptom-Specific Group Therapy (SSGT) model (Shelley, 2006) with each session addressing a symptom of complex PTSD (see Chapter 7). The purpose is not to present a case study of all 12 modules, but rather to highlight a variety of techniques and experiences in the many groups that we were able to conduct. The interdisciplinary collaborations of music therapists, psychologists, social workers, and psychiatrists, as well as trainees contributed examples and experiences that we can draw from, several of which are described here.

Music Therapy in Trauma Treatment

First Groups: Coming to a New Understanding

Our first interdisciplinary collaboration using verbal and musical elements in trauma treatment was piloted in 2000 by a social work intern and a music therapy intern who were both interested in trauma treatment (see Chapter 5). The group was composed of women on an inpatient unit who had documented trauma histories. The interns reported that the women had instantly bonded over their shared traumatic experiences. Many had had their children taken away from them and they were able to share the pain of this loss in the group. The music seemed to have deepened their experience, culminating in the women embracing each other as they sang "Bridge Over Troubled Water" (Simon, 1970). When discussing this very first session in supervision with the interns we felt it was a success.

What followed however, was a surprise to all of us - and a disappointment. For the next session only a few of the group members came back. In subsequent sessions the women who had participated initially never got together as a whole group again. We were discouraged. What had gone wrong? There was much to be learned from this experience. In the Trauma Committee the interns brought their concerns and in discussions that followed we surmised that the music had swept the group up into an emotional place they were not equipped to handle. Many aspects of an improvisation-based music therapy group could trigger service users' feelings of loss of control, abandonment, or helplessness. "For the women's group the free aspect of it allowed them to travel through boundaries much too fast for the group's position in its developmental stage" (R. Fleetwood, personal communication; 21 April 2020). The need for more containment and structure was evident. There were no barriers and no tools to say, "Stop, let's not go there!" Their defence against overwhelming emotions was simply to not return to the group.

This group experience and our subsequent discussions in the trauma committee became an important learning experience in our work developing group interventions. Interns contributed to this work through their presentations to the Trauma Committee (L. Oliveri, personal communication, 2012) and their presentations at national conferences (Rhodes &

Langdon, 2011). In our search for a way to use the expressivity of music while maintaining structure and safe boundaries, we began to experiment with the SSGT model for trauma (mentioned in Chapter 7) using music therapy techniques.

The music therapist began co-leading with a psychologist who was part of the trauma committee, incorporating verbal discussions with musical experiences related to the topics. Music therapy interns expressed a special interest in working with trauma survivors and were drawn to the facility since, as part of their internship, they could regularly attend the trauma committee meetings. Our early trauma groups were called 'empowerment groups' so as to not stigmatise participants as having experienced trauma. When we continued that practice by calling our groups the 'music empowerment groups', it was interesting that group members insisted on calling them 'trauma groups'. "That's my group!" they proudly announced as we gathered the group together. As Judith Herman states:

> The traumatised person is often relieved simply to learn the true name of her condition … She discovers that she is not alone; that others have suffered in similar ways. She discovers further that she is not crazy; the traumatic syndromes are normal human responses to extreme circumstances.
>
> (Herman, 1997, p. 158)

An important aspect of a music therapy group is building community. In a group, the common rhythms and shared songs can quickly create a sense of belonging. In the groups we conducted at our facility, improvisation using percussion instruments such as drums, maracas, tambourines, and claves and melodic-percussion such as marimba-like instruments was common. The music therapist would often play guitar, piano, percussion, or use voice. Harmonic, rhythmic, or vocal accompaniment provided an underlying support. The elements of music – regular rhythms, phrasing, refrain to a song, etc., also provided predictability. We now experimented with combining these aspects with topics from the SSGT model.

Structure of Model

As described in the example of working with relationship and trust (see Chapter 7), for each topic there is a verbal component and a musical exercise that is usually pre-planned. Music is used as a frame with a warm-up and a closing activity or song. The warm-up serves to acknowledge each participant, identify moods and themes, and support the coming together of the group.

The specific topic and the symptoms of traumatic experience are addressed verbally and at times might be written and posted on the wall for reference by all throughout the group. The topic is discussed without individual group members sharing their trauma histories. Tools are presented to work with the topic. A musical exercise works with a particular aspect of the module with the purpose of highlighting or deepening this experience. The music helps to connect the body and the emotions to what might otherwise be a cerebral experience. The music also serves as a container for overwhelming emotions.

The closing is mostly done with music – often an uplifting song – helping group members return to what is familiar and predictable. The songs usually have their own container in the returning again and again to the refrain.

Establishing Music Therapy Rituals for Safety and Containment

Before we could begin to present the SSGT modules we needed to address safety and containment. As part of this process, we found ways to create community and establish a sense of predictability. It is imperative to implement musical elements of structure each week in order to promote trust and safety, to help alleviate anticipatory anxiety and to establish a predictable ritual.

Infants have been found to have astonishing powers of discrimination for subtle features of musical sounds and melodic forms, especially as these are represented in the inflections of a mother's voice …These features are evidently manifestations of a fundamentally innate process of emotional physiology, by expression of which a primary level of intermental communication is established between human subjects.

(Trevarthan, 2001, p. 8)

The effects of physical abuse and deprivation on the developing child are sometimes assessed entirely in terms of the physical damage inflicted on the body, but violence and cruelty is always accompanied, or preceded, by disruption to the affective patterns of caregiver-child or caregiver-infant interaction, and these psychosocial or psychiatric aspects should be taken into account in planning intervention.

(Trevarthan, 2001, p. 26)

This appears to have relevance in our adult trauma informed groups. At the start of each group session a hello-song is presented providing an acknowledgement through melody, words, and movement. This primary singing of their names and reflection of their feelings attempts to heal this disruption and create a feeling of safety at the start of each group.

First Ritual is a Hello Song
https://soundcloud.com/psychosis_and_trauma/hello-song

I composed a hello song (Kijek, 2022) on the guitar, which we sang at the beginning of every group. I used a simple harmonic progression of I, IV, V (A, D, E cords). Sliding up to the A cord I used a muting technique, giving it a funk type rhythm. This gave it a fuller, chunkier sound on the acoustic guitar. The progression was very predictable, repetitive and holding. Austin (2008, p.146) writes that using simple two and three chord progressions is holding and creates a sense of security. The upbeat, funky dance rhythm I used was a great icebreaker, created a fun atmosphere and helped to entice the group members to join in and play along with the percussive instruments we provided including maracas, tambourines, claves, and a xylimba (small 5 bar marimba-like instrument). The melody was simple and catchy. The lyrics to the hello song are listed below:

"Hello [group member's name] … it's nice to see you today.
Hello [group member's name] … it's nice to see you today.
Ooooooooooooooo, Ooooooooooooo … how ya doing today?"

I often began with the group member who I sensed needed to feel the most held and grounded by the music based on their posture, body language, facial expressions, gestures, behaviours, eye contact, etc. All of the therapists sang together to each group member. The group member responded to the question by speaking or singing how they were feeling. Then they were asked to pick the next person in the group we would sing to. The hello song engaged the group members, grounded them in reality, fostered social interaction between group members and established a consistent and predictable beginning of each group.

This hello song became our musical check-in. It became a wonderful assessment tool to gauge how the group members were feeling in the moment based on their responses. During the first few groups, most of their responses were superficially pleasant (i.e., "OK", "fine", "good"). By the 2nd session, group members were singing along to the hello song. After a few weeks, I started to model that it was acceptable to have a negative response. I sang that I was feeling tired. "Ooooooooooo, I'm so tired today." As the group continued and trust slowly built, the song became a safe container for the group members to share more honest feelings. They began to feel more comfortable to share negative feelings as well such as sadness, loneliness and nervousness.

With this song the group members came alive when hearing their names. It was almost magical to witness. Their postures changed, their faces lit up, some looked like they were beaming. Like the little girl that finally receives the attention she's been craving. Singing their names each week reaffirmed and validated their sense of self and helped to establish trust and safety in the group.

Throughout the 12-week course more choices can be provided, asking group members how they would like to have their names sung. They could have a choice to hear their names soft, medium or loud. This can foster a sense of empowerment and provide insight about what feels comfortable for each member in the moment. In order to explore wider ranges of emotions with their instruments, music therapists, using their supporting instruments, can present different dynamics, tempi and meter, modelling crescendos (building up the music louder and faster) and decrescendos (bringing the music back down softer and slower). Although it might be difficult at first for the group members to follow, they begin to progress towards the end of the 12-week group. It can be illustrated how playing the instruments softly might represent feeling pensive or even sad or playing loudly could represent feeling anxious or angry. The work on these music therapy techniques can be continued as well during group improvisations.

The Second Ritual Involves Breathing Exercises

Diaphragmatic breathing exercises are utilised as a second ritual, often used after the verbal component to help ground the group members. This is also used at any time that group members become triggered. Deep breathing can be utilised not only in the group but independently as a healthy coping skill. It can be explained that breathing can help to regulate strong emotions and reactions stating that breathing can calm you down if you are feeling scared, anxious or angry. It can also be explained that breathing can help people feel connected to their body if they feel disconnected to it (dissociation), and can even help them fall asleep if they are having trouble sleeping at night. For more detailed information on the diaphragmatic breathing exercise and how it was taught, see the module on 'Bodily Manifestations of Trauma' (p.196).

The Third Ritual Consists of Uplifting Closing Songs

Each week, group members are asked to select a song of empowerment as the closing song to end the group. This can be accompanied by the therapist. Familiar songs are tricky because a happy song for one group member can be a sad song for another. A song can trigger a group member in so many ways. Although several different songs have been tried, the most requested seem to uplift the group members: "Lean on Me" (Withers, 1972), "Stand by Me" (King, Leiber, & Stoller, 1961), and "Three Little Birds" (Marley, 1977).

One or sometimes all of them can be played at the end of each group. Group members often look forward to singing these songs once the verbal content of the group is finished. Having these three rituals: a familiar hello song at the beginning of each group, deep breathing exercises, and closing songs at the end of each group helps to build safety and containment.

Singing Familiar Songs

There are important aspects to consider when choosing familiar songs. Bailey (1984) states that singing familiar songs, especially during the initial sessions, can help to establish a rapport and a trusting relationship with service users. As they choose familiar pre-recorded songs, they can experience a locus of control, a sense of safety and comfort (Zatulovsky, 2002). When a person sings a song that has meaning to them, it validates their feelings and reflects who they are. Bruscia writes:

> Songs are ways that human beings explore emotions. They express who we are and how we feel, they bring us closer to others, they keep us company when we are alone … songs weave tales of our joys and sorrows, they reveal our innermost secrets, and they express our hopes and disappointments, our fears and triumphs.
> (Bruscia, 1998, p. 9)

When a group member selects a song, it can also serve as an assessment tool. A therapist can gain insight into the inner life of the group member by looking at the mood and theme of the song as well as the lyrics (Y. Zatlovsky, personal communication, October 2004). Song themes can reveal a person's needs, concerns and moods. Bailey (1984) writes that "people choose to hear and participate in songs which support their needs and which convey the mood and messages they want to hear" (p. 7).

However, music therapists need to take great care when selecting a song, taking into account each client's issues, potential triggers and the lyrical content. This brief example illustrates how a song of comfort for one group member triggered another group member to feel a lack of support.

Marleen requested "You've Got a Friend" (King, 1971). The song theme is about reaching out to a friend in a time of need and the friend being there to comfort and support you. This song is commonly played in music therapy sessions to comfort and support our clients. I sang and played the song on the guitar and some of the group members sang along. I noticed Linda's affect completely change. She appeared sad and gazed out the window. She left the room briefly. After the song, Linda came back and sat down. As we verbally processed the

190

lyrics of the song, Marleen proudly stated that she felt "blessed" because she has so many friends. Both the song and Marleen's response triggered Linda's issues of isolation and abandonment. Linda blurted out "I have no friends! They only want stuff from me!" Linda was initially triggered by the lyrics of the song, and when Marleen boasted about all of her friends, this was magnified. Linda realised that she didn't have any true friends. Although Linda needed support in this moment, she didn't have the confidence to ask for it. This was a great learning experience for all of us. Although familiar songs are amazing containers for feelings, the lyrics can easily trigger trauma survivors (B. Scheiby, personal communication, March 2005).

Pre-Group

In 2004 we began with a pre-group (as was done in the verbal groups; see Chapter 7) prior to conducting the 12-week sessions for the Women's Music and Empowerment Group. This gave each service user a chance to decide if they would like to be part of the group. Due to some anticipatory anxiety and apprehension about the group, the pre-group helped service users to gain a sense of control. We wanted to make sure group members were empowered to choose the group or to decline. At times music can be experienced as overstimulating to some service users. During the pre-group it can be explained that people react differently to different types of music and that we encourage feedback and reflection about their experiences. For example one person may feel triggered by beating a drum, another may be distressed by loud sounds. We explain that we welcome discussions about the music and want to make sure everyone is comfortable by keeping this dialogue open and being willing to encourage the group members to honour individual needs. Some people may simply say, "I don't like music" or "These instruments are for kids" or "Music gives me a headache." The pre-group also gave the selected service users the opportunity to meet all of the group leaders and try out the group before actually committing to join the entire 12-week group. The trauma committee carefully selected service users using various assessment screenings. Our ultimate goal was to have six group members. Everyone who joined the group received a journal to record their personal experience and a handout about the group.

During this pre-group we focused on reinforcing safety and implementing more structure by trying a 1960s folk song, "Alice's Restaurant" (Guthrie, 1967) and using it as a fill-in song (P. Jampel, personal communication, March 2004). A fill-in song is a common music therapy technique used to explore feelings where the group members fill in the blank line with their responses. The song helps to engage the group members, establish group cohesion and ground members in the here and now experience. With the line "You can get anything you want", group members can fill in their requests.

Food is typically a safe and non-threatening topic and was usually a great icebreaker to begin a first group. It is also a wonderful assessment tool to gauge how the group members are able to identify and express their needs. The song has a simple, predictable blues-like chord structure and the approach shows the group members' level of comfort based on whether they participate or not. In other groups, the song had often been a favourite and was frequently requested in groups.

During the first group, it was explained that you could have ANY-THING you wanted from Alice's restaurant, like a genie granting your wish. Any type of food you like or really anything you wanted. All you needed to do was to place your order.

I played the first verse on the guitar and modelled this by singing to all of the group leaders. "You can have ... at Alice's Restaurant." I asked each group leader one at a time what they wanted from Alice's restaurant and sang the verse with their response. "You can have [response – e.g. spaghetti and meatballs] at Alice's Restaurant." The group members listened with curiosity to the group leaders' responses. Building safety and trust was our most important goal with this group. Therefore, the group members were given the option to order something only if they felt safe enough to do so. We were astonished that most of the women in the group were silent and did not ask for anything at all! In fact, three of the women remained silent and didn't engage at all in the music therapy directive. We then pointed out that the group members did not only have to ask for food, but they could also ask to be in a place that feels safe. "If you want to fly away, you can. If you want to go away from here to a place where no one will bother you, you can even ask for that" (F. Margolis, personal communication, 2 March 2005).

Again, there was silence. We suspected from this experience that most of the women in the group were not in touch with their own needs, so they were not able to express those needs to us. Traumatised children repeatedly do not get their needs met and can even feel guilty for having their own needs. Some are afraid to express themselves because it doesn't feel safe to do so. This early in the group trust and safety were not yet established.

It is of interest to note that over the next few weeks once trust was established, the song was often requested and became a completely different experience. For example, to our surprise, one of the group members who had initially been completely silent, looked up with soulful eyes and asked, like a child would ask their mother, "can we PLEEEEEEEEEEEEEEASE sing Alice's Restaurant?" This time, every group member was able to verbalise their own needs and order their favourite foods within the safe container of the song! Some of the group members were now smiling, giggling and appeared to be enjoying the experience. Clearly, the sense of safety and even fun had been created in the group.

Looking at Specific SSGT Modules

The following presents the way music is used to work with particular modules of SSGT. We are not presenting entire sessions but rather the musical work within several of the topics. In 'Affective Numbing' we see how the incongruence of affect and inner experience is revealed and worked with in music. With 'Self-Injury', the focus is on the tools of self-care with a 'Self-Love Drum Improvisation' (Aamon Yeldell, 2022). The 'Bodily Manifestations of Trauma' module uses breathing and toning techniques to provide tools for trauma survivors to gain coping skills and reconnect with their bodies. In 'Re-scripting Nightmares', the therapist uses the piano to both recreate the nightmare and encourage the group members to find new endings. Finally, in 'Trust and Relationships', a fill-in song provides a place for words to be expressed freely without needing to be explained.

Affective Numbing

A person first has to be able to recognise that s/he is having a feeling and be able to identify the feeling. Next, s/he has to learn ways to tolerate and survive the experience of feeling. This often involves becoming able to modulate or control the intensity of feelings. Finally, the person must be able to integrate feelings by connecting them to other parts of his or her experience so that s/he can understand what evokes feelings and what the feelings tell about needs and experience.

(Saakvitne, Gamble, Pearlman, & Lev, 2000, p. 61)

In this module we focus on the identification and experience of emotions. The group leaders explain that it is common for trauma survivors to have difficulty identifying and experiencing their emotions and they may feel 'numb'. They may have learned to stuff down their feelings during the time of the trauma. As they learned to not only block out negative feelings, they also missed out on positive feelings like happiness, joy and fun. A verbal topic introduces feelings with a handout given to group members that illustrates various emotions such as angry, sad, and anxious. Also discussed are the various shades of feelings, explaining that not all feelings are dichotomous; they are not just black and white. There is a whole grey area in between. Miller (1981), Montello, (2002), and Austin

(2001) write that neglect, abandonment, physical, emotional, and sexual abuse from a primary caregiver can cause parts of the young, developing personality to become fragmented. The 'true self' that feels emotions becomes replaced by a 'protective false self', much like wearing a mask to the world (Austin, 2001).

The overall goal for group members is to use music as a tool to help them identify a feeling or emotion. This brief music therapy example was a breakthrough for Susan because she was able to briefly get in touch with her feelings and her 'true self'.

I created five basic emotion flashcards (happy, sad, angry, scared, and anxious) to be used in musical improvisations. Each card had a drawing of an emotion on the front and the name of the emotion on the back. Each group member took a turn selecting one of the cards that displayed an emotion they wanted to express on their instrument during their group improvisation.

Susan chose the 'Happy' card. The music therapists and remaining group members helped to support Susan by playing their instruments together. Susan beat the drum with a mallet with an extremely fast tempo and the rest of the group tried to match her intensity. As I tried to follow and support Susan's playing on the guitar, I experienced a feeling of anxiety. I felt as if I couldn't strum fast enough to keep up with her beat. There were no spaces; no place to breathe. She ended her playing abruptly. Afterwards, I asked Susan how she was feeling and with a huge smile on her face, her response was "not good." One co-leader pointed out that "sometimes we put on a happy face to the world when we really aren't feeling happy". I asked Susan what she needed now and she shrugged her shoulders. I encouraged her to play where she left off. This time, I matched her intensity and gradually moved the music into a softer and slower pace. I modelled softer and slower on the guitar. The other group members also slowed down their playing. We were all impressed that Susan was able to follow my cue. After playing we asked Susan how she was feeling in the music. She answered, "nervous." Although Susan may have wanted to feel happy, she was able to recognise and verbalise that she was really feeling nervous. Meeting Susan where she was in the music by 'matching' her rhythm and then bringing it down softer and slower helped her become aware of what she was initially feeling and how it changed. Susan responded that she felt better when she played slower. She related that she was able to hear the other group members slowing down and that helped her feel less nervous. Susan's improvisation helped her to gain insight and integrate her emotions with her affect, which was a first step towards gaining some experience and insight into this process.

Self-Injury

For this module we begin the group with a discussion of self-injury, discussing ways people hurt themselves mentally, emotionally, and physically. People may say negative things about themselves or blame themselves. One may remain in an abusive relationship. One may cut or burn oneself to gain a sense of control or to feel something when one is dissociating from one's body. Following this a discussion can develop of how to break the cycle of self-harm with an example of catching oneself making a negative comment to oneself and instead acknowledging that one has made a mistake and that it is okay.

This discussion can lead to the topic of how to nurture, self soothe, and take care of oneself. When one has experienced abusive or neglectful childhood experiences these skills may not have been learned. As the discussion continues some group members are encouraged to share ways they comfort themselves such as watching a favourite TV show, listening to soothing music, or doing some art work.

Self-Love Drum Improvisation
https://soundcloud.com/psychosis_and_trauma/i-am-music-excerpt

I have planned an activity using the drum and voice as a support for affirmations (Aamon Yeldell, 2022). With the drum I recreate the sound of the heartbeat and the womb. "From the eighth intrauterine week, the organism lives in an envelope of rhythm … There is the sound of the maternal heartbeat and vessels … and superimposed on this is the different rhythm of the fetal heartbeat …" (Leedy, 1969, p. 55). Next, I add on my voice. "The voice is like a bridge that can connect the mind to the body and heal splits between thinking and feeling. When we sing, we can give voice to and find relief from intense pain, fear, and anger" (Austin, 1998, p. 316).

After our discussions about self-injury and self-soothing, I take the djembe drum and create a steady rhythm. I tell the group we will be creating affirmations for ourselves. I ask the group members to think of things they like about themselves. I model this by beginning: "I am kind-hearted." I repeat this several times in a kind of mantra accompanied by the drum. Now I encourage others to join. At first the other therapist models with, "I am a good listener." Soon the group members come up with affirmations of their own. I repeat each one adding it to the first. It becomes a string of words with the accompaniment of the steady drumbeat. By keeping the drum going as consistently as possible during the group, I am in effect re-creating the womb, unconsciously sending messages of safety in order to tap into our bodies, facilitate flow, and build cohesion. There is a space between the phrases filled in with just the sound of the drum "I am kind-hearted … I am a good friend … I am caring." The drum beat establishes a feeling

of trust and being protected. My voice is reassuring and the affirma-
tions are echoed back and absorbed by the group. My sense is that the
feeling in the room is one of intimacy and healing.

Bodily Manifestations of Trauma

Diaphragmatic Breathing

As mentioned previously, diaphragmatic breathing exercises can be taught to the group members to be utilised as a healthy coping skill. This can become a ritual at the end of the verbal component and a resource especially if the group members are triggered, to help ground and feel a connection to their body. The following explains in more detail the diaphragmatic breathing exercise. Group members are encouraged to try to practise the breathing exercise on their own if they have a nightmare or flashback, if they feel anxious, stressed out, or experience insomnia.

Each inhalation through the mouth is illustrated with an image of sipping something delicious through a straw. They are asked to imagine they are slowly sipping a straw and filling their belly like a balloon, savouring the flavour on the inhalation. To make it even more concrete, each member of the group can be asked to share what their favourite beverage is to drink. The music therapist can share their own favourite. They are asked to exhale slowly and completely and to push out all of the stale air (Austin, 2008, p. 27). Each exhalation can be modelled sounding the letter "fffffffffffffffff" and asking the group to notice the gentle vibration on their lips (D. Austin, personal communication, January 2005). The group members can also be invited to stand in a circle and to slowly bring their arms all the way up on each inhalation and all the way back down to their sides on each exhalation. This can help them to feel the connection to their body and to fully grasp the breathing exercise. At the same time the music therapist can play soothing instrumental music in the background (Langdon & Kijek, 2022).

Soothing-Instrumental-Breathing-Exercise
https://soundcloud.com/psychosis_and_trauma/
soothing-instrumental-breathing-exercise

Toning

Survivors of sexual abuse can experience a sense of disconnection from their bodies because they experience their bodies as not safe. They often feel isolated and have difficulty being intimate or merging with others:

[Toning] creates a safe place within one's own body. Through toning through the web of harmonies, members can create safe places by themselves, feeling others' existence through tones. By doing so, they can feel intimacy with other human beings in a non-intrusive way. The toning process breaks the isolation.

(Kwon, 1997, p. 43)

Toning is "the conscious use of sustained vowel sounds for the purpose of restoring the body's balance" (Austin, 2008, p. 29). The group members are encouraged to push out stale air, release negative emotions and reconnect with their body. Similar to the breathing exercise described above, the group members are asked to inhale slowly and deeply through the mouth. This time they are encouraged to exhale with a gentle humming sound, "mmmmmmmm" and to notice the vibration on their lips. Then this can be expanded allowing the gentle hum to become a vowel sound. The exhalation can be intoned to the elongated sound "ahhhhhhhhhhhhhhh" or "ooooooooooooooo", or other vowel sounds. Keyes (1973) describes how toning can release blocked energy in the body, helping to heal physical pain and illness. She writes:

[By] toning or chanting ... we are able to bring oneness to our divided nature. We are made whole. When one feels discouraged, inadequate, frustrated, fearful, any negative condition, the transforming change begins the moment one ... breathes deeply and sends the voice out.

(Keyes, 1973, p. 44)

Group members connect with their own voice and with each other. This can become an intimate part of the group where group members make more eye contact with each other as their voices join. The group members often seem to enjoy this and sometimes smile or laugh.

Working with Nightmares

"Posttraumatic nightmares are a hallmark of PTSD and distinct from general nightmares as they are often repetitive and faithful representations of the traumatic event" (Forbes, Phelps, & McHugh, 2001, p. 1). Working with nightmares often is difficult and triggering for participants. The topic can be introduced by sharing and discussing tools and various strategies such as grounding (e.g. naming three things to touch, see, or listen to). A breathing exercise might be shared, noticing one's breathing to feel the connection to the body. The creation of music is powerful and needs to be used with great care. Music has the power to lead us into different feeling states through the use of dissonances and harmony, high and low pitches, and changes in rhythm. Grounding can also be achieved by the use of steady rhythms and harmonic elements. These aspects provide a way of modulating affect.

One can enter into an uncomfortable feeling and then find resolution. This can be done to 'rescript' a nightmare and gain a sense of control. The following is an example of handling a sensitive topic after trust had been established over several weeks.

> *In one module entitled 'Re-scripting Nightmares' we explored the potential of music to have an effect on nightmares. Can the content of recurring nightmares be changed with musical interventions? One group leader posed the question of what the sound of a nightmare would be like. The music therapist proceeded to play the keyboard with the pipe organ setting making a sound with many dissonant intervals. The music sounded like it could come out of a horror movie. Several of the group members shared how scary it sounded. The music therapist began to narrate how he imagined a nightmare. He played the music louder and faster while telling the group members that he was trapped and afraid he would be unable to escape. Then he suspended the music for a moment and began to improvise quietly. The rhythm was slow and steady. The group members seemed relieved listening to the peaceful sound. He shared the image of a setting which felt safe and comfortable. Following this the group members engaged in a verbal discussion on how sound and imagery can affect and change their feelings of terror from a scary nightmare to arriving at a peaceful place. The emphasis is on the way in which strong negative emotions can be transformed. This appeared to communicate safety and predictability which allowed a group member to have the courage to explore this difficult topic. He described a recurrent nightmare he had. After checking in with the group members to see if this was all right the music therapist began to play the scary music again. Group members were encouraged to join in the improvisation this time, playing faster and louder. After a short period, the music therapist slowed down the music and changed it to a slow and gentle sound asking the group member who had shared his nightmare what his safe place was. The music decreased in volume and had a steady rhythm. After more discussion and reactions to this technique, other group members were eager to rescript their nightmares. After each member presented and worked musically with a nightmare the music therapist encouraged them to find a safe and comforting place. At the end everyone was encouraged to breathe deeply and slowly and finally to share what the experience was like (Takeda et al., 2007).*

Relationships and Trust

The 'relationship and trust' module, briefly described in Chapter 7, is the last segment of the 12-week module. The group usually begins with the hello song as the musical check-in, followed by a short group improvisation. The theme of Relationships & Trust is then presented verbally with some prompts from the SSGT manual (Shelley, 2006). Group members are asked to define trust. It can be explained that trust is something that is earned over time such as in friendships. Group members can be asked to reflect on any progress that has been made over time in the group. The importance of setting boundaries in relationships is discussed explaining that children who endure physical and/or sexual abuse from their caregivers may grow up without a basic sense of trust. Because they were betrayed by an adult who was supposed to protect them from harm and nurture them, they may feel completely unprotected from their environment (van der Kolk, 1987; Herman, 1997). Krugman states that "these children learn that a person who loves you, will also physically hurt you" (Krugman, 1987, p. 135). Unfortunately, these deep wounds are carried over into adulthood. This profoundly affects their ability to trust and have healthy, intimate relationships.

After the open discussion, songwriting can be used as a music therapy intervention. In this case the group members composed a song which they entitled, "Trust."

> I created a simple and predictable I, IV, V chord progression in the key of C major. The key of C is an easy key for most non-musicians to sing in. Austin (2001) writes that the simplicity of using only two or three repetitive chords is holding and creates a sense of safety and security. I softly arpeggiated C and F chords back and forth, creating a 'holding environment' (Priestley, 1994). The G chord became the turnaround for the predictable return back to C home base. I encouraged group members to create their own melody for the line they composed in order to help foster self-esteem and validate their feelings. The group members who were comfortable with the theme contributed the following positive phrases:
>
> "Trust can build relationships" and "helps you join with other people." Karen, who was abandoned as a child and then moved to several different foster care homes throughout her childhood, stated that 'trust' was too abstract a word and she didn't understand it. One of the co-leaders attempted to change her phrase to make it more positive. However, I strongly felt that Susan's words should be used verbatim in the song because it was an honest reflection of her feelings about trust. I also didn't want her to feel she had to conform to the other positive statements in the song. Her phrase became "Trust is abstract," allowing her experience of trust to reverberate through her melody and words without needing to be explained.
>
> During the post-group, the group members were given a typed copy of the song, which they sang together with great pride. The song gave

them something tangible they could save and cherish from the group
while also giving them closure from the 12 week group experience.

Conclusion

Combining the frames of the SSGT modules with innovations of musical expression encourages and supports survivors through difficult conversations and challenges in their journeys toward healing. The pre-group allows service users to express any apprehensions they may have about using music as a modality for a trauma informed group and allows them to decline attendance in this group if they so choose. Despite the challenges of topics such as self-injury and nightmares, live music with guitar, drum, and voice provides safety. The norm of reviewing experiences and checking in allows service users to alert the music therapist if something may be triggering and help the group to assist in creating a safe experience. Individual follow-up can be provided as needed. In conjunction with the verbal interactions, the music therapy interventions (hello song, self-love affirmations, etc.) provide mirroring and holding. Using musical interventions allows for healing and reparation of aspects group members may have lacked in infancy and early childhood while also fostering self-esteem and empowerment. The music improvisations, vocal toning and breathing exercises help to ground and hold the group members, giving them space to individuate while allowing them the ability to return to the safety of the group holding. The physical act of playing music supports the integration of the physical and emotional aspects, bringing new understanding to the verbal discussions of the topics. In this way group members are able to gain valuable insights and access their feelings while working on gaining awareness of their symptoms and the connection of these to trauma as well as discovering pathways toward healing.

References

Aamon Yeldell, S. (2022). Self-love drum improvisation. Retrieved from https://soundcloud.com/psychosis_and_trauma/i-am-music-excerpt (accessed 27 May 2021).

American Music Therapy Association. (2021). Archives of the American Music Therapy Association. Retrieved from www.musictherapy.org/about/history (accessed 21 October 2021).

Austin, D. (1998). When the psyche sings: Transference and countertransference in improvised singing with individual adults. In K. E. Bruscia (ed.), *The dynamics of psychotherapy* (pp. 315–333). Gilsum, NH: Barcelona Publishers.

Austin, D. (2001). In search of the self: The use of vocal holding techniques with adults traumatized as children. *Music Therapy Perspectives, 19(1)*, 22–30.

Austin, D. (2008). *The theory and practice of vocal psychotherapy.* Philadelphia, PA: Jessica Kingsley Publications.

Bailey, L. M. (1984). The use of songs in music therapy with cancer patients and their families. *Music Therapy*, *4(1)*, 5–17.

Borczon, R., Jampel, P. & Langdon, G. S. (2010). Music therapy with adult survivors of trauma. In K. Stewart (ed.), *Music therapy and trauma: Bridging theory and clinical practice*. New York: Satchnote Press.

Bruscia, K. E. (1998). An introduction to music therapy. In K. E. Bruscia (ed.), *The dynamics of music psychotherapy* (pp. 1–15). Gilsum, NH: Barcelona Publishers.

Cadesky, N. (2022). Group work with adults in short-term inpatient psychiatric treatment and recovery. In L. E. Beer & J. C. Birnbaum (eds), *Trauma-informed music therapy: Theory and practice*. New York: Routledge.

Cui, M. H., Agyeman, M. O. & Knox, D. (2016). A cross-cultural study of music in history. *International Journal of Culture and History*, *2(2)*, 65–69.

Davis, W. & Hadley, S. (2015). A history of music therapy. In B. Wheeler (ed.), *Music therapy handbook* (pp. 17–28). New York: Guilford Press.

Forbes, D., Phelps, A., & McHugh, T. (2001). Treatment of combat-related nightmares using imagery rehearsal: A pilot study. *Journal of Traumatic Stress*, *14(2)*, 433–442.

Guthrie, A. (1967). Alice's restaurant. From the album Alice's Restaurant. Warner Brothers.

Herman, J. (1997). *Trauma and recovery*. New York: Basic Books.

Keyes, L. E. (1973). *Toning: The creative power of the voice*. Marina Del Rey, CA: DeVorss Publications.

Kijek, G (2022). Hello song. Retrieved from https://soundcloud.com/psychosis_and_trauma/hello-song (accessed 27 May 2021).

King, B. E., Leiber J., & Stoller, M. (1961). Stand by me. Single. Atco.

King, C. (1971). You've got a friend. From the album Tapestry. Ode A&M.

Krugman, S. (1987). Trauma in the family: Perspectives on the intergenerational transmission of violence. In B. van der Kolk (ed.), *Psychological trauma* (pp. 127–147). Washington, DC: American Psychiatric Press.

Kwon, H. (1997). Music therapy with mentally ill adults who have a history of child abuse. Unpublished master's thesis, New York University, New York.

Langdon, G. S. (2022). Music therapy in the treatment of complex trauma in mental health. In L. E. Beer & J. C. Birnbaum (eds), *Trauma-Informed music therapy: theory and practice*. New York: Routledge.

Langdon, G. S. & Kijek, G. (2022). Soothing instrumental breathing exercise. Retrieved from https://soundcloud.com/psychosis_and_trauma/soothing-instrumental-breathing-exercise (accessed 27 May 2021).

Lecourt, E. (1993). Music therapy in France. In C. D. Maranto (ed.), *Music therapy: International perspectives*. Pipersville, PA: Jeffrey Books.

Leedy, J. J. (1969). *Poetry therapy: The use of poetry in the treatment of emotional disorders*. Philadelphia, PA: J. B. Lippincott Company.

Marley, B. (1977). Three little birds. From the album Exodus. Tuff Gong.

Miller, A. (1981). *The drama of the gifted child*. New York: Basic Books.

Montello, L. (2002). *Essential music intelligence: Using music as your path to healing, creativity, and radiant wellness*. Wheaton, IL: Quest Books.

Nordoff, P. & Robbins, C. (2004). *Therapy in music for handicapped children*. Gilsum, NH: Barcelona Books.

Pelosi, F. (2010). *Plato on music, soul and body*. Cambridge: Cambridge University Press.

Priestley, M. (1994). *Essays on analytical music therapy*. Phoenixville, PA: Barcelona Publishers.

Rhodes, D. & Langdon, G. S. (2011). *Making the case for the use of words and music in trauma treatment*. Presentation at Advocacy, Therapy, and Leadership, the National Music Therapy Association National Conference, Atlanta, GA.

Saakvitne, K. W., Gamble, S. J., Pearlman, L. A., & Lev, B. T. (2000). *Risking connection. A training curriculum for working with survivors of childhood abuse*. Maryland: Sidran Press.

Shelley, A.-M. (2006). *Men's trauma manual*. n.l.: Anne-Marie Shelley. Retrieved from www.lulu.com/en/en/shop/dr-anne-marie-shelley/mens-trauma-manual/paperback/product-1yvmnwe.html?page=1&pageSize=4.

Simon, P. (1970). Bridge over troubled water. From the album Bridge Over Troubled Water. Columbia Records.

Stewart, K. (ed.). (2010). *Music therapy and trauma: Bridging theory and clinical practice*. New York: Satchnote Press.

Sutton, J. P. (ed.). (2002). *Music, music therapy, and trauma: International perspectives*, London: Jessica Kingsley Publications.

Takeda, K. E., Muenzenmaier, K., Battaglia, J., Langdon, G. S., & Kobayashi, T. (2007). *Syndrome Specific Group Therapy (SSGT) for complex PTSD: A cognitive behavioral group intervention adapted to music and art therapy*. Paper presented at the Male Survivor International Conference 'Relief, Recovery, and Restoration Helping Men Heal from Sexual Abuse', New York.

Trevarthan, C., & Aiken, K. (2001). Infant intersubjectivity: Research, theory, and clinical applications. *Journal of Child Psychology and Psychiatry, 42(1)*, 3–48.

van der Kolk, B. (ed.). (1987). *Psychological trauma*. Washington, DC: American Psychiatric Press.

Wigram, T. & De Backer, J. (ed.). (1999). *Clinical applications of music therapy in psychiatry*. London: Jessica Kingsley Publishers.

Withers, B. (1972). Lean on me. From the album Still Bill. Sussex.

Zatulovsky, Y. (2002). Concealed voices: Aspects of grief in pediatric oncology patients. Unpublished master's thesis, New York University, New York.

13

INTERWEAVING WORDS AND MUSIC IN A MUSIC-VERBAL THERAPY TRAUMA GROUP

Gillian Stephens Langdon

Sometimes when I read over my notes from the past I feel like I am drowning. I'm overwhelmed and confused. What were we doing? Was any of this useful? Did any of this generate change? As leaders of a trauma group we let ourselves enter a space that is fraught with feelings, images, memories, behaviours stemming from abuse, neglect, and pain. Words echo still in my memory of the group. "He hit me and pushed me to the ground. My mother says if I stay with him I'll end up like her." "My father, he's a jail bird – puts his hands all over me." And the song with the refrain, "I just want to go home ..."

Experiencing a group is so much more complex than writing about it in an organised way. When we write we eliminate the aspects that are uncomfortable, incomplete, or which challenge our image as therapists. We pick and choose the moments that make sense and particularly the moments with clear outcomes.

> We see that every Music Therapy session is a journey ... It seeks only health and provides certain artistic forms which help participants travel to that health. We cannot write a script for another person's life, especially those at risk ... As therapists, we guide the journey, guard and support the participants and aid them in identifying meaningful themes ... We must tune ourselves to see and hear the response which is most difficult to observe – the inner response.
>
> (Kenny, 1982, p. 122)

Introduction

In this chapter we will describe the evolution of our music-verbal therapy trauma groups which had begun in the early 2000s (see Chapter 5). Having

DOI: 10.4324/9781003055914-16

become familiar with the symptoms of complex trauma and the power of musical interventions, my co-leader and I began to explore a more process-oriented way of working, starting in 2009. Rather than following the specific module topics, as documented in Chapter 12, we wanted to take up directly topics that came from the group process itself. This way of working is reminiscent of what in music one might call 'free jazz'. In the *Jazz of Physics*, Stephon Alexander (2016, p. 15), a physics professor, writer, and jazz saxophone player, writes, "As I matured musically and came to understand the rules of harmony and the basic forms in the standard jazz tradition, I discovered that free jazz does have its own internal structure and is an extension of the jazz tradition."

With our new way of guiding the music-verbal therapy trauma groups we developed a more flexible approach which was still grounded in a firm foundation of the specific needs of trauma survivors for safety, tools for grounding oneself, techniques for self-soothing, self-care, and positive relationship building (see Chapter 7). We maintained the structure of having a beginning, a middle and a closure. Now the start of the group came from the group's musical initiative or from verbal cues and discussions. The middle focused on topics that emerged and could be explored through verbal and/or musical elements. Closure was often created through a familiar song.

Description of Groups

Group members ranged in age from 18–60 years. Many had been experiencing psychosis and had been in and out of psychiatric care for years. Some were transferred from a children's hospital and some had been incarcerated. Many had histories of violence towards themselves or others. We developed groups for men and groups for women. Admittance followed our usual process with a referral from the trauma committee or the treatment team, and was followed up with an interview by one of the group leaders (see Chapter 7). Groups were held in a variety of locations: on specific units or in a central area to which the co-leaders escorted group members from different units to join. Escorting the group members was time consuming but it allowed trauma informed interventions to be available to a broader group of survivors. In addition, the room we were able to use provided the use of an acoustic piano and a wide variety of instruments. The intention was that the group meetings would provide a setting where the individual strengths and creativity of the group members could thrive.

The new music-verbal therapy trauma group model we piloted offers more flexibility than the more structured model described in Chapter 12. It provides room for spontaneous musical interaction and expressive imagery guided by the immediate needs of the members and created from the present fabric of their lives. Each group member arrives at the group from the world they experience immediately prior to that moment: a fraught phone call with a relative; an expectation of a favour from a friend; witnessing an altercation on the unit. Each person comes in with their own feelings: crying, excited, anxious, silent. At times the group can begin with a musical improvisation that is initiated without having to verbally announce or explain what it is about.

We base group discussions on members' concerns, interweaving exploration of symptoms and strategies as they arise. At one time a group member might come in and, without a word, just hit the drum. The music therapist can immediately mirror this sound on the piano and while supporting the intensity of the sound, create structure and grounding. This can be provided through the use of bass lines and rhythmic forms allowing group members to experience the expression of intense feelings without going out of control. Discussions might follow a musical improvisation and songs can be created based on themes that emerge verbally. At other times the group might begin with a discussion which becomes the foundation for a song or improvisation. Throughout these groups various musical forms are utilised and include free musical and rhythmic improvisation, fill-in songs, and rap with its unique ability to connect words and music in 'freestyle'.

Creating a safe environment is extremely important in trauma informed music-verbal therapy groups as described in previous chapters (Chapter 7 and Chapter 12). A closed group, in which the same members participate in each week's session, builds trust, connection, and safety. Safety is also reinforced by providing respect as a norm in the group, focusing on trauma symptoms rather than details of the events, and by recognising that everyone is free to express themselves in music or words or both or none without being judged.

It is also important for the group leaders to feel safe. Having experienced the structured Symptom Specific Group Therapy (SSGT) (Shelley, 2006) groups as described in Chapter 12, we now felt more confident and flexible in handling specific issues related to trauma. We were better prepared to understand and respond to dissociated states and affect dysregulation, and knew how to assist in grounding. "The predictable rhythms, forms (e.g. verse and refrain) of music, in addition to a feeling of safety, help survivors modulate their emotions during hyper-aroused states. The physicality of playing an instrument or singing helps with grounding ..." (Langdon, 2015, pp. 348–349).

Examples of Our Group Work

Described below are six fictionalised examples based on the many situations we encountered. Through them, we see the interweaving of words and music in the context of different circumstances. Except for the last example, they all take place in the context of a music-verbal therapy trauma group. The focus of each example is on a particular group member, but occurs with the support of the music and interchanges within the group. In the first example a woman experiments with revealing her authentic self for the first time in a group context. In the next example a man who has a lengthy history of hospitalisation due to his threats of violence uses an improvised song to find his way through his paranoia and anger toward another group member. A young woman is anticipating her first unsupervised outing after years of hospitalisation in the third example. The song and the music help her to experience a feeling of confidence. The next example demonstrates the way in which words and music are interwoven, bringing the group member into a safe place of sharing. Following this, a vignette is presented where music is used to recruit what Porges describes as the 'Social Engagement System' (Porges, 2010), which will be elaborated on later. In it we see a woman who has experienced a lengthy hospitalisation deal with intense feelings about living in the community once again. And, finally, a young man is able to come to terms with elements of his past through musical support and grounding while he creates a freestyle rap.

Example 1: Emerging of Feeling and Gaining a Sense of Self

Olivia had spent years institutionalised. I had been working with her for quite some time when she joined the women's music-verbal therapy trauma group which was a closed group of mixed ages. Several of the members were looking at the possibility of discharge from the hospital. In this group Olivia encountered a place of acceptance and modelling of the give and take of relationships through music and words.

She was often seen standing talking to herself in the hallway and occasionally would shout out "leave me alone". In music therapy she always played the xylimba (five note, wooden melodic-percussion instrument) in the same perseverative way, up and down the instrument, hitting the notes in a fast tempo with no changes or dynamics. I attempted to support her playing and encouraged a broader range of expression through guitar or piano but there was no change. It felt like, although she was continuing to be 'compliant' by playing, the playing itself was totally disconnected. I remember in supervision sharing that I felt like a kind of jailor whom she would pay with her notes.

In individual psychotherapy Olivia began to speak of her chaotic experiences of moving from one foster care home to another after being abandoned at a young age. It was clear through her descriptions that there had been little room for her to experience a sense of self. She continued to attend the women's music-verbal therapy trauma group where we began to witness small changes.

As the group begins to enter the room, one group member picks up a bass guitar and begins to explore a bass line. Olivia is standing at the

206

piano. She reaches out and starts to play a simple three note melody. Her body begins to move ever so slightly to the music. As the other group members sit down and the music comes to an end, they clap. Here is an improvisation – and independent of the staff!

In the next session, after a discussion about what each group member wants, a foundational harmonic structure is provided by the music therapist and each member is asked to put into the song what they want. When it comes to Olivia's turn she says she wants to be a flying fish. I picture her flying out of the water, her colours flashing in the light and then, just as quickly diving back to hide in the ocean.

These are little moments in what would be a long journey ahead in Olivia being able to express her needs and grow in self-expression.

Example 2: Affective Lability – Negotiating Strong Feelings

The real power of music lies in the fact that it can be 'true' to the life of feeling in a way that language cannot; for its significant forms have that ambivalence of content which words cannot have. Music is revealing, where words are obscuring, because it can have not only content but a transient play of contents. It can articulate feelings without becoming wedded to them.

(Langer, 1980, pp. 243–244)

There were times when a group member might enter the group with a sense of conflict with another member. In this case we could use an improvised song to work out some of the feelings before entering into a discussion. For example, one of the group members might mumble, "Annoyed". Without entering into a verbal discussion, the music therapist might initiate a song created by stringing together a series of words. There is no need for the words to make any rational connection to one another. For example, the result might be "love … I don't know … angel … guilty". The harmony and rhythm hold this together.

Anton often stands at a wall and talks about how the people on the other side of the wall are talking and laughing about him. Occasionally he has angry outbursts. In the check in song Anton adds his phrase, "On the suspicious side," while glaring at Philip. I initiate a song stringing together words. Anton struggles to find his words for the song. He tries out "determination" and the group sings along. Then he changes it to "predicament", and finally settles on "lenient". Each word is sung by the group members allowing Philip to 'try on' the various feelings as the song progresses. This working out – or should we say 'playing out' – lays a good foundation for a subsequent discussion of relationships and ways of expressing strong emotions.

Example 3: Transitions – Creating Confidence in Mind and Body

As a young woman begins to make the transition from hospital to community, feelings of inadequacy and helplessness can arise. Working with words and music can be a way to discover and support a new relationship with these challenges. For example, when the topic of discharge comes up a group member might be reluctant to share their fears or be unaware of their feelings after having experienced a long hospitalisation.

After a discussion, Sandra reveals that she is going on an unescorted pass for the first time. Another group member adds, "I'm going to visit a residence soon." Sandra is slumped in her chair as usual. Her shoulders are stiff and she seems generally tense. When asked where she would go, she responds, "I just want to take a walk." The music therapist begins to reflect these words in the music, with a rhythmic pattern accompanied on the guitar. As the music develops the music therapist begins to exaggerate the rhythmic pattern. A G major to C major rock progression is presented over a G pedal tone to illustrate a confident sort of strut. This adds a feeling of 'attitude' to just wanting to take a walk. The music seems to create a message of 'Hey, I'm here, taking this walk!' Sandra sits up, her spine straightening. She seems to exude a new sense of pride. Her chest is raised and she has a large grin on her face. This physical experience appears to support what Ogden, Minton, and Pain (2006, p. 211) describe as a "somatic anchor for feeling competent – an anchor that [can be] learned to simulate voluntarily when feelings of inadequacy [arise]."

Example 4: Interweaving Words and Music Unlocks Valuable Conversations

Jesse walks into the room and sits in silence. It is the second week in a row that the usually exuberant young man has been silent. Although the group reaches out, he continues to be unresponsive. We try singing his name. A group member asks, "What happened Jesse?" I am wondering what his inner experience feels like. He has been transitioning to a community residence. As the group ends, Jesse walks out without a word.

The following week Jesse has just returned from an unescorted pass. He is the first one to enter the room and as he passes by the piano where I am sitting, he reaches out and plays two notes in the high register of the piano. Immediately I echo with two ascending notes in the middle register as if asking a question. He answers with two more notes. As the rest of the group enters, he sits down and plays two beats on the drum nearby. Soon the beats become more pronounced and a regular rhythm begins to emerge as the other group members join in. The volume increases and the piano sound becomes more chordal and rhythmic with more open chords incorporating some dissonances. Jesse's body is fully engaged now. He is sitting up and both his arms are involved in the creation of the sound. His body is moving to the rhythm.

The music comes naturally to a close and in the silence that follows everyone seems to breathe into this space. Looking down, Jesse murmurs, "I can't do it." One of the group leaders asks quietly, "What's happening?" Jesse responds, "It's my brother. He just got out of jail and he's selling drugs. Every time he finds me. He wants me to join him. He wants to drag me back to my old world." "What did you do?" asks another group member. "I told him no. But I'm afraid of him." Another group member joins in. "I know what that's like. My father is always doing drugs. He gets violent with me." "I know. I just can't do this," Jesse responds. "How did you get away from him?" one of the group leaders asks. "I went back to the residence. I told them what happened." One of the group leaders responds, "That's so important. We spoke of safe places the other week. Knowing where to be safe; how to ask for help." Another group member joins in. "Jesse, you're doing it. You're making a change!" Looking up with the hint of a smile Jesse says, "Maybe you're right."

More discussion about safe places ensues. As it becomes time to close the group, I ask what song we might end with. They decide on "Lean On Me" (Withers, 1972).

Example 5: Reconnecting – Music and the 'Social Engagement System' in Stephen Porges's Polyvagal Theory

Since melodic music contains acoustic properties similar to vocal prosody, music may be used to recruit the Social Engagement System[1] ... [F]or some clients, especially those who have been traumatized, face-to-face interactions can be threatening and may not elicit a neuroception of safety. In these circumstances, the Social Engagement System can potentially be activated through vocal prosody or music while minimizing face-to-face interactions.

(Porges, 2010, p. 12)

---

[1] "As mammals evolved from more primitive vertebrates, a new circuit emerged to detect and to express signals of safety in the environment (e.g., to distinguish and to emit facial expressions and intonation of vocalizations) and to rapidly calm and turn off the defensive systems (i.e., via the myelinated vagus) to foster proximity and social behavior. This recent neural circuit can be conceptualized as a Social Engagement System" (Porges, 2009, p. 41).

As Deb Dana (2021) explains, "Polyvagal Theory, in shorthand, is the science of connection." In the following vignette we see Evelyn's anger overwhelm her when she recalls traumatic experiences from the past. These cause her to shut down, her verbal abilities lost. The song continues with the guitar accompaniment in a steady rhythm as the refrain is sung, "Where, where, where do we go?" With the support of the music Evelyn's body reengages as can be seen in her rocking, and her tambourine rhythm which is now in sync with the guitar. She hears the therapist and the group members continue to sing and this returns her to a feeling of safety. It is the tone of the vocal music and the breath as well as the steady rhythms and predictable phrasing of the song that help create a feeling of safety for her when these traumatic reminders have surfaced. As she repeats the refrain, she is now able to find a pathway to the 'Social Engagement System', reconnecting to the group. Evelyn is now able to risk verbalising her wish.

Evelyn is preparing to be discharged after being hospitalised for several years. She exhibits grandiose delusions and sees herself as being a famous television star. On the unit she has established herself as a self-confident person without any vulnerabilities. In music therapy she always plays the tambourine in a kind of half-hearted way with no relation to the group rhythms. As discussions of the future emerge, the theme for a song is developed. The music therapist begins to create the refrain of "Where, where, where do we go?" (Langdon, Perry, Angel, & Garroway, 2014; Perry, 2021). Group members begin to share their wishes which are incorporated into the song. Evelyn sits leaning back in her chair in her usual way. When it is her turn the music therapist sings the refrain and, while waiting for Evelyn's response, the music therapist vamps on the chord progression on the guitar. Suddenly Evelyn leans forward and begins, "No one lets me have what I want. They're always telling me what to do. That's what got me in here in the first place. They're always taking from me!" Her speech quickens as her face turns red with anger. Then suddenly she stops with her mouth open. She is speechless. But the music continues. Slowly Evelyn begins to rock with the group's rhythm, repeating the question, "Where, where, where do we go?" and finally responding, "I want to go to a residence ...where I can be free." The group sings back her response, as her tambourine locks into the rhythm. As the group echoes her response Evelyn is able to hear her words validated. She is able to spend a little time 'trying on' her response within the safety of the musical structure of the rhythm, verse, and chorus. https://soundcloud.com/psychosis_and_trauma/where-where-where-do-we-go

Example 6: Challenges and Opportunities of Working with Rap

Part of the very structure of rap... is its attentiveness to social reality, its deep (in-your-face) existential urban chronicalisation of pain, drug use, murder, poverty, anger, disappointment, feelings of rage, and narratives of loss and regret ... [R]ap narratives are also filled with themes regarding the importance of family, positive role models, perseverance/resiliency, warnings/cautionary tales, positive self-image, healthy choices, change, and planning for the future.

(Yancy & Hadley, 2011, p. xxvii)

In embracing this form in a trauma sensitive way, the music therapist can support important expressions of intense experiences, helping service users to share difficult emotions. Rap has the ability to communicate and engage with deep suffering and trauma. Many service users find expression in the form of rap music or spoken word. What follows is a description of the ways to support and work with rap in a trauma informed way.

In a music-verbal therapy trauma group there is a continual dance within the freedom of the creative expression and the needs for safety and grounding. This can be even more challenging when the form is a freestyle rap (improvisation). The challenge for the music therapist is to be open to the creativity and freedom of this medium while finding a way to provide support. "Utilising rap music in therapy when indicated is a culturally sensitive approach to treatment. Culturally sensitive treatment recognises, values, and respects the cultural aspects of clients" (Elligan, 2011, p. 35). At times rap is presented in a designated music-verbal therapy trauma group or it may be shared during a regular music therapy group. The survivor may arrive with a pre-composed verse and ask for a particular beat. This rhythm can be presented as a setting on a keyboard or created by the music therapist based on their description of the sound or a particular hip hop artist's style. In some instances, the survivor may bring their own accompaniment created on their electronic device. Percussion and melodic percussion instruments are available to the group members who can play along with the beat.

After the verse is presented over this musical or rhythmic foundation the group member may continue to create words in a freestyle flow where the rapper is creating and rhyming words spontaneously. This state of 'flow' allows unconscious material to bubble up while the conscious mind is working hard to create rhymes and a sense of coherence to the rap. Sometimes this material begins to overwhelm the survivor and cause them to stare off into space and perhaps dissociate. It is imperative that the music therapist create a place of holding and safety. The challenge is to find ways to insert structure and support while not interfering with the unique musical and verbal material.

One of the ways to accomplish this is for the therapists to take a word or phrase from the spoken word and repeat it here and there throughout the rap. In musical terms this is called a 'hook'. The hook serves many purposes. Most obvious is linking the rapper to the present moment. The first introduction of the hook may cause the rapper to look up at the therapist. In some examples the therapist or co-leader can chant in rhythm with the music, "What's the hook? What's the hook?" drawing the group into co-creation of this support. In my experience this is usually welcomed by the rapper as it demonstrates that they are being heard and welcomed. As the group picks up this hook, the rapper may perceive themselves surrounded by a feeling of affirmation and holding.

The group leaders need to be vigilant in providing this hook at key moments to help the rapper keep connection to the present moment. If the group member appears to be dissociating or beginning to stare off into space, the therapist can bring them back through singing this hook and through emphasising the beat. The availability of the drum for the rapper to play also provides grounding. The physical motion links the body literally to the ground through the connection of the drum to the floor. The therapist's voice helps to bring the survivor back to a place of predictability, safety, and regulation. This can serve, for example, to bring rage and resentment in an angry rap into a more manageable place.

Chris is a survivor of years of childhood abuse at the hands of various caretakers in the numerous foster homes he lived in. He has a history of losing control, sometimes leading to threats of violence. He hardly attends any of the groups. However, he has become a regular at the weekly 'open mic' group. This group is an open group available to anyone attending the clinic. Service users sit in chairs around the perimeter of the room. Anyone who wants to come up to the mic is welcome to. They don't need to be performers per se, they just can come up to the mic and let the music therapist know what they need whether it be a beat from the keyboard, a recording they have brought, an accompaniment, or just the space to rap or sing.

This week Chris stands up. He requests a beat with a strong, clear rhythm. He wants to freestyle. He begins rapping about his day at the residence. He is coming up with some interesting rhymes. As he goes forward he begins to speed up and we can decipher the phrase "two-faced liars." Now his rap is beginning to sound more like a rant and it is hard to make sense of what he is saying. His face is turning red. I catch the phrase, "They don't trust me ..." It is clear he needs help in grounding. I don't want to interrupt him so I begin to chant, "What's the hook? What's the hook?" He looks at me a little startled but continues. A group member throws out the words, "Trust in me." I repeat this using it to punctuate certain phrases during the rap and several of the members who are sitting around the circle pick it up. "Trust in me. I want you to trust in me." Chris' rap begins to slow down a bit and he is becoming more coherent. As the rap comes to a close we hear him say, "Yeah! Trust. I need trust." The group claps and he gives a great bow.

Chris has been able to express his frustration and feel heard. He is no longer alone with this. He is also able to find a way, with the musical support of the group, to return to the rhythmic structure and to modulate from the intensity and out of control expression into a more manageable state where he can actually experience the support of his peers and even grasp the positive message. Sometimes a breathing exercise can be done for further grounding.

Before recognising the needs of trauma survivors for structure and safety in freestyle rap, I would sit in amazement at the feats of verbal and rhythmic dexterity – a supportive by-stander. I remember in one outpatient group a young man began to rap about a death he had witnessed on the street. The intricacy of his words, rhythms, and rhymes was breathtaking. The group followed him with absorbed attention. At the end of the rap, he was gazing off into space, clearly disconnecting from the group and seeming to be dissociating. His friend, sitting beside him, saw this and appeared to recognise where he was and may indeed have understood what he was feeling. He reached over and swiped his friend on the head with his baseball cap. "Come on man!" he said laughing until the rapper looked up and laughed – a rougher sort of grounding than we incorporated later.

Conclusion

A more process oriented music-verbal therapy trauma group allows for the spontaneous interplay of words and music to engage, hold, create, and heal. The co-leaders have the freedom to move between words and music to connect with and support group members. Throughout, the co-leaders are guided by their knowledge of the many challenges experienced by survivors of severe and pervasive trauma.

Whether it is a fill-in song created from a discussion, a musical phrase that unlocks a silent pain, or a hook that grounds a survivor engaged in an emotional rap, this integration of words and music allows the survivor to express the inexpressible, experience safety, find community, and discover ways of sharing amongst peers.

References

Alexander, S. (2016). *The jazz of physics*. New York: Basic Books.

Dana, D. (2021). The polyvagal theory in therapy. Retrieved from www.youtube.com/watch?v=JXGy7M4kvaY (accessed 27 May 2022).

Elligan, D. (2011). Contextualizing rap music as a means of incorporating into psychotherapy. In S. Hadley & G. Yancy (eds), *Therapeutic uses of rap and hip hop* (pp. 27–38). New York: Routledge.

Kenny, C. (1982). *The mythic artery*. Atascadero, CA: Ridgeview Publishing Company.

Langdon, G. S., Perry, R., Angel, J., & Garroway, J. (2014). *Hip Hop healing wounds in trauma recovery*. Presented at the Male Survivor 14th International Conference 'Evolution From Hurting to Healing', New Jersey.

Langdon, G. S. (2015). Music therapy for adults with mental illness. In B. L. Wheeler (ed.), *Music therapy handbook* (pp.341–353). New York: Guilford Press.

Langer, S. K. (1980). *Philosophy in a new key*. Cambridge, MA: Harvard University Press.

Ogden, P., Minton, K., & Pain, C. (2006). *Trauma and the body: A sensorimotor approach to psychotherapy*. New York: W. W. Norton & Co.

Perry, R. (2021). Where where where do we go? Retrieved from https://soundcloud.com/psychosis_and_trauma/where-where-where-do-we-go (accessed 27 May 2022).

Porges, S. (2009). Reciprocal influences between body and brain in the perception and expression of affect: A Polyvagal perspective. In D. Fosha, Siegel D., & M. Solomon (eds), The healing power of emotion: Affective neuroscience, development & clinical practice (pp. 27–55). New York: W. W. Norton.

Porges, S (2010). Music therapy and trauma: insights from the Polyvagal Theory. In K. Stewart (ed.), *Music therapy and trauma: bridging theory and clinical practice* (pp.3–15). New York: Satchnote Press.

Shelley, A.-M. (2006). *Men's trauma manual*. n.l.: Anne-Marie Shelley. Retrieved from www.lulu.com/en/en/shop/dr-anne-marie-shelley/mens-trauma-manual/paperback/product-1yvmnwe.html?page=1&pageSize=4.

Withers, B. (1972). Lean on me. From the album Still Bill. Sussex.

Yancy, G. & Hadley, S. (2011). Introduction: give 'em just one mic: the therapeutic agency of rap and hip hop. In S. Hadley & G. Yancy (eds), *Therapeutic uses of rap and hip hop* (pp. xxiii–xlii). New York: Routledge.

14

DEVELOPING STRUCTURED ART THERAPY GROUPS TO TREAT COMPLEX TRAUMA

Toshiko Kobayashi and Kimberly Michaud

Introduction

In this chapter we will introduce a trauma informed approach (see Chapters 7 and 8) in art therapy for people who suffer from complex trauma and psychosis. Art therapy is one modality within the umbrella of creative arts therapies, which includes music, dance/movement, poetry, and drama. The use of art therapy as a tool for trauma focused interventions offers unique therapeutic qualities and creates a potential for versatile and effective treatment.

A Short History of Art Therapy Treating Trauma

The arts have played an important role throughout human history. Based on recent excavations, Palaeolithic art making found in caves dates back to the dawn of civilisation (Cassone, 2021). At the turn of the nineteenth to twentieth century in Europe, psychiatry was becoming more prominent in the field of medicine. Hans Prinzhorn (1886–1933), a psychiatrist who practised during this period, collected a large amount of his patients' artwork and published *Artistry of the Mentally Ill* (Prinzhorn, 1995). This book greatly influenced the understanding of human expression in artmaking and later inspired the development of the art therapy field. In Great Britain "the use of art as a vehicle for therapeutic expression" was described by El-Mallakh (2021, p. 205).

One of the early pioneers of art therapy, Margaret Naumburg, a trained psychotherapist, began using art as a therapeutic modality to diagnose and treat patients in the 1940s. Her seminal work, *An Introduction to Art therapy* (Naumburg, 1950) describes in detail the treatment for children with severe life experiences. Another pioneer, Edith Kramer (1977, 1993) published *Art Therapy in a Children's Community and Art as Therapy with Children*, which is still used today for training art therapy graduate students (Reinsbakken, 2017).

In 1969, the American Art Therapy Association (AATA), a national organisation, was founded. Over the past two decades, especially in the aftermath of 9/11, the demand for trauma informed mental health care has grown significantly. Art therapy has become more widely acknowledged as an important treatment modality and it was recognised and licensed as such under state laws in 2005.[1]

In the wake of the COVID-19 world health crisis, art therapists have found innovative ways to practise art therapy through virtual portals as many mental health treatments have moved online. It is likely that we will see an increased need for trauma informed therapies to meet the needs of people affected by the pandemic over the next few years. We can anticipate that this will influence the trajectory of the field of art therapy.

Developing a Structured Trauma Focused Art Therapy Group

When an art therapist joined the trauma committee (see Chapter 5) in 2003, she was eager to explore a trauma focused art therapy approach that would be effective for people with psychosis. In the trauma committee (TC) the art therapist learned about interventions for trauma survivors including the Sanctuary Model (Bloom, 1997; see Part I). She also found that there were two manuals that had previously been developed, which the members of the TC were currently using. One of the manuals was educational: *Understanding and Dealing with Sexual Abuse Trauma* (Muenzenmaier et al., 1998). The other one was *Symptom Specific Group Therapy for Complex Post-traumatic Stress Disorder* (Shelley, 2006). Inspired by the music therapist, a long-time TC member, who was already facilitating music-verbal therapy trauma groups, the art therapist began to be interested in developing a trauma focused art therapy group.

It was a novel challenge to create the 12-week trauma focused art therapy protocol by incorporating these two manuals. Subsequently two different groups were developed, the Trauma Symptom Specific Art Therapy (TSSAT)/cPTSD Group Protocol [1] and the Symptom Specific Expressive Origami Therapy (SSEOT). Both groups followed the same newly developed protocol and the format for the session procedure. The only difference was the use of the main media as the base of the directives, with the former being traditional art therapy and the latter origami. It required trial and error and creative thinking for those who were involved in the process. Members of the TC, the creative arts therapists, and the art therapy students played essential roles in the development of these groups.

One outstanding advantage of art therapy is that each artistic expression created by a participant remains afterwards as a tangible object for service users and service providers, who can then go back to review the original

---

1   New York State is one of a growing number of states that have a separate license for art therapists – Licensed Creative Arts Therapist (LCAT) – since 2005.

work and discuss development. Artwork can assist with a deeper understanding of psychosis for both clinicians and service users (Killick, 2017). In addition, the artist can show their work to other people as an independent object. These images have symbolic and figurative meanings associated with memories and feelings that have the potential to facilitate verbal discussions. This figurative expression can disclose unspoken (and unspeakable) experiences of traumatic events. It is important to understand that a person's truth is not necessarily a universal truth but a 'figurative truth', as Garrett (2019) explains in his book *Psychotherapy for Psychosis*. People with psychosis can have their own version of reality possibly created to survive traumatic experiences. Art therapy has the potential to assist service users to realise memories figuratively in the form of images of traumatic experiences. This can help with processing those traumas.

Adaptation of the Trauma Symptom Specific Art and Origami Therapy

The adaptation of the Trauma Symptom Specific Art Therapy (TSSAT) and subsequently the Symptom Specific Expressive Origami Therapy (SSEOT) models were developed by the lead art therapist based on a variety of creative activities. For the TSSAT we used more traditional art therapy techniques such as drawing, collage, and clay modelling. For the SSEOT we used origami exclusively. All activities were selected to target the symptoms of complex-Post Traumatic Stress Disorder (cPTSD) (e.g. nightmares, flashbacks, and dissociation) and were educational in nature (see Chapter 8). Each group provided service users with the description of the symptom and coping skills to deal with it. (e.g. grounding by creative expressions, behaviour scripts, and relaxation techniques.) Finding a corresponding art and/or origami project for each symptom could not be rigidly defined and required constant flexible adaptations.

The primary objective of the TSSAT and SSEOT was to incorporate art therapy while integrating CBT principles and providing information about the symptoms of cPTSD. The most important treatment intention was to assist service users to cope with their stressful life circumstances; and, to support them as they began to recognise the difficulties related to this journey of trauma exploration.

Therapy groups were designed to assist participants gain insight into their own experiences related to emotional and/or physical trauma, and the ongoing effects of this trauma. By allowing for the subtle examination and understanding of symptoms associated with cPTSD, participants were provided an opportunity to learn both how their symptoms may be related to their trauma, and to identify effective coping strategies for cPTSD symptoms. When exploring these symptoms, participants began to grasp the role their traumatic experiences have had in shaping their lives. This process helped to de-stigmatise and normalise feelings. At the same time, many of the group members began to develop self-confidence and motivation to express their creativity autonomously. Making the connection between the symptoms of trauma and their own behaviour was empowering and initiated a process towards change.

In structuring the groups, the art therapists determined the amount of time for each aspect of the group (e.g. making artwork, processing artwork, reflection time while drinking tea). Choice of location was also important to consider. It was essential that maximum comfort and predictability could be provided for participants as they started to explore their trauma related symptoms. Principles of adaptation of the TSSAT and CBT were introduced to assist group members in exploring the links between thoughts, feelings, behaviours, and actions in relation to art making. This was designed to enhance the participants' understanding of how their trauma may have adversely affected not just their thoughts, behaviours, and feelings but also their perceptions of the self, others, and the world. It is important to note that there were slight alterations to all directives based on the membership of the groups. Providing a safe and respectful environment was a top priority in the art therapy room and aided in the development of group cohesion. After each session the art therapists (supervisor and students) reflected on the treatment process. Emphasis was placed on emotional reactions including transference and countertransference.

Participants were men and women at or over the age of 18 who were diagnosed with psychotic disorders and had trauma histories. Prevalent symptoms were dissociation, visual and auditory hallucinations, and delusions. The most typical diagnoses were schizophrenia and schizoaffective disorder. It was uncommon to find any PTSD or trauma history noted in their charts (Muenzenmaier et al., 2014). Histories of incarceration and multiple psychiatric hospitalisations were also prevalent.

One challenge for group leaders was to attend to both the individual needs of group members and to the group process. The goals included creating a non-threatening safe space for building trust, for normalising the therapeutic process, and to encourage free expression and creativity. This safe, supportive environment functioned to assist participants with developing

Table 14.1. Structure and setting of each 60 minutes session of Trauma Symptom Specific Art and Origami Therapy.

Relaxation movement/stretching/exercise (5 min.)

- Discussion of one of 12 trauma symptoms of c-PTSD (5 min.)
- Instruction of the art project relating back to the symptom discussion (5 min.)
- Art making (25 min.)
- Sharing artwork with the group (10 min.)
- Journal writing/reflection with tea and snacks (5 min.)

---

self-expressions and with forming human connections within which to share their creativity. It was crucial for the therapists to understand the potential for each participant to develop a coherent integration of physical, mental and psychological functions. Because artwork can be visually powerful and presents an unpredictable potential for triggers, the safety of all group members was important to avoid re-traumatisation.

Part A: Description of the Trauma Symptom Specific Art Therapy Group

Below is an example of one of the series of the 12 TSSAT sessions.

Table 14.2. Trauma symptom specific art therapy group (TSSAT) protocol for adults. Trauma assessment is done prior to group participation for each individual. Additional session of 'tea party' provided at the end of 12 weeks. These directives, recommendations, and suggestions are flexible and can be determined at the beginning of the session.

No.	Symptoms	Art directive	Summary of art directive
1	Nightmare	Sacred circle drawing	Discussion about good and bad dreams. Draw a large circle and draw anything inside and outside of the circle.
2	Flashback	Peaceful image drawing	Are there any intrusive images we experience? Pick a peaceful colour and draw.
3	Avoidance	Collage	Are there things that we avoid thinking about? Choose unpleasant images from magazines and paste them on a piece of paper.
4	Dissociation	Jigsaw puzzle	Are there times in which we realize that we've been spacing out. Choose images for a collage and cut it up into a jigsaw puzzle, then play with pieces.
5	Hyper-arousal	Monotype print (1920s: Rorschach)	Discussion on self-soothing techniques. Drop blots of paint on a piece of paper, fold and then unfold.
6	Affective lability and impulsivity	Origami model	Discussion of methods of self-control. Observed demonstration of folding an origami claw.
7	Affective numbing	Mask making	Finding (or identifying) our feelings. The mask is made from a paper plate and two rubber bands for ease of wearing.
8	Self-injury	Self portrait	Identifying impulses for self-harm (either in the past or currently). Draw a self-portrait using a small mirror.

(Continued)

No.	Symptoms	Art directive	Summary of art directive
9	Substance abuse & addiction	Scribbles	Discuss substance use as a way to self-medicate. Scribble on a blank paper with eyes closed. Then find any images within the scribble.
10	Self-concept	Inside–outside image	What do we show on the outside vs. how we feel on the inside. Fold paper in half to form a book. Draw a picture on the cover to represent the outside image you present, and a picture on the inside to represent inside feelings.
11	Bodily manifestation	Clay modelling	Discussed bodily expression of thoughts and feelings – create a human figure from clay.
12	Relationship and trust issues	Round robin	Trusting ourselves and others. Each person gets a piece of paper to draw on. Then, pass the artwork to the person sitting next to you. This is repeated every 5 minutes so that everyone gets to draw on each paper.

Trauma Symptom Specific Art Therapy Sessions

Following are the details of six of the 12 art therapy sessions, simplified into step-by-step verbal instructions with variations allowed for individual freedom and creativity including the use of other art materials and media. Weeks 1, 2, 3, 4, 11, and 12 are highlighted and summarised for efficacy of the art exercise, the interest and reaction or lack of reaction by service users, and the focus on the symptoms.

In order to provide a sense of the impact of the group experience on participants we will follow the progress of one fictionalised participant, William, who represents an example of many group members. William was most often alone and could be seen holding avid conversations with himself. He was diagnosed with Paranoid Schizophrenia in his late teens, which did not allow him to finish high school or to attend college. His childhood was troubled and he exhibited disruptive behaviours in school leading to an early expulsion from high school. Although dishevelled in appearance, William was a polite man and tended to obey the rules set up by the unit. William attended every group and appeared at the door eager to participate. While in groups he did not engage in conversations with himself but was involved in the group process to the extent possible for him.

Week 1: Examining Nightmares

Reflecting on dream content (nightmares or repetitive dreams). Art making does not require the participant to be fully aware of the relationship between the nightmare and trauma; rather, it gives space for participants to explore their feelings and reactions to the content.

Participants were given paper with a circle outline. They were asked to draw on the inside or outside of the circle, in order to consider coping methods in regard to their nightmares. Most of the participants were not ready to do so.

William was reluctant to discuss any experience with nightmares. He drew a face that looked similar to his own. The face seemed to have defiant expression, a sad mouth. He did not verbally explore what this meant to him.

Week 2: Examining Flashbacks/Intrusive Thoughts, and How to Create Safety

Participants were provided with information about these topics and discussed common triggers for bad memories and flashbacks, including sensory material such as smells, places, sounds, and touch. The art directive sought to offer a calming respite from intrusive traumatic memories. Participants were given paint in a variety of colours and asked to pick a colour they liked and/or felt was peaceful to them and then create a painting. While painting can be a soothing activity, it can also be provocative and messy, which may induce memories of childhood (Muenzenmaier et al., 2014). As clients were painting, the art therapists verbally explored coping skills for flashbacks, including grounding techniques such as breathing and shifting focus (using the breath as a relaxation point, and changing the thought from a negative to a positive one).

William did not use paint but chose a marker instead and drew a heart. to and wrote a message in it. He alluded to something his grandparent gave him as a child. While William could not explain how this might keep him safe, this might have been his representation of a safety charm.

Week 3: Avoidance

Participants took turns discussing something that they avoid such as noise, crowds, people, and school. They were informed of adaptive avoidance techniques that restrict emotional growth – such as withdrawing and/or avoiding people/relationships due to mistrust and emotional pain.

Participants were asked to make a collage of things they avoid and/or images that were not pleasing. The goal of this art directive is to practise uncovering unpleasantness and to develop a greater tolerance for things / situations that we avoid.

> *William selected images such as flowers and butterflies and used a bright colour border along the paper's edge. He appeared to be integrating the opposite of avoidance into the selected images. William's choice of nature images showed a defence toward the intrusive themes that the art activity presented. William seemed to have come up with his own solution for holding on to his defence measures, demonstrating a healthy self-protection.*
>
> *The therapists felt that participants could benefit from working on developing trust and safety before they are ready to address deeper issues.*

Week 4: Dissociation

Participants explored the concept of dissociation and were asked if they had ever experienced dissociation or feeling spaced out. It was explained that the spectrum of dissociation ranges from daydreaming / selective amnesia to more severe and symptomatic forms such as dissociative identity disorder. The brain's role in dissociation was explored as a mechanism to protect us from absorbing unendurable trauma. Participants were provided with a list of positive grounding exercises to bring back the self to the here and now.

Grounding exercises can use the five senses to achieve the goal of grounding, such as touching something tangible near you, using diaphragmatic breathing techniques, sucking on candy, or chewing gum, smelling a candle or something familiar, or calling a friend.

The instruction was to create a jigsaw puzzle using collage. The first step was to create the collage. When finished, participants were invited to cut their collage into puzzle pieces and finally to re-assemble those pieces. The main idea was to mirror the process of wholeness through creating a collage then cut the collage into fragments to mirror disassociation, and finally to put the pieces back together to generate wholeness again. This art exercise was designed to engage group members in the experience of fragmentation and integration symbolically and physically at the same time.

Some participants disclosed experiences of domestic violence, neglect, and betrayal as adults and children. Group facilitators steered participants away from sharing too much detail. This was to provide safety and reduce extreme emotional reactions.

One group member decided to cut his artwork into a puzzle and enjoyed reassembling it. However, they asked for glue and pasted it back together on a clean sheet of paper to make it permanently whole again.

William made his collage of four separate images, glued down with no overlap. The four images were seemingly unrelated (a table, a flower, an animal, a ball). Every image appeared to be important for him, however he was not ready to talk about his choices of images. By observing his collage, he showed contentment although he was not ready to express this verbally.

Week 11: Bodily Manifestations of Trauma

In this session, group members were encouraged to explore their personal bodily manifestations of trauma. It was explained that trauma can cause physical and emotional distress. Stress management skills were then reviewed. Positive and negative coping mechanisms and self-soothing activities were discussed (e.g. positive skills include diaphragmatic breathing, meditation, and listening to music, while negative coping strategies include rocking side-to-side, binge eating, using substances).

Participants were asked to work with clay and were encouraged to knead, pound, and play with the clay as a possible tool for reducing stress. Most participants were able to create a figure, except for two participants choosing instead to create clay flowers. Interestingly some used several different colours in one figure, (e.g. one red arm, one blue arm, two green legs). In contrast to earlier weeks, where participants showed greater hesitancy and resistance to self-disclosure, all participants demonstrated a willingness to create.

William created a figure with some body parts distorted. This was a visual example of how he may have felt about his body. His experience with awareness of bodily trauma appeared to manifest itself in a literal sense through the artistic representation of himself.

Week 12: Relationships and Trust Issues

In this final session of the TSSAT Group, the discussion centred on self-trust as well as trust of group members and facilitators.

Participants were asked to create a group mural using individual drawings to create a patchwork mural. We implemented a round robin approach to achieve this goal. Each participant was given a piece of paper and asked to draw for five minutes then pass their drawing to the person on their right. This continued until all participants had drawn on each of their neighbour's drawings. All were asked to respect the drawings of others and use them as inspiration and to build on the existing imagery. Participants stayed mostly on their section of the artwork, but notably they were willing to pass the paper around and allowed others to share the collective/creative space, which could have been experienced as invasive. All participants respected their peer's boundaries without any complaints.

William started his drawing with several fragmented images (e.g. a figure with several body parts missing). This may have been a continuation of the previous sessions' exploration (bodily manifestations of trauma). Another participant filled in the body parts of William's figure and used circles to incorporate William's broken image into the collective (collaborative) artwork. This interaction shows how these two participants found a way to trust one another. Trust was revealed in their proficiency with uniting a whole body. William allowed others to integrate his fragmented image and then place it into the larger mural.

Once all drawings were completed, all artwork was put together in a large patchwork mural on the wall. William's drawing was placed in the centre of the mural. Everyone conversed and shared the process while viewing the mural and drinking tea. We all chatted as a group of artists, reflecting on the group mural and our experience of the past 12 weeks for the remaining time. Both the group members and facilitators appeared relaxed and seemed to enjoy sitting together in a somewhat informal group situation.

Part B: Developing Symptom Specific Expressive Origami Therapy (SSEOT)

The core concept for using origami as therapy was formulated through my wish to find a non-intrusive way to communicate with people who were affected by trauma. I became confident that origami could be used as a powerful therapeutic tool when I visited and lived in several different countries while using origami with persons who were affected by trauma. This reinforced my idea and became my lifework. I was able to actualise Expressive Origami Therapy (EOT), which I originally named Enrichment Origami Art Therapy (EOAT) (Kobayashi, 2004; Azarani, 2012).[2]

EOT was formulated while visiting refugee camps, impoverished areas, and experiencing 9/11 myself as a Project Liberty crisis counsellor with FEMA in New York City. The four pillars of EOT principles are (1) safety, (2) maintain good health, (3) family and community support, and (4) fulfilment (Kobayashi, 2004, 2007, 2010a, 2010b; Kobayashi et al., 2007).

I learned that my innovative ideas for using origami as a therapeutic tool worked very well with people who have limited resources and varied cultural backgrounds. The Educational Manual (Muenzenmaier et al., 1998) helped to focus my ideas for healing with origami into the structured protocol that I titled SSEOT. Some service users found origami to be more structured and contained, and less restrictive as compared to traditional art therapy. One

2 While I was studying art therapy at NYU, two professors, Edith Kramer and Ikuko Acosta encouraged me to use origami as a tool of art therapy (1999 to 2021).

of the main principles of EOT is encouraging autonomous creativity – "in fact, everybody has it (creativity) because it's a human thing. It's just that people employ their creativity in different ways" (Atwood, 2020). Everyone is free to include the use of varied art media such as crayons/markers/scissors, etc. Origami appeared to become a grounding structure providing the base upon which to add free expressions. Growing up in a Buddhist culture, it seems to me, all creativity and individual expression start with 'sati'.[3]

Origami as a Tool of Art Therapy

Origami, the art of folding paper to create figures and shapes has been practised for centuries, mainly in Asian countries. Although it is widely believed that origami is Japanese, in fact, paper was invented in China (Hunter, 1947) and most East Asian countries still practise origami today. Japanese people were able to elevate the art of origami in a new and unique way. Origami has been used for ceremonial occasions, such as birth, marriage, funerals, cultural traditions and rituals. Origami is also used for community bonding and stress reduction and is associated with wellbeing for a variety of populations (e.g. monks, merchants, the elderly, and the children).

Intriguingly it seems, trauma focused therapies have basic principles in common with origami. Gotama Siddhartha (563–483 BC) taught the importance of 'sati (notice/aware/observe)' more than 2500 years ago and it has been widely practised in Asia. One of the oldest texts, *Sutta Nipata* or *Buddha's Teachings* (Bodhi, 2017) was written in Pali, the spoken language of that period. This text refers to the word 'sati', which was understood as to notice and be aware, which is important in gaining enlightenment. Nowadays 'sati' is translated as 'mindfulness' in English. Its popularity has been attributed to both Thich Nhat Hanh (2014), and his student Jon Kabat-Zinn (2013), who introduced his Mindfulness Based Stress Reduction Programme in the 1970s in the West. Origami is one of the long practised mindful activities. All creativity and individual expression start with 'sati', as one of the most precious functions learned by our fingertips and brains since the invention of paper.

Adapting TSSAT to Origami Therapy

After experimenting with the first TSSAT group, we noticed positive changes occurring with group members; including a greater willingness to work in a cohesive group, greater insight into their thoughts and behaviours, and the responsibility of showing up for groups without reminders. It made sense to explore more variations of trauma focused art therapy using different media

---

3 'Sati' is a word in the ancient spoken language of Pali used in India (i.e. be aware, notice, and put your mind to it).

for populations with a variety of levels of functioning and diagnoses. Consequently, there was an opportunity to implement SSEOT on the trauma unit (see Chapter 8). While administering the SSEOT, the 12-week sessions' overall format was the same as described earlier, but instead of art directives, origami projects were developed. The process of developing SSEOT was a unique struggle since this was the first attempt to adapt origami activities as a predominant media for trauma care. SSEOT supports mind and body integration through origami activities to assist in recovering these most basic needs for all of us, and was developed for participants who were unable to maintain a safe place to live, good health, family/communal support, and autonomous decision making. These four points are the basic principles of EOT.

As origami requires close physical proximity between participants and therapists and because it was the first time experiencing folding origami for most of the people, we limited the number of participants to 10. However, we were unable to form a closed group due to the growing numbers of people who were interested in joining the group. Some people were not ready to follow the origami directives and instead chose to sit and observe. We faced a dilemma in how to deal with these observers. We decided to welcome all participants who were interested in the group. Chairs were squeezed in along the table and along the wall. Interestingly, after a while those observers started to actively participate. Through this learning process SSEOT became a viable form of therapy.

SSEOT Sessions

In the following summary we describe two SSEOT sessions and follow the progress of two of the group participants, Ken and Ellen. Ken and Ellen represent fictionalised vignettes, representative of all group members. Ken was actively psychotic and reported that he was a close acquaintance of the president. He had attended two years of college prior to having been diagnosed with schizoaffective disorder in his early twenties. Ellen described herself as a bride of God. She was perceived as manipulative and demanding. Feelings of grandiosity were suggested by her imagined closeness with God. It seemed that based on this perceived relationship she placed herself above her peers. In groups both Ken and Ellen disregarded their peers' conversations and trivialised their issues. Both had an occasional visitor, but often reported afterwards that they were jealous of them.

Week 9: Substance Abuse and Addiction – Folding
"My Yacht" and "My Boat" Origami Models

Two floating models were chosen. Participants were advised to create an environment for boats on a piece of construction paper. Boat models are a traditional model in Japan and Asia and the Yacht is popular in the United

States. One participant drew a figure holding some drugs and alcohol. This provoked other people to discuss their memories of substance use. They expressed that drinking too much resulted in losing control. It was a meaningful moment when they opened up and shared a discussion about substance abuse issues. It should be noted that the group leaders also expressed their own difficulties (e.g. eating healthily instead of instant foods). Group members then also expressed their interest in living healthier.

Ken put a shape on a piece of construction paper and attached it to his yacht. He then cut a human figure from black origami paper and put it on the boat. He was not ready to talk about his origami work, but he smiled with contentment. Someone mentioned that the person might be in danger from alcohol. Ken said that the person did not drink much and just touched his origami boat and left the room before tea was served. One of the facilitators followed him and asked him if he would stay for the tea. He refused, but returned on another day and joined the group for tea time.

Many participants requested more variations of floating origami models and stayed for a while, joking and laughing. Enabling group members to approach serious issues indirectly is one of the unique qualities of art making/ origami.

Week 12: Folding Origami 'My House' and Creating a Village

In one of the group projects, all participants successfully followed instructions and demonstrated the ability to add their own creative fold to 'My House'. They then chose to use a variety of art media to decorate their houses (i.e. markers and crayons). Each house was unique in its own way; with various windows, doors, chimneys, and more. Each house was a different size and shape, demonstrating a variety of mastery with the folding technique. Some participants drew animals and people in their house.

Finally, a large piece of paper was introduced, and participants were asked to create a collaborative collage of their houses. Each participant pasted their own house onto the paper, and then drew trees, flowers, etc.

Ellen was the first to draw a road connecting her house which she proudly announced to the group. This led others to attach their houses to the road, and some created their own roads. Everyone then added more details such as stick figures in the empty spaces. They articulated the names of these stick figures later to the group leaders. The finished mural was proudly named "Retreat" when completed and displayed on the wall.

The step-by-step process of folding paper seemed grounding, as demonstrated by lowered defences within the group, and their ability to participate companionably. Feelings and memories of the past and future expectations were casually shared. Participants worked together and formed a supportive community while creating the origami artwork, something they appeared to appreciate and were possibly experiencing for the first time. This was visually realised on the final village mural "Retreat". It seemed the naming inferred their wish to go back to the community safely.

Summary

In summary, the origami projects following EOT were particularly constructive to group members and assisted them with making a series of independent choices. In addition to being empowering, working together on group projects also facilitated positive connections and enjoyable group interactions. The following are some of the important aspects of working with origami. First, almost anything can be created in a symbolic shape with origami and during each session the participants added a new object, sometimes at their own specific request. Secondly, additional materials such as colouring materials can be added. Thirdly, folding boxes, flowers, and action models such as 'flapping butterfly' were playfully enjoyed which fostered trust and companionship. Fourth, origami models became popular gifts and ornaments for a holiday tree and seasonal decorations. Fifth, origami is safe. "You cannot harm anyone and yourself with paper/origami!" Sixth (and lastly), origami involves simple physical activity using the fingertips, which directly activates the sensory and motor cortex in the brain (Kobayashi, 2019).

Discussion

Overall, the adaptation of TSSAT and SSEOT worked well. Group members were treated with respect and were able to explore trauma at their own pace. The discussion of cPTSD symptoms normalised their experiences and led to reductions of guilt and shame. Participants developed creative awareness and an art sharing community within the larger institution. Individual participation was encouraged by this newly formed community group.

Using these protocols provided a non-confrontational and non-threatening approach promoting an understanding of how trauma manifests in the body and mind. While the recovery process takes active participation, using art therapy allows space for limited verbal involvement. This suggests that art making can be invaluable for healing. As the therapy groups evolved, members who were mistrustful and quiet in the beginning developed relationships with their peers and with group facilitators.

Changes in participants were noted by art therapists and staff members, some of those changes were:

- Acquired enhanced inter-relational skills.
- Improved participation in programmes.
- Finding positive motivation to explore creative activities, which resulted in less destructive behaviours.
- Enhanced creativity resulted in improved self esteem.
- Greater group cohesion resulted in creation of a supportive community.
- Instillation of hope to move forward.

Creating safety cannot be mentioned enough, as a safe environment invited service users to express themselves creatively, which then fostered emotional growth. The safe environment also allowed for trust building, which was a fundamental experience for persons with psychosis and trauma. The use of art in conjunction with the subtle exploration of trauma symptoms provided participants with the opportunity to understand their traumatic experiences in a non-threatening manner and allowed for honest introspection. After the ground layer of creative expressions had been explored, group members were motivated to discuss and share their feelings of adverse traumatic experiences. This provided an additional layer of healing.

Conclusion and Future Plans

Art therapy was not initially taken seriously as a trauma focused treatment by staff members. This was due to a limited understanding of art therapy as a clinical treatment both within the mental health system and among service users. After completing the 12-week series, the treatment team began to notice and respect the results. This programme was a great opportunity for staff to witness and understand how TSSAT and SSEOT can be effective. In this series of sessions, we were successful in the sense that recipients were motivated to attend all 12 groups whenever possible. Some participants even asked for makeup sessions if they were unable to attend a scheduled group. This demonstrated a motivation to take responsibility for their own healing journey.

It has also become clear that TSSAT has certain limitations for following the original workbooks due to the fact that the workbook was based on verbal communication. Moreover, it was challenging to translate CBT principles into an art therapy protocol. Also, for certain service users who were emotionally dysregulated the task of folding paper could be difficult.

Being aware and taking notice in a compassionate, mindful manner and cultivating empathy among the group participants and providers were important principles during the art therapy sessions. Art making is genuinely based on autonomous urges to express and create, which is an essential aspect of the above-mentioned treatment models. Successful adoption of SSEOT suggests there is potential for using other expressive and creative activities as tools for trauma processing. This opens possibilities for innovative treatment approaches within the creative arts therapies realm.

Next steps: Several interning students graduated and became credentialed art therapists. They are now working as art therapists and are able to adapt these protocols to their current populations. This protocol has been used with populations who are trauma survivors, have issues of substance abuse, and/or a history of mental illness. Extending the adaptation to young adults and an ageing population will be explored next.

There is also the need to develop programme evaluations and outcome research for the different populations based on data collection and validated measures for both protocols.

Reference

Atwood, M. (2020). Q&A Margaret Atwood. *AARP/Bulletin, 61(10)*, 4.

Azarani, T. (2012). *Therapeutic applications of the origami and the creative arts in the treatment of disaster relief, trauma, and severe mental illness.* Conference presentation, APA 64th IPS, New York, 4–7 October.

Bodhi, B. (2017). *Sutta Nipata: An ancient collection of the Buddha's discourses and its canonical commentaries.* Somerville, MA: Wisdom Publications.

Bloom, S. (1997) *Creating sanctuary: Toward the evolution of sane societies.* New York: Routledge.

El-Mallakh, R. S. (2021). William A. F. Browne: Earliest documented use of rehabilitative art in Great Britain. *arttherapy: Journal of the American Art Therapy Association, 38(4)*, 205–210.

Cassone, S. (2021). Archaeologists have discovered a pristine 45,000-year-old cave painting of a pig that may be the oldest artwork in the world. *ArtNet News*, 14 January. https://news.artnet.com/art-world/indonesia-pig-art-oldest-painting-1937110.

Garrett, M. (2019). *Psychotherapy for psychosis: Integrating cognitive-behavioral and psychodynamic treatment.* New York: The Guilford Press.

Hanh, T. N. (2014). *Fear: Essential wisdom for getting through the storm.* San Francisco, CA: Harper One.

Hunter, D. (1947). *Papermaking: The history and technique of an ancient craft.* New York: Dover Publications.

Kabat-Zinn, J. (2013). *Full catastrophe living: Using the wisdom of your body and mind to face stress, pain, and illness.* New York: Random House.

Killick, K. (ed.). (2017). *Art therapy for psychosis: Theory and practise.* London: Routledge.

Kobayashi, T. (2004). *Enrichment Origami Art Therapy with the people at Lower Eastside.* Tokyo: Index Press.

Kobayashi, T. (2007). Use of origami for children with traumatic experiences. In S. L. Brooke (ed.), *The use of the creative therapies with sexual abuse survivors* (pp. 102–120). Springfield, IL: Charles C Thomas Publishing.

Kobayashi, T. (2010a). Origami on children who have experienced traumatic events, Enrichment Origami Therapy. In K. Stewart (ed.), *Music therapy & trauma, bridging theory and clinical practice* (pp. 153–173). New York: Satchnote Press.

Kobayashi, T. (2010b). *Potential of origami as therapy.* Tokyo: Seishin Shobo.

Kobayashi, T. (2019). *Brain Therapy Origami.* Tokyo, Japan: Boutique-sha.

Kobayashi, T., Chen, P.-R., Park, E. H. & Saito, T. (2007). *Syndrome specific group art therapy (SSGT) for complex PTSD patients. Conference presentation,* AATA 38th Annual Conference, Albuquerque, NM, 14–18 November.

Kramer, E. (1977). *Art therapy in a children's community.* New York: Schocken Books.

Kramer, E. (1993). *Art as therapy with children.* Chicago, IL: Magnolia Street Publishers.

Muenzenmaier, K., Schneeberger, A., Castille, D., Battaglia, J., Seixas, A., & Link, B. (2014). Stressful childhood experiences and clinical outcomes in people with serious mental illness: A gender comparison in a clinical psychiatric sample. *Journal of Family Violence, 29(4),* 419–429.

Muenzenmaier, K., Sampson, D., Norelli, L., Alexander, K., Stephens, B., Huckeba, H. (1998). *Understanding and dealing with sexual abuse trauma: An educational group for women. a manual for mental health professionals.* Albany, NY: Trauma Initiative Publication,.

Naumburg, M. (1950). *An introduction to art therapy.* New York: Teachers College Press.

Prinzhorn, H. (1995). *Artistry of the mentally ill.* Vienna, Austria: Springer-Verlag. (Original work published in German, 1922.)

Reinsbakken, M. (2017). The grandmothers. Retrieved from www.artbeatarttherapystudio.com/the-history-of-art-therapy-in-canada-too-eh/march-01st-2017.

Shelley, A.-M. (2006). *Men's trauma manual.* n.l.: Anne-Marie Shelley. Retrieved from www.lulu.com/en/en/shop/dr-anne-marie-shelley/mens-trauma-manual/paperback/product-1yvmnwe.html?page=1&pageSize=4.

15

FOLDING AND UNFOLDING

Expanding Trauma-Focused Art Therapy

Toshiko Kobayashi, Amara Clark, Eunhong Park,
Ping-Rong Chen, and Kamila Agi-Mejias

So many people in our society walk around with deep traumas. I myself have had my own traumatic experiences, both personal and intergenerational. Even before my art therapy training, I often explored and expressed my trauma in artistic form, my favourites being paintings, found-objects art, ceramic, and origami.

My Japanese upbringing was deeply influenced by Asian philosophies (e.g. Confucianism, Taoism, and Buddhism), and led me to ultimately develop Expressive Origami Therapy.

The main motivations that brought me to study art therapy had two focal points. One was to develop origami as a tool of art therapy for treating psychological trauma. The other point was my curiosity in how the body and brain work together when working creatively. As an artist I knew from my experiences that the physicality of art making is connected to my state of mind. As an art therapist I also observed that service recipients seemed to experience changes physically and mentally after attending a series of art therapy treatments. I have started to understand that art therapy can influence neuroplasticity (Hass-Cohen & Carr, 2008). After my own recovery from brain surgery, I experienced this first-hand.

I was seeking effective trauma care (treatments) pertinent to individual needs, noting that there was great diversity in the functioning levels of service users who were in different stages of recovery. My background also influenced my therapeutic relationships, particularly regarding transference and countertransference issues. Balint, a Hungarian physician and psychoanalyst, valued the relationship with his patients in his book *The Doctor, His Patient and the Illness* (Balint, 1957) rather than focusing simply on their diagnosis. This idea of 'human to human' therapeutic relationship resonated with me.

As I studied art therapy further, it appeared to me that the profession of art therapy requires consideration of cultural sensitivity

DOI: 10.4324/9781003055914-18

(Hocoy, 2002), and therefore it is important to be aware of systemic issues, biases, prejudice and racism that may be embedded in the surrounding culture of the art therapy environment. In addition, I became aware that there is a need for diversity in terms of gender (see Chapter 11) and ethnicity in the profession of art therapy itself (Yerrakadu, 2018). This led me to develop my art therapy practice based on four keywords, 'inclusive', 'culture sensitive', 'horizontal relationship', and 'gender free'. I expanded my practice following these four keywords with staff and with my art therapy students alongside service recipients.

I believe in art as therapy as Dalley's book *Art as Therapy* explores (Dalley, 1984). But another important matter is how I also understand 'art' as 'arts', which includes all forms of artistic endeavours. For instance, an example of traditional practice in Japan is the 'tea ceremony'. This ceremony includes the way tea is prepared and served, the arrangement of the room, and the performance of the host and guests. All these components are considered part of the whole art form. Additionally, I consider this practice as therapeutic and important in building connections and establishing safe relationships.

I also think that artists' movements devoted to bringing the arts and medicine closer in the western world are extremely important. McNiff's 'art as medicine' (McNiff, 1981, 1992, 2004) and Malchiodi's 'medical art therapy' (Malchiodi, 1999) are a few examples of this influence.

Attending the Trauma Committee meetings was informative and expanded my view as an art therapy supervisor. I felt that students would benefit from discussion which often involved different perspectives and viewpoints. I felt that these meetings in which there was emphasis on structure and flexibility complemented my therapeutic approach which is based on altruistic ways of living. Thus, I encouraged art therapy students to attend the meetings as well.

In order to make art therapy available to more service users I developed group sessions. I also involved art therapy students. This way we could offer a wider range of individual and group therapy sessions. Modifications to the programme were gradual and based on what we learned as we went along. Staff from different departments were involved and collaborated in this endeavour.

In the end I was very fortunate to have had the opportunity to work with and learn from service users, mental health staff, peer counsellors, and the art therapy students whom I taught. I am grateful to have been a member of the trauma committee. I started understanding trauma as a universal phenomenon that can have an impact on each of us. It can happen to anyone anytime, anywhere.

Introduction

By 2004 and after having facilitated Trauma Symptom Specific Art Therapy (TSSAT) and Symptom Specific Expressive Origami Therapy (SSEOT) (see Chapter 14) art therapy became more widely accepted as a treatment choice not only by the treatment team but also by the service users. The following year, the administration encouraged the art therapy supervisor to assign students to units that did not have art therapists available. At the same time the goals of TSSAT and SSEOT were expanded. Initially the major goals of the groups discussed in Chapter 14 were to provide information about the effects of traumatic experiences and teaching effective coping strategies. We found it was necessary to broaden aspects of our approach to adapt to service users' complex individual needs. For example, information about trauma was introduced when a member expressed concerns and/or the need to deal with trauma relevant information during group sessions verbally or in their individual artwork. The goals now focused on heightening service users' self-awareness, self-confidence, and interpersonal skills. These issues are important for individuals who have experienced both trauma and psychosis and can also improve reintegration back into the community.

The groups described in this chapter do not follow the tightly structured manual outlines that were discussed in Chapter 14. This allows for a more individualised approach and greater flexibility in the context of a group structure. In this way the differences between the art therapy sessions described in Chapters 14 and 15 are similar to the differences in music therapy sessions described in Chapters 12 and 13.

By being able to choose their preferences, service users can get involved in different therapeutic activities such as gardening and origami. These experiences can help in creating a safe environment in which individuals can express themselves and have opportunities to be heard.

Expanding and Adapting Trauma-Focused Art Therapy

In this part we highlight the most important factors to consider in the development of trauma focused art therapy groups. This serves as a contextual background for the following three sections of the chapter in which we outline our art therapy approaches and present fictionalised vignettes.

In running groups there were many practical concerns and limitations to consider: group location and length, criteria used to select participants, and number of people in the group.

Finding a Voice

Many of the service users we worked with had experienced psychosis, had been diagnosed with schizophrenia and / or schizoaffective disorder, and had also experienced traumatic events in their lives, including institutional trauma. In our programme, group dynamics, flexible individualised treatment plans and effective art therapy approaches to treat individuals with an array of complex trauma symptoms were a major focus. Often, people who have experienced a trauma have not yet articulated these circumstances. By finding a voice for an unspoken trauma in figurative expressions, art therapists can assist people *in the process of artmaking.*

Flexibility of Structure and Finding Balance

With this new way of working, we explored trauma-focused art therapy approaches by keeping many aspects of the structure seen in TSSAT and SSEOT but balancing this structure with flexibility. In this way we were able to adapt these protocols to survivors' individual needs including the current stage of treatment, physical and cognitive abilities, current outstanding symptoms, and the preference of attendees. Emphasis was placed on both group dynamics and individualised treatment goals.

Horizontal Relationships Promoting Autonomy

Another core concept of trauma care is to build mutual collaboration between participants and treatment providers, a 'horizontal relationship' (Henriques, 2013). The goal is to create an inclusive, respectful, supportive environment where group members are free to express themselves through both figurative expression and verbal communication without inhibitions. This encourages voluntary freedom of expression and autonomous artistic decisions based on a sense of self.

Promoting Free Expression and Creativity

Art making is an organic process, evoking the realm of phenomenology. We live as beings who love to learn and create.

> When we cover a piece of paper with doodles, ...or when we plant flowers in our gardens, one quality is common to all of these quite different activities, ...the need for activity, it is a final, irreducible psychological fact – an urge in man not to be absorbed passively into his environment, but to impress on it traces of his existence beyond those of purposeful activity.
>
> (Prinzhorn, 1995)

The act of interpreting ideas into visual art pieces provides a unique healing opportunity. Art making has the potential to transcend the limitations presented by verbal language (Buk, 2009). It is not always possible or desirable for group participants to follow the group directives exactly as demonstrated. While administering the TSSAT group (see Chapter 14) it was not always possible for service users to translate verbal language into artmaking. The central idea for trauma-focused art therapy is to allow for free expression. Offering opportunities for autonomous decision making and allowing for participants' requests are important aspects of recovery for trauma survivors.

Safety

A critical consideration for art therapists is to establish a safe and comfortable art therapy environment (Killick & Schaverien, 2013; Killick, 2017) that allows participants to discuss their artistic expressions with others whom they feel comfortable with. Safety includes ensuring that the art materials and tools pose no physical threat. Art therapists also provide a place where the art products are physically contained and saved safely between sessions. This allows the service user to feel safe to leave their artwork in the art therapy room. These considerations are important for increasing feelings of safety and for building trust.

Containment

Creative activities require the participation of physical, emotional and mental activation of the brain. The process of art making can feel uncomfortable, even fear-inducing. Unfamiliar projects and art materials can also be triggers. Group members may be easily triggered by the use of seemingly innocuous tools such as scissors and materials such as paint and clay. When the individual is triggered by their own art, dynamics in the group may become unpredictable. There is a necessity to provide a symbolic and physical sense of containment (Bion, 1962). Observing the group dynamics during each phase, in each new context, requires close attention which tools and materials can be used. Containment can be provided by something as simple as folding paper, outlining and/or framing the artwork. Storing individual artwork in a safe place (as mentioned above) and having the artwork available for later review, is a practice that also provides containment.

Art Therapy Process of Creating and Deconstructing

Art therapy is a process of creating and deconstructing (doing and undoing), adding and subtracting. We start each session by viewing the artwork created in prior groups. We ask group participants for their impressions and whether their art is finished or unfinished. They can decide if they want to continue working on the same piece, perhaps repainting and / or adding or subtracting images. Making art is a physical process that involves eye-hand motor coordination and fosters neuroplasticity. Doidge (2007, 2015) emphasises the potential for neuroplasticity by strengthening the neural pathways (see Chapter 1). Art therapists started to discuss the importance of strengthening the neural pathways through artmaking (Hass-Cohen & Carr, 2008, p. 30). Kobayashi (2019) suggests that the process of folding origami also can promote changes in the brain.

Open and Closed Groups

An important consideration was whether to form open or closed groups. While closed groups are important for effective trauma work, excluding members meant limiting how many individuals could receive art therapy treatment. People showed a wide range of ability and willingness to participate. Some were eager to participate in individual and/or group work, while others preferred to sit and observe the group session. An ideal closed group trauma treatment environment was not practical. As a result we began using an 'open art therapy group' approach (see below).

Engaging Individually within a Group

Due to a need to include the larger number of service users, the solution we devised was to conduct 'open studio' type art therapy groups with multiple co-leaders. This allowed clinicians to engage several participants individually within a large group setting. This approach was necessary due to the diverse functioning levels of group members. All therapists needed to be prepared for unexpected personal requests, behaviour changes triggered by the artmaking, and direct discussions of traumatic experiences that might have the potential to trigger other service users. The multi co-leader 'open studio' type art therapy group was a strategy that allowed us to establish a mutually inclusive treatment environment with limited resources and provide more consistency.

Cultural & Personal Reflections

The individual therapist's understanding and perspective matter a great deal. Individually, service users and service providers have their own cultural background and they carry unconscious biases. Judith Rubin (1987), one of the early developers of art therapy as a formalised therapeutic intervention, named one of her art therapy documentary films, *Art Therapy Has Many Faces* (2008). In fact, art therapy has as many faces as the number of art therapists who implement it. Each art therapist brings their own training, approach, and practices, as well as their own cultural and personal understandings. At the same time, each recipient has their own unique life experience that brings them to therapy encounters. It is important to recognise that the assumptions we make about art and psychological growth are also "culture bound" (Hocoy, 2002, p. 141).

In terms of expanding cross-cultural communication, McNiff emphasises "The specific art object is a tangible meeting point" (McNiff & Barlow, 2009, p. 105). The art therapy supervisor and the trauma committee invited a diverse group of art therapy students to bring their cultural and personal backgrounds into their experiences of learning and providing art therapy. It was important for therapists to be aware of the diverse population in an urban public institution, e.g. immigrants, refugees, and socio economically challenged populations. Our aim was to develop an empowering environment for the diverse service users and create a non-judgmental and non-threatening therapeutic milieu (Hoffman, 1982). Art therapists were making continuous efforts to be aware of their own biases regarding images, colours, and situations and to be open to different expressions in the art of service users.

Inclusive & Cross-disciplinary Approaches

In addition to the collaboration of the art therapy supervisor and art therapy students we welcomed the participation that was provided at times from psychiatrists, psychologists, social workers, nursing staff, peer counsellors as well as other creative arts therapists. In order to provide art therapy treatment effectively, it was necessary to increase the amount of 'helping hands' with art projects. Kramer (1986) referred to as the 'third hand' was a useful concept which was integrated beyond art therapy. At the same time, this contributed to mutual understanding and respect, creating a basis for developing more secure and inclusive relationships. Creating this effective therapeutic milieu for service users and providers was indispensable.

Art Therapy Group

In the following section we present one art therapy student's staff box and four fictionalised vignettes that demonstrate the way in which we worked. We show how the emphasis throughout is on the importance of developing a safe and trusting connection between service users and therapists. In order to expand the reach of trauma care to treating individuals with a range of life experiences, including survivors from the prison system, we found it valuable to use a variety of media (e.g. gardening, origami) reflecting service users' preferences.

Developing Communication and Visual Language through Artmaking

The group started out as a temporary open studio art therapy group and later developed into a closed group. Some group members who were people of colour described traumatic experiences related to racism both outside and inside institutions. Individuals' complex and multi-layered experiences of trauma also included incarceration, long term hospitalisation, and childhood trauma. As we grappled with attempting to establish a sense of safety with sensitivity to our potential role in ongoing dynamics of power and oppression, we utilised art to provide structure, direction, and containment while we sought to inhabit a collaborative role with group members.

Several group members had a history of visual art making (Toledo Museum of Art, 2022; Malissa, 2011) and began to attend regularly. Some described how experiences of trauma increased mental confusion and made it difficult to differentiate between paranoia and a real need for self-protection. Participants struggled with anxiety, paranoia, hyper-vigilance, and loneliness and had difficulty socialising and relating to others. Group members' past experiences with art allowed for discussion of a positive shared identity but also a sense that past creative endeavours now felt out of reach. Some of their memories were of artwork being judged, lost, or minimised and this initially seemed to impact participants' ability to feel comfortable using art to connect to self and others. Due to the group members' interest in developing their artistic skills, the group began to centre around directives that introduced new art materials and / or techniques each week.

In an early session, group members were given options of photos of animals to choose from and were asked to draw an environment for the animal with everything the animal might need. Kendal, who prior to the group had been disengaged and was sleeping in an isolated chair, started to express himself verbally and elaborated in detail about his picture… He drew a den for his wolf in an isolated forest with several protective structures around it. It was noted that Kendal and several of the participants were communicating verbally about their art, when historically they had had great difficulty participating in verbal therapy groups, at times sleeping, described as responding with delusions to prompts, or becoming agitated by questions. Many had also been described as isolated and unwilling to engage with treatment providers outside the art therapy group.

One group member, Luis, seemed initially hesitant and unsure how to start projects, standing and swaying in the room rather than sitting down right away. In addition to being diagnosed with schizophrenia, he had had many experiences of trauma throughout his life. He very rarely spoke and at times it was difficult to understand his verbal communications. When pastels were introduced, Luis seemed very interested and began to draw spontaneous loose scribbles, talking to himself, singing, and then becoming agitated and vocalising loudly. An art therapy student placed several small pieces of pre-cut thick paper *on the table next to Luis, and he began to use one small shape after another quickly, creating a pile of small pastel drawings, and seemingly calming down enough to focus on his artwork.*

Group members expressed discomfort and fear toward more regressive art materials, such as paint, and processes that were less structured such as free drawing or when offered multiple choices of materials. There was a consensus among the members that structured directives were preferred, possibly because these directives promoted a feeling of safety. The group members took on a significant role in deciding the continued format of the sessions in ongoing reviews of the group experience facilitated by the art therapy students.

The theme of group safety continued to be discussed, especially in regard to the felt danger of exploring images. Jordan drew images of devils which he spoke about at length in the group. Knowing this was an image that individuals may associate to in a variety of ways, some of which may feel triggering or flooding, the art therapy students struggled to find a way to allow for both expression and containment for Jordan and his fellow group members. After meeting with the art therapy supervisor, the art therapy students introduced a more structured group discussion about the strength of certain symbolic images, acknowledging the likelihood of both widely recognised and subjective meanings. The discussion also focused on letting the group members know that the art therapy students may pause discussions to check in with everybody regarding how safe each member felt. Participants were able to share their reactions to Jordan's drawings which seemed to help Jordan to gain a new awareness that each person had different reactions to his art.

Over time group members became increasingly engaged with one another. In one session the art therapy students handed out small containers filled with cut out words for "word collages". Group members sifted through the words while chatting. When Kendal picked up the word "sorrow", he nudged the person next to him, Darren, and indicated that Darren may want to use this word. Darren quickly responded "No, that word does not fit into my picture". Kendal examined the word for a long time, looking at his partially formed collage of words glued down to his paper and then back at the word, and then quietly glued down the word "sorrow", where it immediately became a part of a larger picture. With collage, Kendal was able to separate and interact with a symbol, a word with meaning, using it possibly in a humorous way, to interact with a peer, and then test it out in his picture before deciding to accept it as an integral part of his whole artwork. This allowed for taking physical action, symbolic play, contextualising, and creating a concrete form in which Kendal could observe his thinking.

As the group was ending, a collaborative art project was planned for the last few sessions. Group members decided they would rather continue to go back to their portfolios to finish and organise their individual artworks instead, a process we had set aside time for mid-group. This suggests that the group members wanted to protect the space they had opened for their individual processes and maintain the sense of balance they had worked hard to find between being together and working individually. Luis chose a large piece of black construction paper and with assistance glued down several small pastel drawings of various shapes and colours. The image transformed from a pile of loosely drawn energetic abstract drawings to an organised, curated, dynamic picture that framed what appeared to be several different states that Luis had been in during the group.

The psychiatrist and music therapist observed the group on several occasions and noted how group members used art therapy to decrease isolation, access motivation, and to articulate and share their internal experiences. The biggest changes in group members' behaviour seemed to be a new willingness to share thoughts and feelings with each other, increased interest in each other's perspectives, as well as an increased willingness to try new materials and ways of creating. Specific behavioural changes included group members acknowledging that another person was speaking, offering feedback and supportive comments about one another's art, verbalising curiosity about narrative, image, materials, intention, or process, and asking questions that implied interest in getting to know one another. Most of these conversations started with conversation about their art and art making and oftentimes stayed within the metaphor. We attributed behavioural changes in group members to feeling empowered, sharing a group identity, and having a positive experience of connection.

Expressive Origami Therapy

The following section consists of written narratives by several art therapy students. Many of the students came from Asia and had previous origami experiences. They collaborated with other Asian staff (e.g. nurses, recreational therapist, and peer counsellors) who also had familiarity with origami. Growing demand for creative arts therapies included a trauma-focused programme using origami as a primary medium in the outpatient treatment programmes (see Chapter 9). The interdisciplinary collaborative work, which had been started in the inpatient services, was now requested by service users who previously had participated in the SSEOT on the inpatient units.

One of the students describes how the origami treatment impacted the service users in the following staff box.

241

I have been familiar with origami since my childhood back home in South Korea. I was happy to find an art therapy internship under the supervision of an art therapist who founded Expressive Origami Therapy. I was interested in observing the level of anxiety in traditional art vs origami sessions because I saw how origami was like a bridge between the participants and art therapists to open conversation and develop rapport through the step-by-step folding process. The participants seemed to feel accomplished during the process of creating various origami models. Origami offers a less threatening hands-on approach to participants who are not familiar with drawing, painting and other art processes (Kobayashi, 2007). Step-by-step origami directives seemed easy to follow, and less inhibiting for the participants.

I made eye contact with each group member, checked how they folded, and observed the group process. When compared to the traditional art therapy group there was significantly more eye contact with me while folding an origami model. This eye contact seemed so important and reminded me of a child wanting to get confirmation from his/her mother whether they were on the right path or not, such as "am I doing good?", "am I doing right?", or "I do not know what to do". Once participants got feedback they moved to the next step. These concrete, step by step tasks appealed to them while creating three-dimensional origami objects. This process seemed to increase the relational bonds within the origami group and decrease the level of anxiety. This was in contrast to behaviours in the community room where interactions and personal communications were limited or non-existent. It is possible that severe trauma affected the formation of core trust relationships in their childhood (Winnicott, 1989, 1953).

Two fictionalised vignettes are presented below. Both vignettes are based on observations by former art therapy students while facilitating the innovative trauma-focused Expressive Origami Therapy group (Kobayashi, 2004, 2010a, 2010b).

The first vignette describes how one participant who appeared to be disconnected and isolated, became more interpersonally connected.

One morning, Dan approached and greeted me in an extremely robotic manner. Although he was looking at me and saying hello to me, he seemed distant, possibly dissociated, speaking in a monotonous voice, and scratching his head. I was somewhat scared by him. Outside of the group I observed him walking around talking to himself. After a few weeks when I met Dan again in the origami group, I was surprised to see that he could clearly follow the instructions of each step. It seemed that origami, a highly predictable and structured art activity, was able to ground him (Kobayashi, 2007; Malchiodi, 2016). As time went on, I noticed Dan was a regular participant in art therapy groups.

In one session, Dan asked me to demonstrate a boat. I thought it would be a positive experience for both of us, but it was completely the opposite. After following all the steps, Dan realised the origami boat I taught was not the boat that he had inferred at the beginning. He became furious. I invited him to describe more about the shape of the boat which he had in mind. He refused, saying it was all my fault that he couldn't have the boat. If I couldn't understand Dan's needs intuitively without any communications, I would become a bad person in his view. A few weeks later, I discovered the origami boat Dan was thinking about was a Japanese boat which another art therapist had folded in a past session. The next time Dan attended the group, I presented him with the Japanese boat and invited him to fold the boat again. During this process, he accepted help with the most fragile step to prevent his origami boat being torn accidentally. At the end, he appeared satisfied with the outcome.

Another time, in an open studio group, when I passed by Dan's table, we had a small discussion about his human figure drawing, when he suddenly pointed out my blonde hair which was different from his

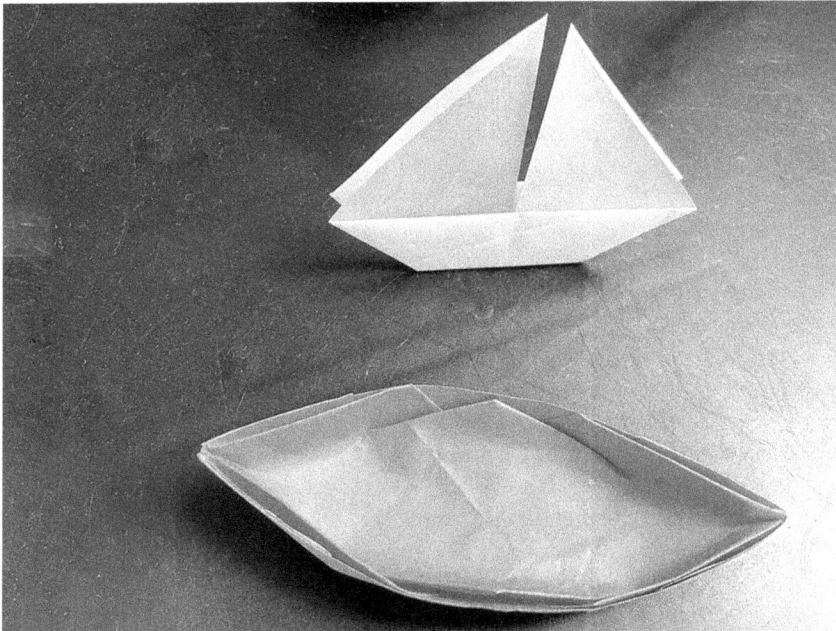

Figure 15.1. Photo of the two types of origami boats.

hair colour. He said "it's beautiful." His tone of voice sounded like it was his first time seeing me and realising that I had blonde hair. I realised that perhaps before this he only saw pieces of me, like a part of my face or a finger, not my entire person, even though I had worked with him one to two times a week for several months. As Dan developed a more mature and sound connection with me; he seemed to have a more integrated image of me.

There was a need to initiate origami therapy groups for outpatients who found it difficult to attend verbal groups. Many of the service users had trauma histories and many spent their time sitting alone. The following vignette describes how group members are beginning to connect and collaborate with each other.

I co-led the newly formed, trauma-focused origami therapy group with a member of staff. The staff member was not only familiar with origami but also knew the service users well. After a month a core group of participants had been formed.

When the group participants were getting more comfortable with origami, a variation of origami known as 'kirigami' was introduced. Kirigami involves a combination of folding and cutting (see Figure 15.2).

At the beginning, the participants seemed hesitant to try kirigami. To encourage their active participation, I demonstrated the steps of creating a piece of kirigami, first. Then, the participants were invited to make one cut on their folded paper then passed the paper to the person next to them. In this round robin approach, each participant made small but consecutive contributions to build the entire, unexpected patterns on the paper at the end. The approach appeared effective in developing trust and creating connections between group members. While cutting shapes they seemed to enjoy the process and were excited to see the outcomes. Eventually, all of them acquired the basic skills of creating kirigami. Most importantly, they had obtained the capacity to observe each other's artworks and then reintegrate some elements into their new creations. I witnessed how the participants gradually developed the identity of an artist and were able to share their unique artworks with each other. After most of the group members had mastered the steps to create kirigami, they started to show their willingness to collaboratively create a collage, using pieces of kirigami. The group seemed to become a great opportunity for them to practise their interpersonal skills and to have a better sense of their own abilities. By the end of the year, the kirigami collage was finished, and the group was hoping to exhibit it. Despite the challenges they had faced during the group process most participants expressed positive feelings about the group which appeared to also remain with them afterwards.

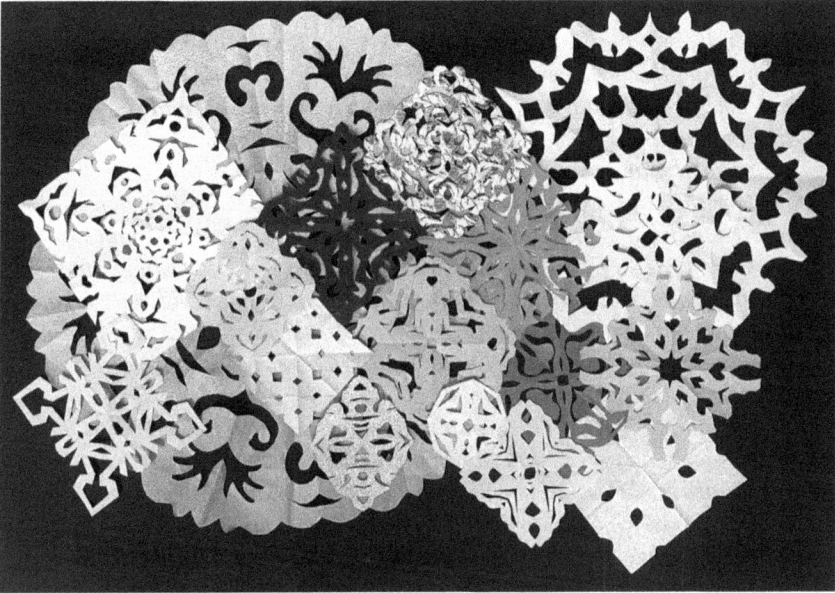

Figure 15.2. A replicated kirigami collage.

Gardening as an Art Form

This fictionalised vignette describes one of the groups that was part of an art therapy pilot programme comparing traditional art therapy with art therapy incorporating gardening. Working with a group of male and female survivors who were not cooperative with most of the programmes on the unit was quite challenging. To collaborate with other staff members was always an important part of the learning process for all art therapy students.

Preliminary Reflection

I was interested in demonstrating that art therapy is an effective treatment modality as it is usually applied, and to see if adding a gardening component would enhance the positive results, and if so, by how much. The two groups consisted of adults between the ages of 18 and 60 who were diagnosed with psychotic disorders most of whom had experienced traumatic life events. Each participant was given a programme evaluation before and after (Silver, 2002).

I decided to look further into gardening when one day someone whom I highly respected mentioned that working with the soil and plants was healing because they are literally the material of our own bodies. This resonated powerfully for me and led me deeper into seeking to combine creative healing processes. I discovered that horticultural therapy was a modality proven to be effective in helping a variety of groups, especially traumatised populations like war veterans and the elderly with dementia (Poulsen et al., 2016).

I discussed this idea with my art therapy supervisor, and she mentioned that there was a time when gardening was part of the programme at many psychiatric institutions.

Over the course of six weeks, my 'art therapy as usual' group was offered materials for painting, drawing, and origami projects and support as needed in an open studio style setting. The gardening study group was offered plastic containers as planters, planting soil, various plants including living marigolds, ferns, various flower seeds such as sunflower and pumpkin, and art materials such as popsicle sticks, plastic figures, coloured foam sheets, stickers, paper for origami additions and markers. The group was instructed how to work with the living plants and seeds and shown images of possible ways to decorate their gardens. Possible suggestions were to create mini amusement parks, gnome villages or mini formal type settings. Everyone participated as suggested. At the end of the series of sessions participants who attended the gardening/art therapy group showed slightly higher ratings in self-esteem and cognition than group members who did art therapy as usual.

Rachel

Rachel, who was extremely disruptive prior to attending the group, was initially discouraged from participating because of her tendency to act out physically and verbally. I was informed that she was not a violent person, but other service users sometimes became aggressive toward her due to their finding her loud behaviour annoying. I tried to dissuade her, but she really wanted to be given a chance to attend.

Surprisingly Rachel followed all instructions, was calm even during the mindfulness relaxation exercise at the beginning of each session, attended all sessions and completed the six-week group. She was pleasant, even extending suggestions and conversing with the other group members in an appropriate manner, which was not her usual behaviour. Her gardening container was one of the most creative. Rachel's container was neat, and she added drawings of a ferris wheel, a carousel and characters. She planted everything without damaging stems and other fragile items. During the group sessions Rachel appeared calmer in, and reportedly outside of, the group.

Summary

The conclusions that I drew are my own anecdotal observations and include the following: Rachel was possibly drawn to participate with this art therapy group for several reasons, perhaps because she had recognised that art therapy groups were different from the normal daily activities, were fun, creative, or calming. Perhaps she over-heard that it had something involving gardening. I had misjudged Rachel as being unable to participate. In fact, she demonstrated the effectiveness of art therapy combined with gardening. One of the most important conclusions was that gardening combined with art therapy had a calming effect on Rachel, something that research suggested might be possible (Clatworthy et al., 2013). I believe that she and the other group members responded well for many reasons, including group rapport, consistency, and relaxing effect by working creatively and with living plant materials. The sense of connection in the group was strong. Watching the tiny seeds sprouting and the living gardens flourishing during the six weeks was seemingly small and yet, I believe, was recognised by all as representing something so much bigger.

Conclusion

In this chapter we have attempted to capture a few examples from our process of expanding a more structured art therapy model (see Chapter 14) to a more flexible and individually focused art therapy approach. One of the important lessons we learned is that active participation and engagement are essential to the process of recovery. To encourage participation, we continued to look for various ways to motivate participants. Many group members showed positive responses to the various media and art therapy interventions including drawing, painting, collage, clay modelling, origami, gardening, crocheting, and other art directives, in both individual and group therapies.

Another lesson we learned is that all participants of art therapy sessions are regarded as artists. As artists, art therapists understand how important the creative process is and its relationship to the artwork. The same is true for service users. One key principle in art therapy is to respect service users and their artwork. This includes not only to recognise and honour their work but also to acknowledge their artmaking process. By creating a safe environment that encourages service users to make use of tangible concrete objects as 'art' they have the opportunity to use symbolism and metaphor to express themselves more fully.

Some of the outcomes for service users included an increased ability for self-expression and making their needs known. Moreover, we saw a decrease of emotional and behavioural outbursts, improvement in relational/interpersonal skills, and enhanced overall ability to participate in treatment. These changes were observed for service users who had attended individual and/or group art therapy sessions, whether in inpatient and /or outpatient settings. These gains also seemed to extend outside of the art therapy groups and were reflected in the ability to develop connections with therapists and peers.

It is important to note some challenges and limitations of inpatient group therapy particularly in public service settings (Yalom, 1995, pp. 449–480). Time limitations and the level of training of therapists, as well as the needs of service users, had to be addressed including the importance of additional supports on the units and during transitions (ibid.). Moreover, since service users may not return to subsequent group sessions due to discharge / decompensation or a voluntary decision not to return, Yalom emphasises the importance of short-term goals for each session (ibid). In our groups we realised that the attention given to each individual is limited and may not be sufficient. This included possible difficulties in accommodating different interests in the choice of creative expressions of each service user.

Being at different stages of recovery required specific assessments for each art therapy technique. We tried to overcome these limitations with the additional help from art therapy students. All students were closely supervised by an experienced credentialed art therapist. This way we were able to accommodate the needs of each service user and extended our outreach and follow up. We also encouraged participants to work more independently which was one of the goals of our creative arts therapies.

In addition, we prioritised time to be set aside for the group leaders after each art therapy group so we could reflect on the process of each session. When time permitted, the programme was additionally reviewed during the weekly creative arts therapies' meetings. Despite the many challenges, it was an exciting time for service users and therapists to work together innovatively.

References

American Art Therapy Association. (2017). About the art therapy association. Retrieved from https://arttherapy.org/about.

Balint, M. (1957). *The doctor, his patient and the illness*. New York: International University Press.

Bion, W. R. (1962). *Learning from Experience*. London: Heinemann.

Buk, A. (2009). The mirror neuron system and embodied simulation: Clinical implications for art therapists working with trauma survivors. *The Arts in Psychotherapy, 36(2)*, 61–74.

Clatworthy, J., Hinds, J., & Camic, P. (2013). Gardening as a mental health intervention: A review. *Mental Health Review, 18(4)*, 214–225.

Dalley, T. (ed.). (1984). *Art as therapy: An introduction to the use of art as a therapeutic technique.* London: Tavistock/Routledge.

Doidge, N. (2007). *The brain that changes itself: Stories of personal triumph from the frontiers of brain science.* London: Penguin.

Doidge, N. (2015). *The brain's way of healing: Remarkable discoveries and recoveries from the frontiers of neuroplasticity.* London: Penguin.

Hass-Cohen, N., & Carr, R. (2008). *Art therapy and clinical neuroscience.* London: Jessica Kingsley.

Henriques, G. (2013). Vertical and horizontal integration in psychotherapy Making sense of integration in psychotherapy. Retrieved from www.psychologytoday.com/us/blog/theory-knowledge/201308/vertical-and-horizontal-integration-in-psychotherapy.

Hocoy, D. (2002). Cross-cultural issues in art therapy. *Art Therapy, 19(4),* 141–145.

Hoffman L. (1982) An historical overview of milieu therapy. In L. Hoffman (ed.), *The evaluation and care of severely disturbed children and their families.* Dordrecht: Springer.

Killick, K. (2017). *Art therapy for psychosis: theory and practice.* London: Routledge.

Killick, K., & Schaverien, J. (eds). (2013). *Art, psychotherapy and psychosis.* London: Routledge.

Kobayashi, T. (2004). *Enrichment Origami Art Therapy with the people at Lower Eastside.* Tokyo: Index Press.

Kobayashi, T. (2007). Use of origami for children with traumatic experiences. In S. Brooke, (ed.), *The use of the creative therapies with sexual abuse survivors* (pp. 102–199), Springfield, IL: Charles C. Thomas.

Kobayashi, T. (2010a). Origami on children who have experienced traumatic events, Enrichment Origami Therapy. In K. Stewart (ed.), *Music therapy & trauma, bridging theory and clinical practice* (pp. 153–173). New York: Satchnote Press.

Kobayashi, T. (2010b). Potential of origami as therapy. *Seishin Preview 107.* Tokyo: Seishin Shobo.

Kobayashi, T. (2019). *Brain therapy origami.* Tokyo: Boutique-sha.

Kramer, E. (1986). The art therapist's third hand: Reflections on art, art therapy, and society at large. *American Journal of Art Therapy, 24(3),* 71–86.

Malchiodi, C. (1999). *Medical art therapy with adults.* London: Jessica Kingsley.

Malchiodi, C. (2016). Expressive arts therapy and self-regulation. Retrieved from www.psychologytoday.com/us/blog/arts-and-health/201603/expressive-arts-therapy-and-self-regulation.

Malissa, M. (2011). Signs and symbols: Art and language in art therapy. *Journal of Clinical Art Therapy, 1(4),* 25–32.

McNiff, S. (1981). *The arts and psychotherapy.* Springfield, IL: Charles C. Thomas.

McNiff, S. (1992). *Art as medicine: Creating a therapy of the imagination,* 1st edition. Boulder, CO: Shambhala.

McNiff, S. (2004). *Art heals: How creativity cures the soul.* Boulder, CO: Shambhala.

McNiff, S., & Barlow, G. C. (2009). Cross-cultural psychotherapy and art. *Art Therapy, 26(3),* 100–106.

Poulsen, D. V., Stigsdotter, U. K., & Djernis, D. (2016). 'Everything just seems much more right in nature': How veterans with post-traumatic stress disorder experience nature-based activities in a forest therapy garden. *Health Psychology Open, 3(1).*

Prinzhorn, H. (1995). *Artistry of the mentally ill*. Vienna, Austria: Springer-Verlag. (Original work published in German, 1922.)

Rubin, J. A. (ed.). (1987). *Approaches to art therapy: Theory and technique*. New York: Brunner/Mazel.

Rubin, J. A. (2008). *Art therapy has many faces*. DVD. Pittsburgh, PA: Expressive Media.

Silver, R. A. (2002). *Three art assessments: the silver drawing test of cognition and emotion, draw a story, screening for depression, and stimulus drawings and techniques*. New York: Brunner-Routledge.

Toledo Museum of Art. (2022). What is visual language? Retrieved from www.toledomuseum.org/education/visual-literacy/what-visual-language.

Winnicott, D. W. (1989) Mirror-role of mother and family in child development. In D. W. Winnicott, *Playing and reality* (pp. 11–118), New York: Routledge.

Winnicott, D. W. (1953). Transitional objects and transitional phenomena – A study of the first not-me possession. *International Journal of Psycho-Analysis, 34*, 89–97.

Yalom, I. (1995) *The theory and practice of group psychotherapy*. New York: Basic Books.

Yerrakadu, C. (2018). Survey of research in multiculturalism in expressive therapies. Retrieved from https://digitalcommons.lesley.edu/cgi/viewcontent.cgi?article=1104&context=expressive_t.

16

TRAUMA INFORMED DANCE/ MOVEMENT THERAPY

Embodied Moving and Dancing

Kelly Long

When I started working at the facility in 2013, I was the only dance/ movement therapist in the building. Many service users expressed disinterest in joining dance/movement therapy groups, and often I was alone in my group room. It was important for me to find subtle ways to encourage movement, like synchronous walking together around the unit or simply playing catch with a stress ball. Once people started moving, they started to express how they felt better and more alert. Over time and with encouragement, people began to expand their movement into expressive dance. By attending the trauma committee, I was able to share ideas and perspectives with clinicians from other disciplines and feel their support for me as a novice therapist.

One of my favourite dance/movement therapy groups consisted of three men, all of various ethnicities, ages, and diagnoses who had experienced stressful experiences in their lives. All three men initially expressed hesitation to join a dance group, fearful of the stigma of being part of a group that one group member perceived as "feminine". One man told me candidly "But I can't dance" when invited to join our group. In time, however, this group became such a supportive and cohesive place of belonging. It was as if we had created our own family. Over time we developed our own family traditions and routines. Once a week we'd meet on the Unit, travel to our group space together, dance, and share snacks. Each group member had their own role-setting up the chairs, handing out the drinks, collecting the garbage at the end of the group, and so forth. It was surprising to me how much trust was developed and how willing these men were to try new things week after week.

DOI: 10.4324/9781003055914-19

Dance/Movement Therapy Techniques
for Trauma Survivors

A living, breathing, ephemeral art form, dance is and always has been a universal language and means of self-expression. Before a human being talks, she moves. From infancy through childhood, human beings learn to master various movements. For example, an infant moves her mouth in a sucking motion and soon acquires the ability to feed. As she grows and develops so too do her movements, as she later learns to grab and hold food to eat. Some months later she further develops her fine motor skills and learns to hold utensils. This movement progresses into the ability to cut her own food, and so on. In the matter of a few years, she now has an entire movement repertoire of latching, biting, grabbing, holding, and intentionally shaping the way she gets one of her most basic biological needs met: eating. These movements not only enable her to survive, but also enable her to develop a sense of mastery, of independence, and of control.

Individuals who have endured complex trauma often lack a sense of mastery of their environment and of their life. Survivors often struggle to feel in control of their lives or of themselves. Trauma itself is an example of a profound loss of control. In complex trauma survivors,

> Symptoms are viewed as the result of adaptive efforts that have gone awry, in which the individual does not have sufficient resources to respond to the trauma stressor ... or to renew adaptive processes ... Moreover, effective responses to traumatic stressors lead to emphasis in particular responses, particularly those related to heightened arousal, narrowing of attentional resources, constriction of emotional and bodily experience to fight, flee, avoid, or defend against the trauma.
>
> (Courtois, Ford, & Cloitre, 2009, p. 85)

In an article about dance/movement therapists who facilitate groups for women incest survivors, one group leader notes "there was a need to develop a balance between 'control with choice'" (Ambra, 1995, p. 19). Movement is a practice and language that offers a way to restore, repair, and rejuvenate a person's sense of self. Movement can empower a person and help to integrate the fragmented elements of a survivor's experience. Dance/movement therapy (DMT) is a process focused on helping a person "regain a sense of wholeness by experiencing the fundamental unity of body, mind, and spirit" (Levy, 2005, p. 1). DMT is a discipline of the field of creative arts therapies that uses a combination of both verbal and non-verbal techniques to help a person heal, cope, and grow. Some techniques used specifically with survivors of complex PTSD include mirroring, grounding, the use of rhythm, metaphor, and focus on embodiment.

Simply put, mirroring is the empathic reflection of another. In DMT mirroring looks like the therapist matching the movement of the person. For example, if an individual raises her arm to the side, the therapist does the same in an effort to move as a mirror image. However, mirroring is far more nuanced than mocking or copying another. Mirroring is non-judgmental.

> In Chacian[1] dance therapy, you mirror the patients' movements. Mirroring, which may occur as part of the empathy process, involves participating in another's total movement experience, i.e., patterns, qualities, emotional tone, etc. Mirroring is often the first step in establishing empathic connections, particularly with patients who are unresponsive to other modes of interpersonal exchange.
>
> (Sandel, Chaiklin, & Lohn, 1993, p. 100)

Mirroring affords a person an opportunity to be witnessed, joined in her movement experience, and empathised with on a kinaesthetic level. Survivors of complex trauma often feel isolated and alone in their pain. Through being mirrored a person is no longer alone. In her article *Embodied Concepts of Neurobiology in Dance/Movement Therapy Practice*, Homann (2010) provides an overview of the discovery of mirror neurons, and offers language dance/movement therapists can use to articulate the value of mirroring in their work. She writes:

> We are constantly in relationship, adjusting our responses to others based on our sense of what is happening in the minds of those with whom we are in relationship. This capacity for empathy provides the foundation for attachment and interrelationship throughout life ... Our capacity for empathy appears to be anchored in our mirror neuron system.
>
> (Homann, 2010, p. 89)

In DMT, mirroring also enables the clinician to gain a greater understanding of a survivor's experience. To see a survivor stiff, fists clenched, twisted in her torso, head hanging forward is an entirely different experience from embodying that posture and moving in it.

> The task of the therapist [is] to constantly mirror in movement and in words what is being seen, and sensed in the movement behavior ... Then, the therapists match perceptions ... primarily through the process of focusing, facilitating an integration of words, emotions, and physical phenomena within the individual; an integration of the intellectual (neomammalian brain), the emotional (limbic or

---

1   Marion Chace, pioneer in dance/movement therapy.

paleomammalian brain), and the physiological (reptilian brain) aspects of the self.

(Chambliss, 1982, p. 26)

Wilhelm Reich (1990) wrote of the concept of "body armor" in his description of how a person's physical shape shifts as an intrinsic defence based on past trauma. By reflecting a survivor's body, a clinician gains an invaluable depth of understanding of that person's lived experience in the here-and-now, as well as insight into her past traumatic experiences that have shaped and altered her body. Movement and mirroring are the vehicle by which a rich and strong alliance between survivor and therapist can begin to form.

Grounding is an essential skill to teach trauma survivors. Grounding can be described as one's "ability to perceive and live in the here and now, and to [one's] contact with the ground" (Meekums, 2002, pp. 64–65). Some of the most effective grounding techniques incorporate the body. Chewing gum, holding an ice cube, washing hands or showering, snapping a rubber band on a wrist, holding something heavy, or simply planting one's feet firmly into the ground are all examples of grounding techniques directly involving the body. In a DMT group, grounding can be achieved in a variety of ways. Self-touch is a simple tool to help a person feel alive in the here and now. Tapping one's lap with her hands, clapping, squeezing and releasing fists or hands, massaging and offering self-soothing rubbing on a scalp, sternum or lower back are all quick, easy ways movement can be used to ground.

Another example is to tap one's toes one at a time, right and left. Tapping while being mindful of the toes inside the shoes, the tightening and releasing of one's lower leg muscles, and the shift of weight from the heel to the entire foot is a simple movement a group can collectively practise together. To tap in sync to the rhythm of a song or to the collective rhythm a group creates together is a powerful way to achieve a sense of connection. Trauma survivors often struggle to match others' rhythms, as they are often dissociated or disconnected from their own body (Ogden et al., 2006). For some, achieving synchronous toe taps to other people is a huge achievement and offers a sense of mastery. In DMT sessions it is often a goal to achieve rhythmic group movement because

> Rhythmic action in unison with others results in a feeling of well-being, relaxation and good fellowship. Even primitive man understood that a group of people moving together gained a feeling of more strength and security than anyone individual could feel alone.
>
> (Levy, 2005, p. 196)

Subsequently, DMT sessions often encourage clients to step in rhythm, clap, snap, or tap various body parts. Even brief moments of audible synchronicity can achieve this sense of strength and security.

254

DMT sessions often utilise metaphor and imagery to facilitate a healing process. For example, dancing with arms stretched out to the side while moving up and down can develop into an image verbalised by the therapist such as a bird. After feeling one's wings extend out and contract in the therapist might encourage the client to explore what it feels like to fly. What does it mean to be able to escape and fly away? What does it mean to be able to see what is happening below from a safe space above? What does it mean to have freedom to fly anywhere you choose to go? What kind of bird are you – a colourful one? A bird who sings or talks? A bird who dives into the sea? Are you a regal majestic eagle, or a tiny fast hummingbird? Are you a woodpecker able to create a safe space for yourself to burrow into and hide? Moving through these types of questions and physically embodying the associated feelings are an enriching part of the therapeutic DMT process. Moving via metaphor enables a trauma survivor to have a corrective experience and reinstates a sense of control.

When metaphor and imagery are shared among a group, the group can achieve a shared experience and sense of belonging:

> Dance/Movement Therapists have a unique perspective when working with victims exposed to traumatic environments...therapeutic approaches that work with the body provide new avenues through assisting victims (of trauma) through a simultaneously physical and metaphorical process.
>
> (Devereaux, 2008, p. 69)

By creating a shared experience that group members actively choose to participate in via dance and movement, a survivor can develop close bonds and sense of safety. Mirroring one another's movements offers an opportunity for shared empathy for each individual as well as for the entire group. Many groups don't mirror at all, but instead dance freely together in ways that elicit joy, fun, and a sense of community. This is a corrective, healing experience for a survivor who may feel depressed, afraid, and isolated.

In my experience I have observed DMT reduce a variety of challenging symptoms commonly experienced by trauma survivors such as auditory hallucinations, visual hallucinations, or flashbacks. When people are dancing and moving together, they express feeling alive. They are involved in a physical process that calls for one to focus on the present moment. When a person is dancing with others, she is both expressing herself and observing others simultaneously. Many group members have reported a reduction of auditory or visual hallucinations while participating in a DMT session. For survivors unable to verbalise or articulate changes in symptoms, a reduction of their symptoms has been clearly observed by a decrease in their talking out loud in response to internal stimuli, by increased eye contact, and/or by a group member responding to verbal instructions or cues she isn't able to commonly hear or respond to. Dancing and moving with eyes open encourages a survivor to be present in both mind and body. In doing so, survivors have reported flashbacks rarely if ever occur during sessions. Group members have also reported a reduction of flashbacks experienced after DMT group or individual sessions.

The Three Step Process

At our facility around 2014, a specialised DMT group process developed after the dance/movement therapist participated in the multidisciplinary trauma committee. Some survivors participating in DMT also participated in art therapy, music therapy, or specialised hybrid creative arts and verbal therapy groups. Discussing how to address the needs of these service users and learning about interventions used in other modalities facilitated a deepened understanding of who the group participants were as multifaceted persons. Trauma committee discussions also enabled clinicians to better understand their own countertransference and resistance, while also helping them to feel supported in their experience of both. By gaining a more holistic understanding of both the group members and themselves, dance/movement therapists can begin to take calculated risks within the group and to experiment in the structure of the sessions. Ultimately a new way to meet the collective group needs of some of the most severely traumatised and profoundly unwell service users can be discovered.

Step 1: Building Safe Connections

People who have been severely traumatised are not always willing to sit in a circle, or to sit in a chair at all. Many times DMT sessions began with a few participants sitting around the perimeter of the room, some standing, one person looking out the window, and another pacing in and out struggling to stay in the room at all. As DMT pioneer Marian Chace would recommend, to truly meet each client where she was, it was acceptable for clients to choose to come and go during sessions (Sandel, Chaiklin, & Lohn, 1993). This was established as a group rule and reviewed with each client individually before the start of the session. It was also okay for clients to choose to only watch, to sleep, read a magazine, or to dance in their own way. A goal of these sessions was to establish a safe place where clients felt comfortable and accepted, regardless of their current limitations or symptoms. It was important to honour this and offer praise for merely being in the room. In writing about some of her sessions with people with serious mental illness at St. Elizabeth's hospital, Chace wrote:

> Even passive participation of watching seems to be more active than one realizes, because many patients respond to the rhythmic

action that they are seeing and the rhythmic sound that they are hearing. One day after Miss X had watched the rhythmic circle for some weeks she finally participated actively. I made the error of telling her that I was happy she could now be with us. She was very hurt and asked me if I had failed to recognize her ... I have been (watching) for weeks. I am stronger now, that is all.

(Sandel, Chaiklin, & Lohn, 1993, p. 201)

Examples like Miss X confirm that simply being present in the room for any period of time is a valuable experience for a traumatised client.

In step 1 of the group process, a tangible prop such as a weighted scarf, a stress ball, or a large physioball is introduced. Each group member is offered a chance to hold and feel the prop in her hands, and if able to do so is asked to verbalise what the prop feels like. The majority of group members tend to describe what the prop looks like by describing the size or colour of the prop, while few if any are able to tap into their felt sense. This indicates group members often rely on their vision to assess the prop and are not yet embodied or able to feel on a body level. Nevertheless, as long as one participant is willing to hold and feel the prop the next progression can begin. Next the prop is passed from one group member to another. Initially the directive asks group members to look at the person they intend to pass to and slowly roll or walk the prop to that person. This challenges participants to begin to focus on being present in the room and aware of their surroundings. If a participant is looking out of the window, she is clearly not ready to be passed to. Other group members are encouraged to respect each participant's varying comfort levels but might try calling the person's name or walking near the person as means of assessing the person's readiness or willingness to join. In this way survivors immediately become co-facilitators of the group, inviting other peers to join the directive. To be a co-facilitator offers a sense of empowerment while simultaneously utilising the coping skill of caring for others. To witness this process is to witness a group of people organically caring for one another in a genuine, non-judgmental, truly beautiful way.

If no verbal cues are required and a participant is already looking at the prop, the group members begin to understand that she is expressing a readiness and willingness, perhaps even a desire, to be passed to. The person receiving the prop is always encouraged to truly receive the prop, not to immediately redirect it, push it away, or pass it along. By physically receiving and briefly holding the prop, the seeds are planted for participants to be open to receiving other therapeutic components such as support, help or feedback. By first introducing this process with an object outside of themselves, it is relatively easy for most participants to accept the prop, stop it from being in motion, and then pass it along. In many groups the passing of the prop progresses from slow rolling on the floor, to then bouncing from one person to another. This requires a greater sense of intention on the part of the group members. Each person must increase her alertness and focus on the prop so as to be ready for a potentially wonky bounce. Additionally, each participant is asked to make a clear choice as to who she is passing to. By doing this, ambivalence begins to fade away and the participants' ability to make decisions strengthens.

When passing props, participants are always encouraged to say the name of the person they are passing to. Sometimes this is a successful way to incorporate breath and sound, other times participants rely on nonverbal communication via eye contact or gesture. If this is successful the next progression in this phase of the group is to ask participants to pass by lightly tossing in the air. Group members are encouraged to maintain safety and strive to be gentle in their passing of an object. It is the responsibility of the group leader to be ready to intercept any prop thrown too hard or in any dangerous way as a means of ensuring safety for all. Furthermore, it's important that no prop used has the capacity to ever cause physical harm to anyone regardless of how hard it is thrown. Remarkably, even some survivors who have been known to exhibit violence rarely require redirection in this directive. By modelling self-control, intentional movement, thoughtfulness and clear decision-making, participants mirror the group leader's careful, spontaneous, playful passing motion. In time group members mirror each other's passing motions until it is achieved by the entire group. After doing this motion a few times group members visibly relish in feeling in control of themselves while also connected to one another. "The dance sessions seem to be a meeting ground where the patients develop understanding of each other as people more freely than in many situations in a hospital setting" (Sandel, Chaiklin, & Lohn, 1993, p. 201). This is evidenced by brighter affect, increased eye contact, increased spatial awareness, decreased body tension, more vertical body posture, and via participants taking up more physical space within the circle. It is very rare for any participants to be on the perimeter of the room or walking in and out of the group room when this movement progression is complete.

Step 2: Developing Movement and Expression

After 10–15 minutes completing step 1, step 2 of the session can begin. In this step group members are asked to sit in a circle in chairs. The chair serves to ground the person, establish a safe space for each individual, and clearly delineates shared group space from individual space for each participant. This is all achieved non-verbally simply via the placement of the chairs but can be reinforced verbally if needed. The chairs also offer a literal means of support for each participant. Many of them express feeling fatigued from the passing of the prop and are more than willing to be seated. Once seated the group leader leads the movement for participants to mirror which begins a warm-up of each muscle group of the body. This is a technique used by DMT pioneer Marian Chace, who "gently guided the patients through verbal narration and dance, into expressive movements which incorporated chest, abdomen, and pelvic areas" (Levy, 2005, p. 25). In her warm-up, Chace understood:

> This extension of movement throughout the body helped to inte-grate the often-fragmented sense of self in the severely disturbed individual. Guiding small movements into total body activity were simple rhythmic movements like swinging, pushing, or shaking. The patient was encouraged to make a more complete commitment to and identification with his or her moving self...The movements aroused in the patients a sense of enjoyment of body action. In ad-dition, they helped to loosen the body and release excess tensions that could impede both the group process and the surfacing of emo-tional material. It is difficult to process emotions if the body is ex-cessively tense.
>
> (Levy, 2005, pp. 25–26)

In the trauma informed DMT session, Step 2 always begins in the same way: by asking clients to sit tall, plant their feet on the ground, and gradually tap toes one foot at a time to the rhythm of the music. Beginning this phase of the group in the same manner each session creates a familiarity and sense of ritual. After becoming familiar with the group process, participants enjoy predicting this step and often verbalise statements like "I know what you're going to do next!" This not only indicates a level of comfort, but also indicates the participants' sense of ownership. This is their group, they know what to ex-pect, they know what to do. That kind of knowledge is very powerful for a sur-vivor of complex trauma who has likely endured a lifetime of unpredictability.

In step 2, sometimes group members are not able to mirror an entire movement. For example, if swinging arms forward and backward is too challenging, a person can be encouraged to simply lean forward and back-ward with their torso or even just their head. Movement can always be mod-ified to accommodate a participant's limitations. Mirroring the essence of the movement in sync with the shared group rhythm is far more important than identically mimicking the entire movement. As the movement process develops into increasingly full-bodied expressive movements, the verbal process develops as well.

> "A movement therapist does not cut off from verbalization; she uses it as a tool along with the movement. It helps the patient become aware of why he is moving, aware he is moving with a purpose. Ver-balization is not used for 'telling' a patient what to do; it is used for helping him know where he is going and why he is going."
>
> (Sandel, Chaiklin, & Lohn, 1993, p. 355).

Imagery both from the participants and the group leader is offered to further clarify and understand the movement. For example, if the movement is a push of the hands horizontally side to side, a group leader might ask "what are we pushing away?" or suggest an image herself like "it feels like I'm pushing something heavy, like a giant bowling ball that won't roll away". The connection between these words and the physical experience of moving significantly strengthens the mind-body relationship. It also helps to connect the movement process to an exploration of emotions that ideally emerge into clear patterns or themes.

When patterns or themes emerge the movement becomes the symbol for what is often unspeakable. "Symbolism in dance therapy provides a medium by which a patient can recall, reenact and reexperience" (Sandel, Chaiklin, & Lohn, 1993, p. 79). Regardless of illness, these symbols serve as a sort of language by which a person can communicate both past and present thoughts and feelings.

> Symbolic expression in dance therapy form the bridge between the patient's internal and external worlds as they transfer energy from one realm to the other in a social context. Patients living in a world of personal chaos and terror find order and meaning in shared symbolic expression. Subsumed by the symbolic significance of the dance, they become part of an event that transcends the self.
>
> (Schmais, 1985, p. 33)

For people with complex trauma, it can be difficult to express painful emotions or memories. Collectively, however, a group of trauma survivors can "express fear, anger, disgust, or sorrow through movement. Movement allows the acting out of feelings which are not 'socially acceptable' in verbal transactions. The sessions also permit patients to play out different roles, such as supporter, performer, leader, etc." (Schmais & White, 1986, p. 28). At times these roles are about the here-and-now group participants, while at other times they are linked to roles in a participant's personal life. Reenactments of various past relationships (parental, sibling, perpetrator/survivor) can subtly emerge via the movement process:

> [These movements] are bounded by time by a specific rhythm and structured in space- by a specific pathway. Incoherent, intangible impulses are channeled into concrete images. Strong feelings are accepted and experienced by the group and the guilt and anxiety associated with these feelings are often reduced.
>
> (Schmais, 1981, p. 105)

This is what enables group members to so freely express difficult feelings despite the painful emotions often attached to these memories. Over time, group members are able to express these emotions with more assertion as individuals. Eventually the process of individuation occurs, and a strengthened sense of self emerges.

> When patients do not have to see or hold on to each other to be together, when they can risk leaving the circle or changing the structure of the session, a feeling of group wholeness is sensed, and they are ready for closure.
>
> (Schmais, 1981, p. 105)

Step 3: Establishing an Individual Sense of Self

In step 3 of the three step DMT process, group members return to focusing on their own body. Instead of focusing on the environment or on others, the focus is on each individual person's physical sensations in the present moment. Simple stretches and breathing exercises are led by the group leader. Often group members are encouraged to touch their own bodies by resting their hands on their sternum, feeling their own hearts beating inside of them. Specific relaxation techniques are utilised to encourage the release of any physical tension remaining in the body. For example, group members might be invited to join in progressive muscle relaxation by squeezing hands into tight fists, then slowly opening their palms to stretch their fingers wide. By first contracting muscles before stretching muscles one can access increased flexibility more than if simply stretching. In addition to stretching, structured breathing techniques are utilised to assist clients in regulating their parasympathetic nervous systems and quieting any inner arousal. For example, they might be asked to breathe in for four counts, hold their breath for four counts, and then exhale for four counts. Step 3 can be facilitated either standing or sitting depending on the needs of the group.

Regardless of a seated or standing position, participants are encouraged to maintain an awareness of their own individual space and not to intrude into others' space. It is during step 3 that issues of separation, abandonment, and loss often emerge. Some service users have difficulty tolerating these themes, especially those with fear of abandonment. Participants should always be encouraged to stay until the end of the session, but if necessary, it's permissible for them to leave the group prematurely to avoid a triggering or re-traumatising situation. Sometimes participants appear restless, struggling to find stillness as the imminent end of the group approaches. These group members can be encouraged to witness others in stillness even if they cannot join in directly. Just as the repeated movement ritual of toe-tapping offered a sense of ownership in step 2, a similar ritual is established in step 3. Each trauma informed DMT group ends with a stretching movement during which outstretched arms reach up the side of the body, scooping up any positive feelings named by group members, hands extend overhead toward the ceiling, then gathering down into one's heart as palms come together in a prayer-like gesture. This is repeated three times, and the group leader verbalises the importance of completing this third motion as an entire group. Remarkably, even some of the most resistant participants join in this motion after observing it twice. This is the reason for the repetition.

Exceptions to the Three Step Process

In my experience, dance/movement therapy groups structured in the three-step process have been an effective trauma informed therapy for service users among various genders, ages, diagnoses, and cognitive capacities. However, there are of course some cases when participating in a group is too painful or dysregulating for a survivor. In this approach, the initial focus is on symptom management, followed by creating narratives, recognising patterns, making connections between internal states and actions, and later incorporating body-oriented work.

One fictionalised example of a client who could not join the trauma informed DMT group due to her hyperarousal and retraumatisation via movement was a service user, 'Alice'. Initially Alice was not ready or appropriate for structured DMT groups. However, despite her acute stress and disorganisation, movement was demonstrated to be an effective intervention.

> In most groups Alice presents as highly impulsive. She runs around the room pretending to shoot people with imaginary guns. She grabs all paper off the walls and tables, and stuffs as many objects as possible down her shirt or trousers. She shrieks and yells various noises while restlessly walking all over the room like a pinball bouncing up, down, back, and forth. Initially when Alice is preparing to leave the Unit for a medical appointment, she begins shrieking, running in circles, and shoots people with her imaginary gun. I proceed to put my hands up and quickly whisper "Don't shoot, I need your help." Alice looks closely at me as if intrigued and approaches me continuing to shoot as she walks closer. I begin to slowly outline my own body with my fingertips, coming close to my skin but not making physical contact. Alice closely watches this drawing-like motion. "I'm drawing a safety bubble to protect me from the scary things outside," I explain. "I'm drawing the lines extra thick so my bubble doesn't pop. I'm making the walls extra strong so I can be safe inside my bubble no matter where I go. Would you like to try to make your own bubble?" Alice nods her head in agreement and begins outlining her wrist and arm with her opposite hand. She listens attentively as I verbally guide her through a process in which she outlines her entire body. We repeat this process several times. Finally, I ask, "Is your bubble strong and sealed?" Alice nods yes. Alice and I test the bubble out. I splash imaginary water

toward Alice and her bubble. "I'm dry!" Alice shouts with a prideful
smile. Alice agrees to be escorted by me to the medical appointment,
and I reassure her if any leaks in the bubble arise they'll be immedi-
ately fixed.

  From that point on going to medical appointments off the Unit was
no longer such a dysregulating, retraumatising event for Alice. Us-
ing a simple body-based intervention of outlining the body with clear
imagery sufficed in providing Alice with a sense of safety and a clear
sense of her own boundaries.

As with all processes, other limitations have also been discovered. For example, in some sessions group members have refused to pass the prop, instead holding it in their possession, thus interrupting the flow of the group.
In some cases, group members have left the room with the prop. Then it is
helpful to have alternative props on hand so the group can continue despite
that individual's resistance to the directive. Another example of a limitation
to the three-step process was discovered when a blind patient joined the
group. In this case the group leader used clear narration of the movement to
guide the participant in how to move. The group leader also modified passing directly in and out of that participant's hands herself, thus allowed the
overall three-step process to be maintained. Other limitations experienced
are with service users on the autism spectrum who struggle to follow verbal directions or read the movement and/or cues of other participants. For
these participants, individual dance/movement therapy sessions or modified
group sessions have been found to be a more effective intervention than
the three-step process groups. Lastly, the three-step process group can be
challenging to join for service users who find it difficult to remain present
in one space for at least a few minutes at a time. Although there is value in
observing the group even for brief minutes, some service users may find the
DMT group overstimulating. Others may be in a floridly psychotic state to
the degree they're unable to remain in the group space. For these individuals, it's important to honour the limitations of the group and instead extend
an invitation to join the session another time.

Conclusion

In conclusion, as the prevalence of trauma among adults with psychiatric diagnoses remains high, the approaches to treatment must continue to evolve.
The creative arts therapies interweave non-verbal and verbal interventions
that assist survivors to develop a sense of mastery of their environment and
of themselves. Using a tailored three step process, dance/movement therapy groups at an urban psychiatric facility enable survivors to advance on
their road to recovery as they strive to return to a meaningful life in the
community. For many clients, the 3-step process group allows service users

to reconnect with their own bodies in an invaluable way. Learning to feel safe in own's own body is a critical piece of the healing process for so many trauma survivors. Similarly, learning to use one's own body as a tool that can assist in self-regulation, self-expression, and connection to other people is a vitally important part of recovery for many service users. Movement, dance, and body-based mindfulness exercises are methods of moving that enable trauma survivors to reclaim personal power in their lives, regain a sense of control, and reinstate a sense of holistic interconnectedness with oneself and the greater world.

References

Ambra, L. (1995). Approaches used in dance/movement therapy with adult women incest survivors. *ADTA Journal of Dance Therapy, 17(1)*, 15–24.

Chambliss, L. (1982). Movement therapy and the shaping of a neuropsychological model. *American Journal of Dance Therapy, 5*, 18–27.

Courtois, C. A., Ford, J. D., & Cloitre, M. L. (2009). Best practices in psychotherapy for adults. In C. A. Courtois & J. D. Ford (eds), *Treating complex traumatic stress disorders: An evidence-based guide* (pp. 82–103). New York: Guilford Press.

Devereaux, C. (2008) Untying the knots: Dance/movement therapy with a family exposed to domestic violence. *ADTA Journal of Dance Therapy, 30*, 58–70.

Homann, K. (2010). Embodied concepts of neurobiology in dance/movement therapy practice. *ADTA Journal of Dance Therapy, 32*, 80–99.

Levy, F. (2005). *Dance movement therapy: A healing art.* Reston, VA: American Alliance for Health, Physical Education, Recreation and Dance.

Meekums, B. (2002). *Dance movement therapy: A creative psychotherapy approach.* London: Sage.

Ogden, P., Kehuni, M., & Pain, C. (2006) *Trauma and the body: a sensorimotor approach to psychotherapy.* New York: W. W. Norton & Co.

Reich, W. (1990). *Character analysis*, 3rd enlarged edition. New York: Farrar, Straus, Giroux.

Sandel, S., Chaiklin, S., & Lohn, A. (eds). (1993). *Foundations of dance/movement therapy: The life and work of Marian Chace.* Columbia, MD: Marian Chace Memorial Fund of the American Dance Therapy Association.

Schmais, C. (1981). Group development and group formation in dance therapy. *The Arts in Psychotherapy, 8*, 103–107.

Schmais, C. (1985). Healing processes in group dance therapy. *American Journal of Dance Therapy, 8*, 17–36.

Schmais, C. and White, E. Q. (1986). Introduction to dance therapy. *American Journal of Dance Therapy, 9(1)*, 23–30.

CONCLUSION

Kristina Muenzenmaier, Mara Conan,
Gillian Stephens Langdon, Toshiko Kobayashi,
and Andres Ricardo Schneeberger

In 2023, we continue to be witnesses to the cruelty and brutality that human-ity is capable of. Still, while maintaining an awareness of global atrocities, we must focus energy on the smaller work that each of us is capable of in the fields of our daily lives. In this book we have shared our journey toward a deeper understanding of trauma and psychosis. Whether survivor, family member, friend, clinician, or administrator, we hope our contributions can be useful and forge a pathway to healing.

Trauma affects not only the individual but also families, neighbourhoods, communities, and countries. It may lead to helplessness, feelings of impo-tence, and re-enactments, as well as have an intergenerational impact often not recognised.

The aftermath of traumatic experiences has received increased attention during recent decades. Trauma is now a part of everyday vernacular and there is less stigma in talking about it. However, the practical application of this knowledge in a large, urban psychiatric facility is often elusive. We need to return again and again to highlight the issues and the systems that impact survivors.

Recognising the current need for guidance and practical approaches for trauma focused work, we have presented our experiences with personal sto-ries and fictionalised vignettes woven throughout the book in order to bring this work to life. Our writing has been a continuation of the collaborative process begun in the trauma committee. As we wrote, we worked together planning the scope of each chapter and the best way to describe the experi-ences of survivors and the work we did together. We discuss therapeutic and educational interventions in individual, group, and family settings as well as efforts to build a safe community for both service users and staff. We have also shared the multicultural, multimodal, and multidisciplinary approach of our programme. The positive outcomes we achieved came through a col-laborative approach with survivors and across the disciplines of psychia-try, psychology, nursing, social work, and creative arts therapies. Through these varied modalities we began to understand the unique needs of each

DOI: 10.4324/9781003055914-20

individual knowing that the ability to listen with humility is indispensable. Crucial to this work has been highlighting service users' resilience and resources, acquisition of new abilities and skills and, most importantly, the development of hope for the future. In addition, it became clear to us that advocacy for social and political change is essential along with the recognition of what can and cannot be changed in the systems in which we worked.

We are indebted to the ideas and commitment of theorists, researchers and clinicians from many different fields who have inspired and informed our work. The developments in neuroscience have opened new territories in understanding the impact of trauma and different approaches to treatment. It is our hope that the combination of non-verbal and verbal therapies adapted to individual needs in a trauma informed context can be expanded. We also recommend creating programme assessments including quantifiable therapeutic outcomes in order to determine the efficacy of the elements of the programme. It is important that evaluations also take into account the survivor's viewpoint of the effectiveness of the interventions.

The multi-levelled support we received was essential in keeping us going despite obstacles. The nurturing approach of committee members towards one another, as well as administrative support, played a major role in continuing work that at times was overwhelming and emotionally stressful.

Most importantly, a strong motivating force has been working together with service users towards increased ability in establishing connection, engaging in creative activities, and expressing thoughts and feelings.

It is our hope that by sharing our story and the outcomes we were able to achieve, the interdisciplinary approaches described in this book can serve as a model for what continues to be a challenge for survivors of psychosis and trauma and those who support them. Most importantly we want to make it known that perseverance and mutual supports in this work can transform hopelessness into a positive outlook for the future for all those who are aspiring to a better life.

INDEX

Indexer: Dr Laurence Errington.

Note: Page numbers followed by "n" denote endnotes.

abandonment and/or rejection issues 171, 177, 191, 261
adverse childhood experiences *see* childhood experiences
affective lability (strong emotions/ feelings) 104, 130, 189, 207, 219, 260
affective numbing *see* numbing
alexithymia 141
Alice (fictionalised vignette) 262–3
Alice's Restaurant (song) 191, 192
Alma (fictionalised vignette) 149–50
American Art Therapy Association (AATA) 215
Anton (fictionalised vignette) 207
Antonia (fictionalised vignette) xlv, 116–17, 130–3
art therapy xxxi, xliii–xliv, 110–11, 215–50; expanding and adapting 234–8; history 215–16; inpatient unit 126–32; outpatient clinic 150–1; structured 215–31; *see also* creative arts
Asian countries, origami in 225; and students and staff from Asia 241
assessment 47–63, 69; guidelines 53–6; hospital-wide 47–63; implementation 50–1; often overlooked in individuals experiencing psychosis 49; political dimensions in US 35; writeup 56–7; *see also* interview
attachment (childhood) xxxii, xl, 30
attention-deficit/hyperactivity disorder, displaying symptoms of 141
Auslander's story/life experience xxxv, 20–30
autonomy, promoting 235
avoidance 13–14, 15–16; art therapy and 219

Balint, Michael 232
behaviours (psychotic), understanding the complex array of 15
biological factors: environmental and xxxiii, 31; genetic and/or xxxiii–xxxiv, 33, 98, 137
biomedical (medical) model of mental disorder 20, 34, 49–50, 120
bio-psycho-social model 20
bisexual people 172, 178
Bloom's Sanctuary Model xxvii, 67, 216
body (somatic...): art therapy and bodily manifestations 220, 228; delusions 12; music therapy and reconnection with body 193, 196; music-verbal therapy and confidence in body 208; responses to stress 141–2; *see also* embodiment
body armour (concept) 254
borderline personality disorder 33, 34, 38; Auslander's 26
bottom up political networking 37
brain and neurobiology xiii; mirroring and 253–4; plasticity 232, 237
breathing exercises 189, 196, 197, 261
Brenda (fictionalised vignette) 3–4, 11–13, 16–17
Buddha (Gautama Siddhartha) 225
burnout 78, 81, 90
Bush's (GW) New Freedom Commission on Mental Health 41

calming oneself, identifying ways of 57
Capgras syndrome 12, 13, 15
care (mental health): changing the dialogue 36–8; continuity of 146; family therapy and systems of 159, 166; trauma-informed (*see*

trauma-informed care); widening the circle of 76–94; *see also* interventions; self-care; staff; therapy; treatment

Carmen (fictionalised vignette) 162–5

CBT (cognitive behavioural therapy) 103–5; art therapy and 217, 218, 229; groups 71, 98, 103–5, 113

Chace (Marion) and Chacian dance therapy 253, 256, 259

change: enacting 118–20; in negotiating life circumstances 106

Charles (fictionalised vignette) 57–8

chart review 53

childhood experiences (adverse/stressful/ traumatic/severe (SCE)) 7–10; disbelief of reports of 34; discussion of existing literature 5–6; gender differences 8; music therapy and 187; music-verbal therapy and 212; New York State, high rates 49–50; potential influences throughout lifespan 9; *see also specific types of experiences*

children: abuse (*see* emotional abuse and neglect; physical abuse; sexual abuse); attachment xxxii, xl, 30; gender issues 171–2; *see also* infants

Chris (fictionalised vignette) 212–13

client *see* consumer

closed groups in art therapy 237

cognitive behavioural therapy (CBT) xli; groups 71, 98, 103–5, 113, 218

cognitive difficulties 141

cohesiveness: group 105, 106, 113; inpatient unit 117–25

co-leadership 111–12, 237; music therapy 186; music-verbal therapy 204, 213

collaborations: art therapy xlv, 217, 227, 235, 238, 241, 245, 247; clinician–survivor 60; interdisciplinary 134, 185, 241; music therapy 185; trauma committee 65, 67, 68, 73, 74; *see also* connecting; dialogue

collage 219, 222, 223, 227, 240, 244, 245

communication in art therapy: cross-cultural 238; development through artmaking 238–41; *see also* dialogue; relationships; verbalisation; voice

community: art therapy and sense of 228; inpatient unit and sense of 125, 126–33; outpatient clinic and sense of 146–53; transition (as outpatient) to 146–7, 165, 208

complex trauma and PTSD xxxvi–xxxvii, 32, 103; art therapy 215–31; dance/ movement therapy 252, 260; group therapy 97–115; political aspects 33–4

confidentiality 81, 85

conflict (group) 207

connecting/forming connections (and reconnection) 51–3, 64–75; dance/ movement therapy 256–8; inpatient unit 130, 134; music therapy and reconnection with body 193, 196; music-verbal therapy 209–10; *see also* collaboration; dialogue

consolidation 129; family therapy 161–3, 165

consultation, inpatient unit 117–18

consumer/survivor/ex-patient (C/S/X) and client/service user: collaboration between clinician and 60; political involvement 36–9; survivor's perspective xxx, 20–30

containment: art therapy 236; music therapy 187

continuity of care 70, 146

control issues on inpatient unit, training 124–5

conversation *see* dialogue

coping (and coping strategies) xxxviii; families 104–5, 157–9

core aspects of trauma treatment programmes xxxvi–xli, xlv

Core Conflictual Relationship Theme 10

countertransference 79, 80, 159, 160, 218, 256

COVID 89, 90, 216

cPTSD *see* complex trauma

creative arts therapies (groups or unspecified) xxxi, xliii, 108–11, 148–51; inpatient unit 123, 129, 130, 132; outpatient clinic 148–51; for staff 90–1

creative arts therapies (individual) 132, 149

creativity in art therapy 235–6; process of creating 236–7

crises *see* incidents

Critical Incident Stress Debriefing (CISD) 85–6

Critical Incident Stress Management (CISM) 86

cross-cultural communication in art therapy 238
culture issues: art therapy 237; in assessment 51–2

Dan (fictionalised vignette) 242–4
dance/movement therapy (DMT) xxxi, xliv, 148, 251–66; exception to three step process 262–3; techniques 252–6; three step process 256–8
Dare to Vision conference (1994) 28
Deborah (fictionalised vignette) 152–3
debriefing 84–6; end of interview 55; incidents 84–6; 9/11 and 87
decision-making in inpatient unit 120; training 124–5
deconstructing in art therapy 236–7
deep (diaphragmatic) breathing exercises 189, 196, 197, 261
delusions 4–16; in fictionalised vignette (Brenda) 11–12; fluidity of transitions between dissociative symptoms and 16; grandiose 11, 12, 15, 16, 210, 226; paranoid (see paranoid delusions); stressful childhood experiences and 9–10
demoralisation 78, 80, 81
de-stress groups for staff 90–1
Diagnostic and Statistical Manual see DSM
dialogue/conversation: body music-verbal therapy 208–9; family therapy 160–1, 163–4; political 36–41; see also communication; verbalisation
diaphragmatic (deep) breathing exercises 189, 196, 197, 261
didactic lectures 88
didactic presentations and skills training 104
discipline specific staff training workshops 89
Disorders of Extreme Stress Not Otherwise Specified (DESNOS) 32, 119
dissociation 5–6, 9; art therapy 219, 222; Auslander's experience 21, 27; in fictionalised vignettes 4, 12–13, 14–15; flashbacks and 6, 133; fluidity of transitions between delusions and 16; outpatient 141
Dissociative Experiences Scale-Taxon (DES-T) 7

drug abuse see substance/drug abuse
drug therapy, psychopharmacological 120, 156
DSM: DSM-III xxxii, 16, 31; DSM-IV 5, 32; DSM-5 5, 17; sexuality and 178; Structured Clinical Interview for (SCID) 7

economic concerns and financial issues 78
educational trauma group 100–5; components xxxviii–xxxix; Understanding and Dealing with Sexual Abuse Trauma: An Educational Group for Women xxxviii, 100, 101, 216
embodiment in dance/movement therapy 253, 255, 257
emergencies see incidents
emotion(s): numbing (see numbing); painful (see pain); working with xl–xli; see also feelings
emotional abuse and neglect 34; gender differences 8
emotional reactions xxxviii, xxxix, 87, 100, 142–3; group therapy 112; inpatient unit 123; outpatient clinic 137, 140, 142–3, 151; strong (affective lability) 104, 130, 189, 207, 219, 260; see also feelings
Employment Assistance Program (EAP) 77
empowerment xxix, xl; family therapy 159, 160, 165; music therapy 186, 189, 191; staff on trauma unit 120
engagement: in art therapy group 237; in family therapy 159–60; music and social engagement system xliii, 209–10
Enrichment Origami Art Therapy 224
environmental factors 171; biological and xxxiii, 31
Evelyn (fictionalised vignette) 210
experiences: life (see life experiences); understanding the complex array of 15; see also re-experiencing
expression: in dance/movement therapy 258–9, 260; free (in art therapy) 225, 235–6
Expressive Origami Therapy (EOT) 225, 226, 241–4; Symptom Specific (SSEOT) 216, 217, 224–8, 228, 229, 230
eye contact: dance/movement therapy 258; origami therapy group 242

Family Intervention for Trauma
Treatment (FITT) model 158
family therapy xlii, 155–67
feelings: emerging of 206–7; managing
142–3; strong (affective lability)
104, 130, 189, 207, 219, 260; *see also*
emotions
females *see* women
feminist perspectives xxxiv, 31, 34
fictionalised vignettes xxix, xli, xlv;
Alice (dance/movement therapy)
262–3; Alma (outpatient music
therapy) 149–50; Anton (music-verbal
therapy) 207; Antonia (inpatient
unit) xlv, 116–17, 130–3; Brenda
(trauma–psychosis relationship)
4, 10–13, 16–17; Carmen (family
therapy) 162–5; Charles (assessment)
57–8; Chris (music-verbal therapy)
212–13; Dan (art therapy) 242–4;
Deborah (outpatient and community
networking) 152–3; Evelyn
(music-verbal therapy) 210; Gina
(outpatient-individual therapy)
138–44; informed interventions and
136; Jeremy (sexual orientation)
172–4; Jesse (music-verbal therapy)
208–9; Jordan (art therapy) 240;
Karen (assessment - treatment
recommendations) 58–9; Kendal (art
therapy) 239, 240; Luis (art therapy)
239, 240, 241; Maribel (sexual
orientation) 169–71, 178; Monica
(trauma and psychosis, dissociation)
14–15; Mr. T (assessment) 52; Olivia
(music-verbal therapy) 206–7; Rachel
(art therapy/gardening) 246, 247;
Ramona (outpatient transition from
inpatient) 147; Sandra (music-verbal
therapy) 208; Sara (transgender)
175–6; Steve (group therapy) 106–8
figurative expression 217, 235
financial issues/economic concerns 78
`first-aid', psychological 89, 90
flashbacks 219; art therapy 219, 221;
dance/movement therapy 256;
dissociative 6, 133; in fictionalised
vignette (Brenda) 13, 16
food: art therapy and 227; child
development and 252; family therapy
and 163; music therapy and 192
fragmentation xxviii, 17; memory
141, 144

France, history of music therapy 184
free expression 225, 235–6
funding issues and economic concerns 78

gardening as art therapy 245–6, 247
Gautama Siddhartha 225
gay people *see* homosexual people
gender differences in adverse childhood
experiences 8
gender identity 12, 174–7, 178, 179
generational transmission of trauma 158
genetic and/or biological factors xxxiii–
xxxiv, 33, 98, 137
Gina (fictionalised vignette) 138–44
grandiose delusions in fictionalised
vignettes 11, 12, 15, 16, 210, 226
grounding 150; in art therapy 221, 222;
in dance/movement therapy 254; in
music-verbal therapy 205; nightmares
and 197
Group Education and Skills Training
(GEST) 103
group process 105–8
group therapy/treatment/psychotherapy
xxxi, 71–2; art (*see* art therapy); CBT
(cognitive behavioural therapy) 71,
98, 103–5, 113, 218; complex trauma
97–115; creative arts (*see* creative
arts); dance/movement (*see* dance/
movement therapy); educational (*see*
educational trauma group); efficacy
of programmes of 99–100; LGBTQ+
170, 178; music (*see* music therapy);
outpatient clinic 144–6; process
103–8; sexual abuse 29, 98, 99, 100,
101; symptom specific (*see* Symptom
Specific Group Therapy); verbal (*see*
verbal therapy)
guilt 164

hallucinations 4–16; in fictionalised
vignette (Brenda) 4, 11–12, 13, 16;
stressful childhood experiences and
9–10
health professionals *see* staff
health-risk behaviours 91; through
lifespan and adverse childhood
experiences 9
hearing voices (voice hearing) 6, 16, 37,
41–2
helplessness (feelings of): music therapy
triggering 185; staff 79, 80
hip-hop (rap) 11–13

historical perspectives xxvii–xxviii, xxxii–xxxiv, 5–6; art therapy 215–16; music therapy 183–4; United States xxxiv, 31–4, 183–4
history (trauma) xxxi, 48, 56; in assessment 56; Auslander's 28; fictionalised vignettes 57–8, 172–3; lack of attention paid to 50; LGBTQI+ people 171–4
History of Physical and Sexual Abuse Questionnaire (HPSAQ) 7, 10
homosexual people (gay men and women) 172, 176, 178; hatred (homophobia) 176, 178
hook (musical term) 212
horizontal relationships 235
hospital and facility-wide dimensions: assessment 47–63; outreach 69
hospitalised patient/inpatient xxxi, xlii, 116–35; art therapy/origami 241, 248; Auslander's experience 20–30; Jennings' (Ann) daughter Anna 38; political issues 37, 38; transition to outpatient/community 146–7, 165, 208; trauma unit (see trauma unit)
hyperarousal 219; cognitive difficulties 141

ICD 10 and 11 32–3
imagery in dance/movement therapy 255, 260
imipramine (Tofranil) 25, 26
incest 5; Auslander's experience 28; dance/movement therapy 252
incidents (incl. crises; emergencies) 70; debriefing 84–6; procedures after 83; on trauma unit 124–5
inclusion (inclusive relationships; inclusiveness) 120; art therapy 238; staff 121–2, 123, 128; trainees at trauma committee meetings 85
individual therapy/psychotherapy 58, 67, 138–44, 152, 162, 164, 206; inpatient unit 129; LGBTQ+ persons 178; music-verbal therapy and 206–7; see also self
infants: movements 252; music and 187
inpatient see hospitalised patient
insight (gaining) 254; in fictionalised vignettes 59, 130, 194; group therapy 200, 217, 225
integration (and re-integration) xxviii; family therapy and 161; programming 129; see also reintegration

interdisciplinary dimensions see multidisciplinary and interdisciplinary dimensions
intergenerational transmission of trauma 158
International Classification of Diseases (ICD 10 and 11) 32–3
international initiatives 32, 37–9
International Society for Trauma and Dissociation (ISSTD) 32
International Society for Traumatic Stress Studies (ISTSS) 32
interpersonal interactions see relationships
interventions xl–xliii; multimodal (see multimodal interventions); trauma committee and 66–9; see also care; therapy
interview (trauma) 53–6; guidelines 55
intrusive pathway/thoughts 221; art therapy and 221; PTSD 13; re-experiencing 12, 13, 140

Jennings' (Ann) daughter Anna 38
Jeremy (fictionalised vignette) 172–4
Jesse (fictionalised vignette) 208–9
jigsaw puzzle 219, 222
Joint Commission on Accreditation of Healthcare Organizations (JCAHO) 65
Jordan (fictionalised vignette) 240

Kabat-Zinn, Jon 230
Kansas (University of), music therapy 184
Karen (fictionalised vignette) 58–9
Kendal (fictionalised vignette) 239, 240
kirigami 244
Kraepelin, Emil 6
Kramer, Edith 215

lability, affective (strong feelings/ emotions) 104, 130, 189, 207, 219, 260
lesbians see homosexual people
LGBTQ+ xxxi, xlii–xliii, 168–80
life circumstances 98, 106; of staff, assessment and 52–3
life experiences: childhood (see childhood experiences); survivor's (Auslander's) account xxxv, 20–30
local initiatives (US) xxxv, 37–40
longitudinal research 6–10
Luis (fictionalised vignette) 239, 240, 241

males (men), sexual abuse under-reported or under-assessed in 52
marginalisation: family therapy and 156, 159; LGBTQI+ 168
Maribel (fictionalised vignette) 169–71, 178
mask making 219
Mastering the Key Connection 39, 67
meaning of experience xxxii, xliii, 134
medical (biomedical) model of mental disorder 20, 34, 49–50, 120
medical records, review (for assessment) 53
medication, psychopharmacological 120, 156
memory 144; fragmentation 141, 144; intact 144
men, sexual abuse under-reported or under-assessed in 52
mental health care see care
mental illness/disorder: labelling emotional pain as 27; medical/biomedical model 20, 49–50, 120; in primary caretaker, gender differences in childhood experience 8; severe (see severe/serious mental illness)
metaphor in dance/movement therapy 255
Michigan State College, music therapy 184
mind: art (incl. origami) therapy and 226, 228; music-verbal therapy and 208
mindfulness 225, 265
mirroring in dance/movement therapy 253, 254, 255, 258, 259
modelling, co-leadership and the potential of 112
Monica (fictionalised vignette) 14–15
movement see dance/movement therapy
multidisciplinary and interdisciplinary dimensions xxxi, xlv, 70–3; collaborations 134, 185, 241; multimodal and 73, 129; New York State 36; training in inpatient unit 123; trauma committee 70–3, 74, 256, 265, 266
multimodal interventions 129, 265; US 70–3
music therapy (group) xxxi, xliii, xliv, 108–10, 125, 149–50, 183–214; history 183–4; inpatient unit 125, 131–3; 9/11 and 87–8; outpatient clinic 149–50; therapist's description of her experience 125; verbal and xxxi, 108, 109, 131, 185, 186–7, 203–14

names, hearing theirs sung 188–9
National Association of State Mental Health Program Directors 41
national initiatives (US) xxxv, 32, 37–40
Naumburg, Margaret (1890–1983) 215
negative and positive symptoms 5, 11
neglect see emotional abuse and neglect
networking: with community agencies 152–3; political 37
neurobiology see brain
New Freedom Commission on Mental Health 41
New York State (NYS) 31–2; assessment 49, 50; child abuse, high rates 49; Office of Mental Health (OMH) 36, 39, 50, 67, 75; Trauma Conference (Mastering the Key Connection) 39, 67; Trauma Initiative and Taskforce 36, 37, 39, 50, 65, 66, 102
Nhat Hanh, Thich 225
nightmares 221; art therapy 219, 221; music therapy 193, 197–8
9/11 events 86–8
numbing (affective/emotional) 193–4; and avoidance of intrusive thoughts 15
nursing station 117, 122, 126, 127

Olivia (fictionalised vignette) 206–7
open-ended questions 54, 55
open groups in art therapy 237
origami (therapy) xliv, 71, 128, 216, 217–19, 224–8, 232, 233; expressive (see expressive origami therapy)
out-patient setting xlii, 136–53; art therapy 244, 248; creative arts for staff 90; educational trauma group 100
outreach (reaching out) 81, 82–3, 92, 118; community agencies and 152–3; facility-wide 69–70; family therapy and 129; incidents and 83, 86; inpatient unit 128, 129; music therapy and 108

pain (emotional/psychological pain): Auslander's 25; labelled as mental illness 27
paralysis (staff) 79

paranoid delusions 13; fictionalised vignettes 11–12, 13, 162
parents (primary caretakers), substance abuse 8, 151
peer support 37, 41, 212
personal reflections, art therapy 237–8
pharmacological treatment (psychiatric medication) 120, 156
phase-oriented family trauma treatment model 158–63
physical abuse: Dare to Vision conference (1994) 28; gender differences in, or witnessing abuse 8; homosexual man's childhood experience of 172; music therapy and 187
Pinel, Philippe 184
political action 31–46
polyvagal theory 206, 209–10
Porges's polyvagal theory 206, 209–10
positive and negative symptoms 5, 11
post-traumatic stress disorder see PTSD
pregnancy (growing a baby), Auslander's 25, 28, 29
pre-group: CBT 104; music therapy 191–3, 200
President's New Freedom Commission on Mental Health 41
Prinzhorn, Hans (1886–1933) 215
programmes (trauma) 76–94; core aspects of xxxvi–xli, xlv; integration of programming 129; staff xxxi, xxxvi–xli, 76–94
pseudo-hallucinations and sexual abuse 5
psychiatric hospitalisation see hospitalised patient/inpatient
psychiatric medication (psychopharmacology) 120, 156
psychodynamic perspectives xxxii–xxxiii
Psychological First Aid Program (PFA) 89, 90
psychopharmacological treatment (medication) 120, 156
psychosis–trauma relationship xxviii, 3–17
psychotherapy see therapy
PTSD 13–14; avoidant pathway 13–14; complex (see complex trauma and PTSD); delusion and hallucination interaction between 13; group CBT 103, 105; intrusive pathway 13; as new concept in DSM-III 31; secondary 79
PTSD Checklist (PCL) 7, 56

qualitative research 6–10

Rachel (fictionalised vignette) 246, 247
racism, systemic xxix
Ramona (fictionalised vignette) 147
rap music 211–13
rape 31, 34
reaching out see outreach
reconnection see connecting
record (medical) review for assessment 53
recovery, redefining 37
recruitment, trauma programme for staff 82
re-experiencing 15, 140–1; intrusive 12, 13, 140
reintegration see integration
rejection and/or abandonment issues 171, 177, 191, 261
relationships (interpersonal interactions) 10; art therapy and 223–4, 235, 242–4; family therapy and 161, 165; horizontal 235; inclusive (see inclusion); music therapy and 198–200; therapeutic (see therapeutic relationship); trust and 16–17, 104, 109, 121–2, 142, 159–60, 186, 198–200, 218, 220, 223–4, 228; see also connecting; group therapy
resilience and family therapy 160
re-traumatisation risk 38, 87, 160, 161; in assessment 50
re-victimisation experiences 97, 98; US women 31
rhythm: in dance/movement therapy 254, 256–7; in music-verbal therapy 205, 207, 208, 209, 210, 211, 212, 213
role-play (clinicians/staff) 124; in assessment 51; role reversal 124
round robin in art therapy 219, 223, 244

safety xxxix, 117–25, 126–33; art therapy 221, 236, 240; dance/movement therapy 256; family therapy 159–60; group therapy 97, 99, 101, 101–2; inpatient unit 117–25, 126–33; LGBTQ+ people 178–9; music therapy 187; music-verbal therapy 205; therapeutic relationship and 16–17; vulnerability vs feelings safe 142; see also Sanctuary Model; trust
Sanctuary Model (Bloom's) xxvii, 67, 216
Sandra (fictionalised vignette) 208

Sara (fictionalised vignette) 175–6
self, gaining/establishing a sense
 of xxxix–xl; dance/movement
 therapy 261; music-verbal therapy
 206–7
self-care (staff) 90–1
self-concept and art therapy 220
self-harm/injury 100; art therapy 219;
 music therapy 193, 195
self-help models 37
Self-Love Drum Improvisation module
 193, 195–6
self-portrait 219
self-worth 143; loss 13
September 11 (9/11) events 86–8
service user see consumer
severe/serious mental illness (SMI)
 32, 36, 52; families and 155–68;
 LGBTQI+ and 174–7
sexual abuse 35, 36, 38; assessment
 and interviewing 54; Auslander's
 experience 25; Dare to Vision
 conference (1994) 28; family therapy
 and 164; gender differences in, or
 witnessing abuse 8; group therapy
 29, 98, 99, 100, 101; hallucination vs
 pseudo-hallucinations 5; homosexual
 man's experience of 172; Jennings'
 daughter Anna 38; music therapy and
 187, 196; trauma assessments and
 52–3, 54, 56; see also incest; rape
sexuality and sexual orientation 170,
 173, 174–5, 177, 178, 179
shame vs feelings of self-worth 143
Siddhartha Gautama 225
singing see songs
skills-training, group therapy 103, 104
social engagement system and music
 xliii, 206, 209–10
somatic... see body
songs (and singing) 128, 188–91; familiar
 ones 189, 190–1; uplifting closing ones
 189–90; writing/composing 109, 188,
 199–200
space, individual, in dance/movement
 therapy 258, 261
staff/health professionals/clinic team
 xxix, 76–94; assessment and the life
 circumstances of 52–3; community
 and 151; empowerment (in trauma
 unit) 120; inclusion 121–2, 123,
 128; training (see training); trauma

programme xxxi, xxxvi–xli, 76–94;
 traumatisation (see traumatisation)
Steve (fictionalised vignette) 106–8
stigma 21, 88; LGBTQ+ and 177, 178
stress: bodily responses to 141–2;
 childhood experiences causing (see
 childhood experiences)
stressful childhood experiences see
 childhood experiences
structured art therapy 215–31
Structured Clinical Interview for the
 Diagnostic and Statistical Manual of
 Mental Disorders (SCID) 7
students see trainees and students
substance/drug abuse 226–7; art therapy
 220, 226–7; by primary caretaker incl.
 parents 8, 151
support group 65, 213
survivor see consumer
symbolism xliii; art therapy and 217,
 222, 236; dance therapy and 260;
 LGBTQI and 176; music therapy and
 xliii; trauma and psychosis relation 17
symptom(s) (psychotic) 56–9; in
 assessment 53, 56–9; Auslander's
 20–30; historical perspectives 5,
 6; positive and negative 5, 11;
 understanding the complex array of 15
Symptom Specific Expressive Origami
 Therapy (SSEOT) 216, 217, 224–8,
 228, 229, 230
Symptom Specific Group Therapy
 (SSGT) xli, 193, 193–200, 205; cPTSD
 103, 110, 185; music therapy 185,
 186, 187, 193–200; music-verbal
 therapy 205
systemic racism xxix

tapping one's toes 254, 259, 261
therapeutic relationship xxix, xxxix;
 countertransference 79, 80, 159, 160,
 218, 256; safety 16–17; trust 16–17,
 104, 109, 142, 159–60, 186, 198, 220,
 223–4
therapy (treatment incl. psychotherapy):
 assessment helping with
 recommendations 58–9; group (see
 group therapy); individual (see
 individual therapy); LGBTQ+ persons
 177–9; programme (see programmes);
 see also care; interventions; treatment
 resistant

Thich Nhat Hanh 225
thoughts: intrusive (*see* intrusive pathway/thoughts); organised *vs* disorganised 144
toe-tapping 254, 259, 261
Tofranil (imipramine) 25, 26
toning techniques 193, 196–7
top down political networking 37
trainees and students: art therapy 91, 216, 233, 238–45, 248; outpatient clinic 137–9; on trauma committee 73, 79
training (staff) 88–9; inpatient unit 122–5; outpatient clinic 137–8
transgender people 174, 175, 176; hatred (transphobia) 176, 177
trauma: assessment (*see* assessment); childhood (*see* childhood experiences); complex (*see* complex trauma); historical realisation of the importance xxxv, 98; history (*see* history); intergenerational transmission 158; programmes (*see* programmes); relationship between psychosis and xxviii, 3–17
trauma committee xxxiv–xxxv, xxxvi, xliii–xliv, 64–75; art therapy xliii–xliv, 216, 233, 238; dance/movement therapy 251, 256; early steps 65–6; influence on interventions of developments within 66–9; inpatient unit and 117, 118, 119, 121, 123, 127, 134, 136; multidisciplinary and interdisciplinary dimensions 70–3, 74, 256, 265, 266; multimodal interventions and 70–3; music therapy 185, 186, 191; outpatient clinic 136, 137, 138, 146, 148, 150, 153; outreach 69–70
trauma conferences 50, 73; NYS Trauma Conference: Mastering the Key Connection 39, 67
trauma-informed care: art therapy xxx, 111, 216, 225, 234; group therapy and 98–9; inpatient (*see* trauma unit); intervention xli, 215, 265; national level in US 41; outpatient clinic 136–53; `trauma focused' approach xxxiv
Trauma Recovery and Empowerment Model (TREM) 99n1, 105
Trauma Symptom Specific Art Therapy (TSSAT) 217, 218, 219–24, 229, 234, 235, 236; adapted to origami therapy 225–6; description of the group 219–24
trauma unit (inpatient) 116–35; safety and cohesiveness 117–25
traumatisation (staff) 70, 77, 78–9, 80, 81, 82, 83, 88–9; direct 78; secondary 79; vicarious 70, 79, 80; *see also* re-traumatisation risk
treatment resistant (concept) 11, 79, 91, 119, 137, 151; *see also* therapy
trust 65–6, 78, 104, 112, 159–60; art therapy and 111, 223–4; group therapy and 109, 111, 223–4; music therapy and 109, 198–200; relationship and 16–17, 104, 109, 121–2, 142, 159–60, 186, 198–200, 218, 220, 223–4, 228; trauma committee and development of 65–6; trauma unit 118, 121–2; *see also* safety
Twin Tower (9/11) events 86–8

Understanding and Dealing with Sexual Abuse Trauma: An Educational Group for Women xxxviii, 100, 101, 216
United States (US) xxxiv, 31–46, 70–3; history in xxxiv, 31–4, 183–4; inner city violence 116; multimodal approaches 70–3; women and political action 31–46

vagus nerve (polyvagal theory) 206, 209–10
verbal therapy (in groups) 72–3, 110, 203–14; music and xxxi, 108, 109, 131, 185, 186–7, 203–14
verbalisation in dance/movement therapy 259, 262
vicarious traumatisation 70, 79, 80
victimisation experiences 19; acknowledged (by others) 67; LGBTQI+ 172
Victims of Crime Act (1984) 31–2
violence: trauma unit 120, 121, 124, 133; US inner cities 116; workplace 78
visual language, development through artmaking 238–41
voice: finding a voice 234–5; hearing voices 6, 16, 37, 41–2
vowel sounds 187
vulnerability: feeling safe *vs* 142; LGBTQ+ 172

war trauma xxxii, 31

WHO and ICD 10 and 11 32–3

women (females) 31–46; childhood trauma (incl. abuse) 35, 38, 100–1; LGBTQI+ 169, 172, 176; political action 31–46; transgender 175, 176; on trauma unit 119–20; trauma-informed care 98; victimisation experiences (US) 31

word (verbal) and music therapy xxxi, 108, 109, 131, 185, 186–7, 203–14

working through obstacles: family therapy 161, 164; inpatient unit 118–20

workplace violence 78

World Health Organization (WHO), ICD 10 and 11 32–3

World Trade Center (9/11) events 86–8

yoga, afterwork 90

For Product Safety Concerns and Information please contact our EU
representative GPSR@taylorandfrancis.com
Taylor & Francis Verlag GmbH, Kaufingerstraße 24, 80331 München, Germany